Cognitive Stimulation Therapy for Dementia

Cognitive Stimulation Therapy (CST) has made a huge global, clinical impact since its inception, and this landmark book is the first to draw all the published research together in one place. Edited by experts in the intervention, including members of the workgroup who initially developed the therapy, *Cognitive Stimulation Therapy for Dementia* features contributions from authors across the globe, providing a broad overview of the entire research programme.

The book demonstrates how CST can significantly improve cognition and quality of life for people with dementia, and offers insight on the theory and mechanisms of change, as well as discussion of the practical implementation of CST in a range of clinical settings. Drawing from several research studies, the book also includes a section on culturally adapting and translating CST, with case studies from countries such as Japan, New Zealand, and Sub-Saharan Africa.

Cognitive Stimulation Therapy for Dementia will be essential reading for academics, researchers, and post-graduate students involved in the study of dementia, gerontology and cognitive rehabilitation. It will also be of interest to health professionals, including psychologists, psychiatrists, occupational therapists, nurses, and social workers.

Dr Lauren A Yates is a Research Fellow at the Institute of Mental Health at the University of Nottingham, UK.

Dr Jen Yates is a Research Fellow at the Institute of Mental Health at the University of Nottingham, UK.

Professor Martin Orrell is Director of the Institute of Mental Health at the University of Nottingham, UK.

Dr Aimee Spector is Reader in Clinical Psychology at University College London, UK.

Professor Bob Woods is Director of the Dementia Services Development Centre at Bangor University, UK.

Aging and Mental Health Research
Series Editors: Martin Orrell and Steve Zarit

For more information about the series, please visit www.routledge.com.

Aims and scope
In the 21st century the world's ageing population is growing more rapidly than ever before. This is driving the international research agenda to help older people live better for longer and to find the causes and cures for chronic diseases such as dementia. This series provides a forum for the rapidly expanding field by investigating the relationship between the ageing process and mental health. It compares and contrasts scientific and service developments across a range of settings, including the mental changes associated with normal and abnormal or pathological ageing, as well as the psychological and psychiatric problems of the ageing population. The series encourages an integrated approach between biopsychosocial models and etiological factors to promote better strategies, therapies, and services for older people. This will create a strong alliance between the theoretical, experimental, and applied sciences to provide an original and dynamic focus, integrating the normal and abnormal aspects of mental health in ageing so that theoretical issues can be set in the context of important new practical developments in this field.

Rationale and readership
The series will be directed at an international audience with series editors in London and North America. The readership will be initially via the library market drawn from many disciplines including academics, researchers, and post-graduate students with particularly strong representation from psychiatrists and psychologists in the field of mental health in older people. Its strong scientific foundation will also make it of considerable interest to basic scientists interested in the biological, psychological, and social aspects of ageing and mental health. Each book would bring together thematically linked chapters aiming to disseminate and further research in ageing throughout the world. The series would appeal to the international market with each book aiming for a diverse representation of authors taking into account the readership in Europe and North America, Australia, and Asia (e.g. China and Japan) and the growing academic representation in South America and other rapidly developing areas. Equally, the chapters would aim for a broad appeal to represent a diversity of settings and cultures where applicable.

In this series

Cognitive Stimulation Therapy for Dementia
History, Evolution and Internationalism
Edited by Lauren A. Yates, Jen Yates, Martin Orrell, Aimee Spector, and Bob Woods

Cognitive Stimulation Therapy for Dementia

History, Evolution and Internationalism

Edited by Lauren A. Yates,
Jen Yates, Martin Orrell,
Aimee Spector, and Bob Woods

Routledge
Taylor & Francis Group
LONDON AND NEW YORK

First published 2018 by Routledge

2 Park Square, Milton Park, Abingdon, Oxfordshire OX14 4RN
52 Vanderbilt Avenue, New York, NY 10017

Routledge is an imprint of the Taylor & Francis Group, an informa business

First issued in paperback 2019

British Library Cataloguing-in-Publication Data
A catalogue record for this book is available from the British Library

Library of Congress Cataloguing-in-Publication Data
A catalog record for this book has been requested

ISBN: 978-1-138-63117-5 (hbk)
ISBN: 978-0-367-36271-3 (pbk)

Typeset in Bembo
by Apex CoVantage, LLC

Contents

Preface vii
MARTIN ORRELL
Contributors ix

PART I
Overview of CST and related approaches 1

1 **Introduction** 3
AIMEE SPECTOR

2 **Cognitive stimulation, training, and rehabilitation: the bigger picture** 11
JAVIER OLAZARÁN AND RUBEN MUÑIZ

PART II
The CST research findings 31

3 **CST: development process** 33
BOB WOODS

4 **Group cognitive stimulation therapy: clinical trials** 49
MARTIN ORRELL AND LENE THORGRIMSEN FORRESTER

5 **Individual cognitive stimulation therapy (iCST)** 69
LAUREN A. YATES

6 **Cognitive stimulation therapy: implementation in practice** 89
AMY STREATER

7 **Involving family carers in cognitive stimulation therapy** 109
JENNY COVE

PART III
The CST process – how does it work? 129

8 **People's experiences of cognitive stimulation therapy: a qualitative understanding** 131
PHUONG LEUNG

9 **Neuropsychological aspects of cognitive stimulation therapy** 153
BRIDGET T.Y. LIU, ANTONY C.L. AU, AND GLORIA H.Y. WONG

PART IV
CST: an international perspective 175

10 **Guidelines for adapting cognitive stimulation therapy to other cultures** 177
ELISA AGUIRRE AND KATJA WERHEID

11 **Japan** 195
KATSUO YAMANAKA, YUGO UEDA, AND CHIHIRO MATSUDA

12 **New Zealand** 207
GARY CHEUNG AND KATHRYN PERI

13 **United States** 217
JANICE LUNDY, DEBORAH HAYDEN, MARLA BERG-WEGER, DANIEL B. STEWART, AND JOHN E. MORLEY

14 **China** 227
ZHAORUI LIU, YUEQIN HUANG, TAO LI, AND GUANGMING XU

15 **India** 237
SRIDHAR VAITHESWARAN, MONISHA LAKSHMINARAYANAN, AND SHRUTI RAGHURAMAN

16 **Sub-Saharan Africa** 253
STELLA-MARIA PADDICK, SARAH H. MKENDA, GODFREY MBOWE, ALOYCE KISOLI, WILLIAM K. GRAY, CATHERINE L. DOTCHIN, ADESOLA OGUNNIYI, JOHN KISSIMA, OLAIDE O. OLAKEHINDE, DECLARE L. MUSHI, AKEEM SIWOKU, BABATUNDE ADEDIRAN, AND RICHARD W. WALKER

Index 265

Preface

Cognitive stimulation therapy for dementia

Cognitive Stimulation Therapy for Dementia has been an incredible journey. Although it was not a journey that Bob Woods, Aimee Spector, and I started, it is a journey that as it continued, has branched out and been adopted by many countries of the world.

I am thrilled to see this book come to fruition and would particularly like to thank Dr Jen Yates and Dr Lauren Yates who joined as co-editors, and as the other authors will know have done very much the lion's share of the organising, managing and editing of this work. Bob Woods has been an excellent friend and colleague for over 20 years and it is wonderful to see how much he has remembered about not only how CST started, but also the rich and intriguing history of its development. It is also good to see Aimee Spector's chapter showing us the multitude of aspects of CST today and the list of countries where it has been adapted and taken root. I was particularly pleased to co-author a chapter with Lene Forrester (née Thorgrimsen) since Lene was a key contributor to the first main CST trial, working closely with Bob, Aimee and I. Whereas Aimee and Lene were the first two CST PhDs, we have now had in total six PhD's completed from the various projects, and all of these authors appear in this book.

Many authors from round the world have contributed chapters, bringing to life CST in many different environments to show us, for example, how CST groups can be developed and run in Tanzania and Nigeria, and how CST can be adapted for the Maori culture in New Zealand. There are also terrific illustrations of how to get CST into practice including developing training programmes. Perhaps the best example of this is from John Morley and his colleagues in the United States who have now trained over a thousand people. In terms of the mechanisms of action of CST, it was very exciting to see a chapter by Gloria Wong and colleagues looking at the impact of brain reserve and cognitive reserve on the clinical effects of CST in practice. Together the book provides a comprehensive illustration of both the quantitative and qualitative impact of CST, the theory and mechanisms of action, as well as a very comprehensive guide to its implementation in practice, and its adaptation for different countries and cultures.

When Bob Woods and I set out our editorial for how reality orientation should be developed and evaluated, we did not have a useful or robust plan for how to potentially get things into practice. Unlike drug companies, we did not have any funding to support publication and promotion of CST as a useful therapy, so Aimee, Lene, Bob, and I produced the first UK manual 'Making a Difference' (Hawker Publications) as a way to help standardise the use of CST and provide clear guidance for staff working in dementia care. Somehow this has worked. With the publication of the maintenance CST manual and DVD, the individual CST manual and DVD, as well as the continued demand for training, CST has developed a life of its own, and continues to flourish and spread.

Bob, Jen, Lauren, Aimee, and I are so grateful for the brilliant contributions from all of the authors from all around the world. This, I think, should be the definitive guide to CST for many years to come. We hope readers of this book will be inspired and encouraged to pioneer and innovate CST for the future.

Martin Orrell
Director of the Institute of Mental Health, Nottingham

Contributors

Dr Elisa Aguirre, PhD
North East London NHS Foundation Trust, London, UK

Babatunde Adediran
University of Ibadan, Nigeria

Professor Marla Berg-Weger, PhD, LCSW
Executive Director
School of Social Work, Gateway Geriatric Education Centre, Saint Louis University, United States

Dr Gary Cheung, MBChB, FRANZCP
Senior Lecturer in Psychiatry Department of Psychological Medicine
School of Medicine, Faculty of Medical and Health Sciences, University of Auckland, New Zealand

Dr Jenny Cove, PhD
Clinical Psychologist
Royal Brompton Hospital, London, UK

Catherine L Dotchin, MD
Newcastle University and Northumbria Healthcare NHS Foundation Trust, UK

William K Gray, PhD,
Northumbria Healthcare NHS Foundation Trust, UK

Deborah Hayden, RN, BSN, OTR/L
Director, Occupational Therapy
Perry County Memorial Hospital, United States

Yueqin Huang, MD, MPH, PhD
Institute of Mental Health, Peking University, China

Aloyce Kisoli, MSc, RN
Kilimanjaro Christina Medical University College, Tanzania

John Kissima, AMO
Hai District Medical Office, Kilimanjaro, Tanzania

Ms Monisha Lakshminarayanan, MSc Psychology (Clinical)
Schizophrenia Research Foundation, Chennai, India

Mr Antony AC Lau, BSc MMedSc
Sau Po Centre on Ageing, The University of Hong Kong

Dr Phuong Leung, BSc, MSc, PhD
Research Assistant
Division of Psychiatry, Faculty of Brain Sciences, University College London, London, UK

Dr Tao Li, MD
Institute of Mental Health, Peking University, China

Dr Bridget Tianyin Liu, BSocSc, PhD
Department of Social Work and Social Administration, The University of Hong Kong

Dr Zhaorui Liu, MD, MPH, PhD
Institute of Mental Health, Peking University, China

Janice Lundy, MA, MHA
Director, Social Work and Geriatric Care Management
Perry County Memorial Hospital, United States

Chihiro Matsuda, MA
Clinical Psychologist
Clinical Psychology Team, Tsurukawa Sanatorium Hospital, Tokyo, Japan

Godfrey Mbowe
Department of Occupational Therapy, Kilimanjaro Christina Medical University College, Tanzania

Sarah H Mkenda
Department of Occupational Therapy, Kilimanjaro Christina Medical University College, Tanzania

John E Morley, M.B.B.Ch
Dammert Professor of Gerontology, Professor and Division Chief
Division of Geriatric Medicine, Department of Internal Medicine,
Saint Louis University, United States

Ruben Muñiz
Fundación Maria Wolff
Madrid, Spain

Declare L Mushi
Institute of Public Health, Kilimanjaro Christina Medical University College, Tanzania

Adesola Ogunniyi, MBChB
University of Ibadan, Nigeria

Olaide O Olakehinde, RNM
IDEA study, Department of Medicine, College of Medicine, University of Ibadan, Nigeria

Javier Olazarán, MD, PhD
Fundación Maria Wolff & HGU Gregorio Marañón
Madrid, Spain

Professor Martin Orrell, PhD FRCPsych
Director/Head Institute of Mental Health
Division of Psychiatry and Applied Psychology, Faculty of Medicine & Health Sciences, University of Nottingham, Nottingham, UK

Stella-Marie Paddick, MRCPsych
Newcastle University and Northumbria Tyne and Wear NHS Trust, UK

Dr Kathy Peri, MHsc, PhD
School of Nursing, Faculty of Medical and Health Sciences, University of Auckland, New Zealand

Ms Shruti Raghuraman, PhD candidate (clinical psychology)
Division of Psychiatry and Applied Psychology, School of Medicine, University of Nottingham, Nottingham, UK

Akeem Siwoku, OT
Department of Psychiatry, College of Medicine, University of Ibadan, Nigeria

Dr Aimee Spector
Reader in Clinical Psychology
Department of Clinical, Educational and Health Psychology, University College London, London, UK

Daniel B Stewart, MSG
Doctoral Student
School of Social Work, St Louis University, United States

Dr Amy Streater, BA (Hons), MSc, PhD
Research & Development Department, North East London Foundation Trust, UK

Dr Lene Thorgrimsen, PhD, DClinPsychol
Consultant Clinical Psychologist/President-elect ACBS UK & Ireland Chapter
BMI Healthcare

Yugo Ueda, MA
Clinical Psychologist,
Clinical Psychology Team, Tsurukawa Sanatorium Hospital, Tokyo, Japan

Dr Sridhar Vaitheswaran
Dementia Care in Schizophrenia Research Foundation (DEMCARES), Chennai, India

Dr Richard W Walker, MD
Newcastle University and Northumbria Healthcare NHS Foundation Trust, UK

Professor Dr Katja Werheid, PhD
Clinical Psychologist and Clinical Neuropsychologist
Department of Psychology, Humboldt University at Berlin, Germany
Klinikum Ernst von Bergmann, Neurology Department, Potsdam, Germany

Dr Gloria HY Wong, BA, MA, PhD
Assistant Professor, Honorary Assistant Professor, Department of Psychiatry,
Honorary Research Fellow
Department of Social Work and Social Administration, Sau Po Centre on Ageing, The University of Hong Kong

Professor Bob Woods, MA, MSc
Dementia Services Development Centre, School of Healthcare Sciences, Bangor University, UK

Dr Guangming Xu, MD
Tianjin Anding Hospital, China

Dr Katsuo Yamanaka, PhD
Associate Professor, Clinical Psychologist
Faculty of Human Science, University of Tsukuba, Tsukuba, Japan

Dr Lauren A. Yates, BSc, PhD
Research Fellow
Institute of Mental Health, Division of Psychiatry and Applied Psychology, Faculty of Medicine & Health Sciences, University of Nottingham, Nottingham, UK

Part I

Overview of CST and related approaches

Chapter 1

Introduction

Aimee Spector

CST: development of the initial concept

CST was effectively 'conceived' twenty years ago. A timely editorial entitled 'Tacrine and psychological therapies in dementia – No contest?' (Orrell and Woods, 1996), presented an invaluable snapshot of the time. At this point, Tacrine (a previously used drug for dementia) and other potential drug therapies were evaluated through large, robust randomised controlled trials (RCTs). In stark contrast, 'psychological therapies', which included specific programmes such as Reminiscence or environmental manipulation, just did not have the evidence base. Research was primarily small scale, uncontrolled, and riddled with methodological flaws; and there were no evidence-based treatments which also had a replicable treatment manual. As a result, clinicians and policy makers were focusing on pharmacological therapies, despite modest benefits and risks of adverse effects, stating that 'gold-standard' evidence was simply not available for psychosocial alternatives. The vision was to develop a novel 'psychological therapy' and evaluate it in a trial adhering to the same methodological expectations of any drug trial. The contest was on!

And this is precisely what happened. Orrell and Woods successfully secured funding to develop and evaluate probably the largest trial of any psychosocial intervention at that time and I was recruited as the lead researcher and PhD student. The aim was to build an intervention based on what we already knew, largely anecdotally, was working. We systematically reviewed the literature on two widely used psychological interventions: Reality Orientation (RO) and Reminiscence Therapy (Spector et al., 1998; Spector et al., 2000), as well as scoping the literature on all the key therapies available. In order to develop the intervention, the workgroup pulled out what appeared to be the best techniques from the more effective therapies, combining these together into one programme. Our work was most influenced by the largest, most scientifically robust, and effective study at the time. This randomised controlled trial (Breuil et al., 1994) was led by a team at the Hopital Broca in Paris, who described their therapeutic technique as 'Cognitive Stimulation'. This differed from the more traditional 'RO', ('the presentation and repetition of orientation-based

Table 1.1 CST sessions

Session 1:	Physical games	*Session 8*	Being creative
Session 2:	Sound	*Session 9:*	Categorising objects
Session 3:	Childhood	*Session 10:*	Orientation
Session 4:	Food	*Session 11:*	Using money
Session 5:	Current affairs	*Session 12:*	Number games
Session 6:	Faces/scenes	*Session 13:*	Word games
Session 7:	Associated words	*Session 14:*	Team games

information'), which previously dominated the literature. Whereas RO had a more repetitive element, Breuil's Cognitive Stimulation approach seemed to have unique properties, more implicitly engaging people in enjoyable group cognitive tasks. Their trial included 56 people with dementia and found significant improvements in cognition when presenting them with tasks such as word association and object categorisation.

Our examination of the literature led to the development of a 14-session programme, designed to run twice a week for seven weeks. This 'dose' of CST was determined by the past literature and by what was feasible within the confines of the research funding and timetable. Both the content and name of the current CST programme was largely based upon the foundations of Breuil et al.'s innovative work, while also including elements of RO, Reminiscence, and multisensory stimulation. Each session was given a theme, with a choice of activities within each to be adapted for the interests and abilities of the group. Table 1.1 provides a summary of the group CST sessions.

Twenty years on: the CST journey

The CST research programme and individual studies will be described throughout this book, but a brief summary follows. The initial CST study (Spector et al., 2003), described in Chapter 4, was a single-blind, multi-centre RCT including 201 participants. It demonstrated significant improvements in cognition and quality of life (QoL) for those participating in the 14-session programme when compared to those receiving usual care. Further, complex economic analysis, which considered the cost of running CST groups in addition to the differences in use of services between the treatment and control groups, showed that CST was cost-effective (Knapp et al., 2006). This early CST work led to many questioning whether such benefits could be maintained over a period beyond seven weeks. Consequently, we developed the 'Maintenance CST' (MCST) programme, consisting of 26 additional, weekly sessions designed to follow from the initial (more intensive) CST programme. This was evaluated through another RCT with 236 people with dementia. It demonstrated that QoL can continue to significantly improve for up to six months if people receive ongoing CST, and that activities of daily living can improve for three months (Orrell et al., 2014).

The qualitative effects of group CST, discussed in Chapter 8, have been evaluated through interviewing 38 people (those with dementia, family carers, and care staff) about the experience of CST groups (Spector et al., 2011). Results showed that positive experiences of being in the group (such as feeling able to talk in a non-threatening environment) were really valued, and that benefits in everyday life were evident, including noticeable improvements in concentration and alertness. The neuropsychological changes have been explored in more detail (Spector et al., 2010; Hall et al., 2013) – see Chapter 9, as have models of implementation (Streater et al., 2016), discussed in Chapter 6. Most recently, we have developed and evaluated a one-to-one, carer-led CST programme (iCST), Orgeta et al., 2015). This 25-week, 75-session programme led to significant improvements in carer QoL and in the relationship between the person with dementia and their carer. However, the primary outcomes (cognition and QoL for the person with dementia) did not change. Uptake of the intervention was low, with an average of 33 sessions being delivered and a quarter of the treatment participants receiving no sessions. This may well have impacted on the findings, which are discussed in Chapter 5.

CST in the UK: how does it feature?

The seminal CST study was possibly the largest published trial of any psychosocial intervention at the time and showed significant improvements in cognition and quality of life. The Department of Health's 'National Institute of Clinical Excellence' (NICE) issued their guidelines for dementia in 2006, specifically referencing the 2003 CST study. NICE stated that

> People with mild to moderate dementia of all types should be given the opportunity to participate in a structured group Cognitive Stimulation programme. This should be commissioned and provided by a range of health and social care workers with training and supervision. This should be delivered irrespective of any anti-dementia drug prescribed for the cognitive symptoms of dementia.

This was the only non-pharmacological treatment recommended for the cognitive symptoms of dementia, and crucially, there were no such recommendations prior to this. The additional economic analysis, led by colleagues at the London School of Economics (LSE), was novel and likely to have had an important impact on NICE's recommendations. In fact, a recent review suggests that this and the more recent economic analysis accompanying the MCST trial (D'Amico et al., 2015) were the only trials of Cognitive Stimulation to formally analyse costs (Streater et al., 2016).

An important step to enable the widespread implementation of CST has been the publication of four training manuals. Following the initial publication of a manual in the United States entitled 'Our time: an evidence based group program to offer cognitive stimulation to people with dementia – manual for group leaders' (Spector et al., 2005), there have been three UK manuals published through Hawker Publications. 'Making a difference' (Spector et al., 2006) describes the initial, 14-session CST programme and 'Making a Difference 2' (Aguirre et al., 2012) includes the MCST programme and a training DVD. Crucially, the 'key principles' of CST (see Table 1.2) were more formally introduced in this second manual. This was driven by clinical feedback, suggesting that the techniques of CST and clarification of how it was both similar and different to other therapies, was needed. 'Making a difference 3' (Yates et al.,

Table 1.2 Key principles of CST

	Key principle	*Description/rationale*	*Applied example*
1	Mental stimulation	Getting people's minds actively engaged, pitching tasks at a level whereby people are suitably stretched yet do not feel deskilled.	Asking people to calculate their score in the 'physical games' session by adding numbers.
2	New ideas, thoughts, and associations	Continually encourage new ideas, thoughts, and associations through making new semantic links with material.	Asking people to think of similarities and differences when shown two or more faces in the 'faces' session.
3	Using orientation, but sensitively and implicitly	Integrating time, place, and person-related information into general discussion and activities.	Tasting seasonal fruit in the summer ('food' session), Christmas word games ('word games' session).
4	Opinions, rather than facts	Always asking for opinions before factual information. Opinions cannot be wrong and are more engaging to discuss.	Asking views on political or topical issues within the 'current affairs' session.
5	Using reminiscence as an aid to the here-and-now	Reminiscence itself promotes well-being, but it also helps orientate people to the present through making comparisons.	Comparing old and new coins or the cost of items in the past and present in the 'using money' session.
6	Providing triggers to aid recall	Recall is aided through providing triggers including a RO board and multi-sensory cues.	Make the date and other orientation information visible during discussion.
7	Continuity and consistency between sessions	Memory is supported through features including keeping sessions in the same room with the same facilitator, and use of a theme song.	Let the group dictate the routine, which may be somebody helping with the tea, another leading the song, another helping to set up.

	Key principle	*Description/rationale*	*Applied example*
8	Implicit (rather than explicit) learning	Subtle tasks which avoid asking direct questions, focusing on facts, and putting people on the spot; enable more implicit learning.	People may learn new things in the 'current affairs' session, yet the informal nature of the discussion does not draw explicit attention to this.
9	Stimulating language	Language skills are stimulated through tasks including naming people and objects, word construction, and word association.	Asking people to describe a word without actually using it in the 'word games' session.
10	Stimulating executive functioning	Executive functioning skills are stimulated through tasks including discussion of similarities and differences.	The 'categorising objects' session uses executive functioning through mental organisation.
11	Person-centred	During CST, people should be valued, treated as individuals, and provided with a positive and supportive social environment.	Always making the activities interesting and relevant to those in the group.
12	Respect	People's views should be valued, recognising diversity of views and opinions.	Encouraging people to express a range of views, which stimulates interesting discussion.
13	Involvement	Sessions should involve everyone, giving each person the opportunity to contribute, and appealing to each person's interests.	Tell the group what the next session will be and let them guide you towards preparing materials which will involve everyone.
14	Inclusion	Everyone should be included, sometimes meaning that quieter people require additional support.	Without putting people on the spot, regularly ask if everyone has had a chance to express their view.
15	Choice	Choice should be offered within activities, to cater for the interests and abilities of the group.	Let people choose their activity in the 'Being Creative' session.
16	Fun	Groups should provide a learning atmosphere which is fun and enjoyable.	Add a competitive element to games (in the 'team games/quiz' session).
17	Maximising potential	People often do not achieve their potential due to lack of stimulation or opportunity. In contrast, sessions should maximise potential.	Offer a task which is sufficiently challenging, without making people feel as if they have failed. For example, add prices to the task in the 'food' session if appropriate.
18	Building/ strengthening relationships	Within a supportive social environment, sessions should strengthen relationships between group members and facilitators.	Encourage participants to meet socially or in another context once groups end, for example within the same lunch club.

2014) presents the individual CST (iCST) programme for family carers, also including a training DVD. A systematic review (Fossey et al., 2014) highlighted the common disconnect between evidence and practice in dementia care, noting that few evidence-based interventions have replicable training manuals, yet so many training manuals are available which have no evidence base. Creating an evidence-based intervention which is now manualised has certainly aided implementation, along with a widely accessed one-day training course and website (www.cstdementia.com).

The use of CST within the NHS appears to have grown continually since its inclusion in the NICE guidelines. In 2007, the National Audit Office reported that CST was being used by 29% of community mental health teams (CMHTs) in the UK. The Memory Services National Accreditation Programme (MSNAP) conducted an audit of their accredited memory services across the UK in 2013, finding that 66% were routinely offering group CST to people following a diagnosis of dementia. This figure was reportedly over 80% in 2015. In 2016, it was announced that CST was to become a necessary standard for accreditation.

International CST developments

The translation and adaptation of CST began quite rapidly following its development in the UK. Work was undertaken concurrently in several countries including Japan, Italy, the United States, New Zealand, and sub-Saharan Africa, to name a few. The World Alzheimer Report (2011) stated that CST should routinely be given to people with early stage dementia. This appeared to be a catalyst for more recent developments, for example in Hong Kong and Brazil, where CST neuroimaging work is taking place. Guidelines on adapting CST for different cultures and languages were developed (Aguirre et al., 2014), drawing on the work conducted in Japan, Africa, and a UK translation into Swahili. The guidelines present a clear process to follow, based on the formative method of adapting psychotherapy, and are presented in Chapter 10. In 2015, the 'International CST centre at UCL' was launched as a platform to support international collaboration. This consists of an information-sharing website (www.ucl.ac.uk/international-cognitive-stimulation-therapy) and regular conferences. Some examples of international CST developments will be expanded upon later in the book. Currently, CST is either being researched and/or used clinically in Australia, Brazil, Canada, Chile, China, Germany, Greece, Hong Kong, Italy, Ireland, Indonesia, Israel, Japan, Nepal, New Zealand, Nigeria, Philippines, Portugal, Singapore, South Africa, South Korea, Tanzania, Turkey, the Netherlands, and the United States.

CST: its future within dementia care

The evidence for CST is strong, both for its potential effectiveness and cost-effectiveness. The latter was investigated further by Matrix Evidence, who were commissioned by the National Institute of Innovations and Improvements (2011).

Their focus was to compare the costs of 'behavioural interventions' with the use of antipsychotics – considering all the associated costs and adverse events. They chose CST as their 'gold-standard' intervention and based the report on the known costs and benefits of CST. The conclusion was that whereas behavioural interventions cost £27.6 million more per year than antipsychotics, the additional investment is offset by nearly £70.4 million in healthcare savings due to the reduced incidence of strokes and falls. Ultimately, the routine use of CST could save the NHS £54.9 million annually through cost savings and quality of life improvements.

The NHS has certainly embraced CST, with it now becoming a standard treatment within memory services. Anecdotally, however, the number of sessions that people receive in practice appears to vary hugely, ranging from six to 14 sessions and often running once a week. With limited NHS resources, many people are looking towards the voluntary sector, for example the Alzheimer's Society, Age Concern and Age UK, to offer CST as a longer-term treatment option. In an ideal world, people would continue to receive ongoing CST until the natural point where they no longer need it or no longer meet the criteria. This begs an important ethical question – we would not withdraw medication from people when we believed that it was working, so why stop CST? Finally, the awareness and use of CST appears to be limited within care homes. Increasing both knowledge and access to CST for these residents should be a future priority, given the improvements it has shown to make and the huge unmet need for cognitive stimulation within such settings.

References

Aguirre, E., Spector, A., and Orrell, M. (2014). Guidelines to adapt Cognitive Stimulation Therapy (CST) to other cultures. *Clinical Interventions in Ageing*, 9, 1003–1007.

Aguirre, E., Spector, A., Streater, A., Hoe, J., Woods, B., and Orrell, M. (2012). *Making a Difference 2: An evidence based group program to offer maintenance Cognitive Stimulation Therapy (CST) to people with dementia.* Hawker Publications, UK.

Breuil, V., De Rotrou, J., Forette, F., Tortrat, D., Ganansia-Ganem, A., Frambourt, A., . . . and Boller, F. (1994). Cognitive stimulation of patients with dementia: Preliminary results. *International Journal of Geriatric Psychiatry*, 9(3), 211–217.

D'Amico, F., Rehill, A., Knapp, M., Aguirre, E., Donovan, H., Hoare, Z., . . . and Orrell, M. (2015). Maintenance Cognitive Stimulation Therapy: An economic evaluation within a randomised controlled trial. *Journal of the American Medical Directors Association*, 16(1), 63–70.

Department of Health. (2006). *National Institute of Clinical Excellence: Dementia guidelines.* https://www.nice.org.uk/guidance/cg42/chapter/1-Guidance#interventions-for-cognitive-symptoms-and-maintenance-of-function-for-people-with-dementia

Fossey, J., Masson, S., Stafford, J., Lawrence, V., Corbett, A., and Ballard, C. (2014). The disconnect between evidence and practice: A systematic review of person-centred interventions and training manuals for care home staff working with people with dementia. *International Journal of Geriatric Psychiatry*, 29(8), 797–807.

Hall, L., Orrell, M., Stott, J., and Spector, A. (2013). Cognitive Stimulation Therapy (CST): Neuropsychological mechanisms of change. *International Psychogeriatrics*, 25(3), 479–489.

Knapp, M., Thorgrimsen, L., Patel, A., Spector, A., Hallam, A., Woods, B., and Orrell, M. (2006). Cognitive Stimulation Therapy for dementia: Is it cost effective? *British Journal of Psychiatry*, 188, 574–580.

NHS Institute for Innovations and Improvements. (2011). *An economic evaluation of alternatives to antipsychotic drugs for individuals living with dementia.* Matrix Evidence. https://www.acss.org.uk/wp-content/uploads/2016/03/NHS-Institute-for-Innovation-and-Improvement-antipyschotic-drug-evaluation-2011.pdf

Orrell, M., Aguirre, E., Spector, A., Hoare, Z., Woods, R.T., Streater, A., . . . and Russell, I. (2014). Maintenance Cognitive Stimulation Therapy (CST) for dementia: Single-blind, multicentre, pragmatic randomized controlled trial. *British Journal of Psychiatry*, 204, 1–8.

Orrell, M., and Woods, B. (1996). Editorial Comment: Tacrine and psychological therapies in dementia – No contest? *International Journal of Geriatric Psychiatry*, 11(3), 189–192.

Spector, A., Gardner, C., and Orrell, M. (2011). The impact of Cognitive Stimulation Therapy groups on people with dementia: Views from participants, their carers and group facilitators. *Ageing & Mental Health*, 15(8), 945–950.

Spector, A., Orrell, M., and Woods, B. (2010). Cognitive Stimulation Therapy (CST): Effects on different areas of cognitive function for people with dementia. *International Journal of Geriatric Psychiatry*, 25(12), 1253–1258.

Spector, A., Thorgrimsen, L., Woods, B., and Orrell, M. (2005). *Our time: An evidence based group program to offer cognitive stimulation to people with dementia – Manual for group leaders.* Freiberg Press, Iowa.

Spector, A., Thorgrimsen, L., Woods, B., and Orrell, M. (2006). *Making a difference: An evidence based group program to offer Cognitive Stimulation Therapy (CST) to people with dementia.* Hawker Publications, UK.

Spector, A., Thorgrimsen, L., Woods, B., Royan, L., Davies, S., Butterworth, M., and Orrell, M. (2003). Efficacy of an evidence-based Cognitive Stimulation Therapy programme for people with dementia: Randomised controlled trial. *British Journal of Psychiatry*, 183, 248–254.

Spector, A., Woods, B., Davies, S., and Orrell, M.W. (1998). Reminiscence therapy in dementia. *Cochrane Database of Systematic Reviews*, Oxford, UK.

Spector, A., Woods, B., Davies, S., and Orrell, M.W. (2000). Reality orientation for dementia: A systematic review of the evidence of effectiveness from randomized controlled trials. *The Gerontologist*, 40(2), 206–212.

Streater et al. (2016). Staff training and outreach support for Cognitive Stimulation Therapy and its implementation in practice: A cluster randomised trial. *International Journal of Geriatric Psychiatry.*

Prince, M., Bryce, R., & Ferri, C. (2011). *World Alzheimer Report 2011: The benefits of early diagnosis and intervention.* https://www.alz.co.uk/research/WorldAlzheimerReport2011.pdf.

Yates, L., Orrell, M., Leung, P., Spector, A., Woods, B., and Orgeta, V. (2014). *Making a Difference 3: Individualised CST – A manual for carers.* Hawker Publications, UK.

Chapter 2

Cognitive stimulation, training, and rehabilitation

The bigger picture

Javier Olazarán & Ruben Muñiz

Introduction

Dementia burden and aetiology

Dementia is one of the major challenges for our societies, with 7% of the European population aged ≥ 60 years affected (Prince et al., 2013; OECD, 2014). Essentially, dementia deteriorates the person's intellectual and functional capacities, which is typically a long and progressively devastating process. In addition, dementia is often accompanied by behavioural and psychological symptoms (BSPD), which increase patient's cognitive deterioration and functional disability along with the suffering of the patient and his/her family.

The complex, heterogeneous, and still not well understood pathological basis of dementia certainly contribute to the lack of available treatments that may cure, or at least stop, the deteriorating process. Alzheimer's disease (AD) is the most common cause of dementia in the population, followed by cerebrovascular disease (either alone or in combination with AD). In the last decades, increasing attention has been paid to Lewy body disease, which may produce a predominantly motor clinical presentation (Parkinson's disease) or a combination of cognitive and motor symptoms (Lewy body dementia). Currently, Lewy body disease is recognised as the third most common cause of dementia, although it is frequently (80% of the affected brains) accompanied by AD (Lewy body variant of AD).

Frontotemporal lobar degeneration (FTLD) is the fourth cause of dementia. This term embraces a set of pathologically and clinically heterogeneous entities, having in common the initial location of disease in the frontal and/or temporal lobes and, accordingly, a clinical presentation of deterioration of executive capacities (i.e. planning, sequence, and control of thoughts or actions), language impairment, and/or behaviour disturbances.

Finally, there is a heterogeneous set of 'minority dementias', which encompasses very rare neurodegenerative disease (progressive supranuclear palsy, Huntington's disease etc.), chronic infections (neurosyphilis, human immunodeficiency virus infection etc.), toxic or metabolic processes, nutrition deficiencies,

Table 2.1 Causes of dementia in the population

Entity	%	*Total*
PRIMARY (DEGENERATIVE) DEMENTIA		55
Alzheimer's disease (AD)	35	
Lewy body disease	10	
Frontotemporal lobar degeneration	8	
Other primary dementias	2	
SECONDARY (NONDEGENERATIVE) DEMENTIA		5
Cerebrovascular disease (CVD)	3	
Other secondary dementias	2	
COMBINED DEMENTIA		40
Mixed dementia (AD+CVD)	20	
Lewy body variant of AD	15	
Other combined dementias	5	

% Indicates rough prevalence in the population

and other secondary dementias (normal pressure hydrocephalus, head trauma, multiple sclerosis etc.) (Ames et al., 2010) (Table 2.1).

While the possible causes of dementia are innumerable, the vast majority of dementias in old people are attributable to AD, vascular disease, and Lewy body disease, which share pathological mechanisms and often appear in combination (Iturria-Medina et al., 2016). Combined dementia is particularly common in very old people. It has been speculated that the different types of pathology would contribute in an additive form to the clinical presentation, but this has not been clearly demonstrated. Consistent correlates between pathological markers and clinical manifestations of dementia have only been established for neurofibrillary tangles (one of the pathological markers of AD) and vascular lesions. In fact, there are descriptions of brains with a substantial level of amyloid-type AD pathology from people who did not develop dementia during life (Katzman et al., 1989) and the opposite has also been observed: some individuals with dementia do not display substantial levels of pathology at *post-mortem* brain examination (Boyle et al., 2013; Kawas et al., 2015). These paradoxical observations may be explained by lack of sensitivity of the detection techniques, but also suggest that psychological and social factors may be decisive in the compensation, and even prevention, of cognitive impairment and dementia.

Clearly, the pervasive, heterogeneous, and complex background of dementia invites us to imagine alternative approaches for treatment, beyond a simplistic biological vision. The concepts of brain reserve and cognitive reserve were proposed to investigate the potential mechanisms of, respectively, brain, and individual compensation (Stern, 2002), which may be elicited by both pharmacological and non-pharmacological interventions. Predictably, the containment of the burden of dementia will come as the result of a sum of efforts from multiple views and disciplines.

Opportunity for psychosocial interventions

There is an empirical basis for believing that psychosocial interventions (Table 2.2) can improve the symptoms and modify the substrate of primarily biological processes. Just as the adapted use of a limb after injury favours its maintenance and function, the stimulation of cognitive capacities may contribute to the improvement of those capacities or at least slow down their deterioration. Modification of the environment and cognitive restructuring are crucial to obtain adapted responses in people with dementia. From the patient's perspective, psychosocial interventions should provide meaningful benefits in terms of improving or maintaining functional ability, enhancing activity and participation, and attaining personally relevant goals despite cognitive deterioration. In addition, psychological interventions can help the patient and his/her relatives to react positively and 'come to terms' with the disease (Wilson, 1997).

Neuropsychological evidence of brain plasticity

Episodic and prospective memory are usually the most prominently affected cognitive capacities at clinical inception of dementia. Episodic memory is defined as the capacity of mentally reproducing past personal experiences, whereas the

Table 2.2 Essential characteristics of cognitive stimulation, cognitive training, and cognitive rehabilitation

	Cognitive stimulation	*Cognitive training*	*Cognitive rehabilitation*
Aim	General cognitive improvement	Improvement of specific cognitive aspects	Improvement of personally relevant functions
Format	Usually group sessions	Individual or group sessions	Individual sessions, usually with family caregiver
Techniques	Reality orientation, reminiscence, semantic associations	Repeated guided practice	Environmental modification, external aids, cognitive and emotional adaptation
Typical components	Orientation board, pencil and paper exercises, sensoriomotor activities, emphasis on social interaction	Standardised tasks, range of difficulties (adaptive), computers may be utilized	Comprehensive assessment, identification of relevant goals

term 'prospective memory' was more recently coined to define the capacity of remembering and timely performing tasks that had to be done (McDaniel and Einstein, 2011). While episodic memory relies on medial temporal structures (hippocampus and parahippocampus), prospective memory relies on medial temporal and frontal regions. The hippocampus and parahippocampus function as neural nodes (or 'hubs'), richly connected with cortical association areas. Possibly, the degeneration of the hippocampus and parahippocampus comes as the long-term result of the dysfunction of the connected cortical areas. The finding that amyloid deposition in the association cortex precedes hippocampal and parahypocampal degeneration supports that view and permits us to speculate that cognitive support during memory creation would not only improve memory, but also might prevent neuronal degeneration.

Neuroplasticity was defined as the ability of the brain to change according to environmental stimulations or after experiencing neurological damage (Wolf et al., 2006). Empirical research has shown that, given appropriate conditions and support and sufficient time, people with dementia maintain the ability to learn and retain some information and skills despite their memory difficulties. Particularly successful are those interventions which are guided under the principle of errorless learning and include encoding and retrieval support. The use of relatively preserved capacities (e.g. semantic memory and motor functions) in the process of facilitating impaired capacities is another predictor of success. People with mild dementia show learning capacity in tasks of explicit memory, reasoning, and other capacities and functions. In the case of advanced dementia, learning ability is limited to tasks of implicit memory and motor skills (Bäckman, 1996; de Werd et al., 2013).

Data from neuroimaging studies

Studies of functional magnetic resonance imaging (fMRI), single-photon emission tomography (SPECT), and positron emission tomography (PET) have shown the existence of changes in the brains of healthy subjects, people with mild cognitive impairment (MCI), and people with AD who receive cognition-focused psychosocial interventions (Hosseini et al., 2014; van Os et al., 2015). In healthy older subjects, an increase in hippocampal perfusion along with a decrease in frontal cortex activation, as compared to baseline perfusion, were observed during performance of memory tasks that were previously trained (van Os et al., 2015). These findings suggest the existence of neuroplasticity in the hippocampus, leading to greater neuronal efficiency.

In subjects with MCI, an increase in hippocampus activation was consistently observed after memory training, as well as activation of different frontal and parietal cortical regions, not primarily related to the trained cognitive functions, which was correlated with clinical improvement. These changes suggest that, in people with mild brain damage, memory training may convey compensatory mechanisms and reallocate cognitive functions to restore the affected functions (Hosseini et al., 2014; van Os et al., 2015).

Functional neuroimaging evidence is also encouraging in people with dementia. In a randomised controlled trial (RCT), Baglio et al. investigated the effects of a 10-week, intense, multi-component stimulation programme in 60 people with mild to moderate AD. Improvement in language, memory, and neuropsychiatric symptoms was observed in the experimental group, along with activation in the superior temporal gyrus, right insular cortex, and thalamus; whereas no changes were observed in the control group, which received usual care. Moreover, significant correlations were found between the magnitude of increased activity in the left superior temporal gyrus, precuneus, and left thalamus and the changes observed in cognitive performance (Baglio et al., 2015).

Förster et al., investigated the effects of a six-month multi-component stimulation programme in a RCT of 15 people with mild AD. Although no clinical effects were detected, the participants in the experimental group showed decreased activity in the lingual gyrus and the left inferior temporal gyrus, whereas participants in the active control group showed widespread decreased activity in prefrontal, parieto-occipital, and parieto-temporal regions. There were no significant changes in the clinical outcomes in this trial (Förster et al., 2011).

In another RCT, a three-month intervention combining reality orientation (RO) and reminiscence was investigated in 24 residents of a geriatric nursing home with vascular dementia. Brain metabolism was measured pre-treatment and post-treatment using PET. The control group received usual care. Increased brain metabolism was found in the anterior cingulate in the experimental group, which correlated with improvement in social and communication scales (Akanuma et al., 2011).

Biological studies and model of response

In the light of observations of neuroplasticity in the brains of people with blindness and other conditions, it has been hypothesised that cognitive interventions may counteract the pathological substrate and mechanisms of dementia (Vemuri et al., 2016a). Hypothetical mediators of neurogenesis and neuroplasticity have been identified in animal models in conditions of physical exercise. In these models, the production of growth factors such as the brain-derived neurotrophic factor (BDNF) was shown to enhance neurogenesis and to play a key role in cognitive improvement (Foster et al., 2011). Whether those or other factors mediate neuroplasticity in conditions of cognitive activity in humans is not known.

A potential modification of AD biomarkers (Pittsburgh compound B retention, brain hypometabolism, and hippocampal atrophy) by cognitive activity and other lifestyle factors was studied in older people with normal cognition and MCI. While the association between high levels of cognitive activity and better cognitive performance was consistent, the attempts of demonstrating reduction of AD biomarkers in subjects with higher levels of cognitive activity or healthier lifestyle failed (Gidicsin et al., 2015; Vemuri et al., 2016b).

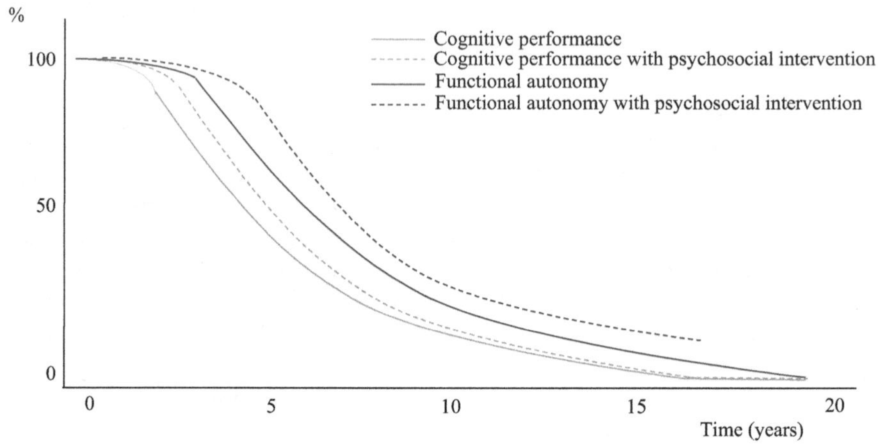

Figure 2.1 Model of response to psychosocial interventions in neurodegenerative dementia

In a study of MRI spectroscopy (^{1}H-MRI) several molecules were measured before and after memory training in a sample of 11 people with MCI (mean age 68, SD 10). Significant decrease in choline-containing compounds was observed in the hippocampus after the intervention (Yang et al., 2016). Since hippocampal choline is usually increased in ageing and AD, those results were interpreted as confirmatory of the existence of brain changes due to memory training (i.e. neuroplasticity).

Overall, the available evidence from clinical, neuroimaging, and biological studies supports a model of response to psychosocial interventions in neurodegenerative dementia showing delay in cognitive and functional deterioration due to reallocation of the neural resources involved in the different cognitive functions, without modification of the lesional load or the total duration of the disease (Figure 2.1). This type of response to treatment is currently accepted as relevant and sufficient in neurodegenerative conditions from both the personal and societal point of view (Pouryamout et al., 2012).

Non-pharmacological therapies: an expanding, versatile field for improving the quality of life of people with dementia and their caregivers

Non-pharmacological therapies (NPT) help individuals with cognitive deterioration and dementia to ameliorate their cognitive capacities and maintain functional autonomy. In addition, NPTs provide patients and especially their caregivers with methods and strategies to prevent and solve behavioural problems, as well as to cope with the functional and emotional consequences of the disease.

NPTs were operationally defined as any theoretically based, nonchemical, focused, and replicable intervention, conducted with the patient or the caregiver, which may provide some relevant benefit. Essentially, an NPT should provide a rationale of intervention design, a protocol to ensure replication, and some empirical data demonstrating relevant benefits. NPT can be focused on the person with dementia, the caregiver, or both. Opportunities for various therapeutic approaches arise when combining different clinical target domains with different target receivers (patients and types of caregivers) (Figure 2.2).

NPT should be designed to optimise or contribute to person-centred care. Agreement and collaboration with the intervention by the recipient (patient, caregiver, or both) is essential for the implementation, and probably for the efficacy of NPT. Carried out under these premises, NPT can break the vicious cycle of experiencing cognitive difficulties, its frequent negative psychological reaction, and ensuing social isolation. The alternative offered by adequately tailored and prescribed NPT is a positive dynamic of cognitive acceptance, emotional stability, social inclusion, and adaptation (Figure 2.3).

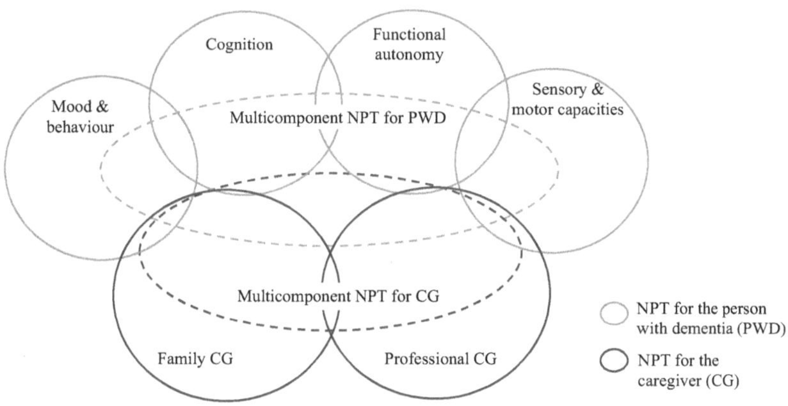

Figure 2.2 Types and focuses of non-pharmacological therapies (NPT) in dementia

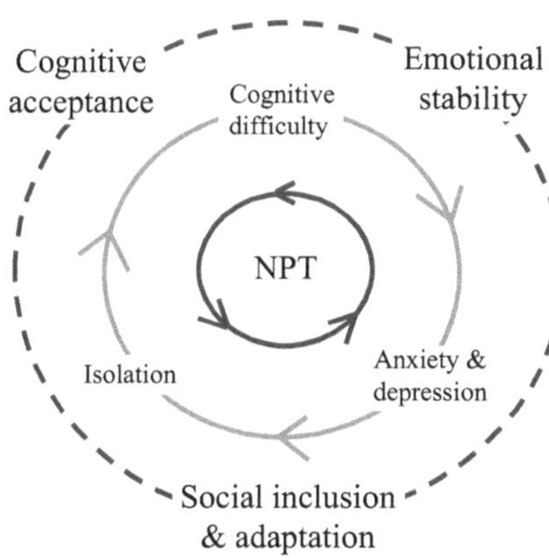

Figure 2.3 Vicious circle of discapacity and social isolation in dementia, reverted by non-pharmacological therapies (NPT)

Areas of potential benefit of NPT are clinical (cognition, functional autonomy, mood, behaviour), as well as psychological and social (psychological well-being, quality of life, delay in institutionalisation, and global cost) (Olazarán et al., 2010).

Cognition-focused NPT

Historical background

The origins of cognition-focused (or cognition-based) interventions for people with dementia can be traced to the RO programmes, which were developed in the United States in the late 1950s. First utilised to rehabilitate severely disturbed war veterans, RO was later used to help psychogeriatric patients 'to activate unused neurological pathways' and 'to find ways to compensate for organic brain damage'. These objectives were pursued in two ways: a) by continually stimulating the patient with repetitive orientation to his environment (i.e. 24-hour RO); and b) by placing them in a group of people where they could meet and compete with other patients so as to be taken out of their isolation (i.e. classroom RO) (Taulbee and Folsom, 1966).

Cognitive stimulation (CS), in its current conception and format, was derived from the former programmes of classroom RO. At the same time, progress in the knowledge of neuropsychological mechanisms involved in memory and other cognitive abilities led to the development of techniques for maintaining or enhancing more specific cognitive functions in people with cognitive impairment and dementia. Those more specific approaches were referred as cognitive training (CT) (also 'retraining', 'remediation', or 'brain training') and cognitive rehabilitation (CR) (Clare et al., 2003).

Cognitive stimulation, training, and rehabilitation: the essentials

CS engages people with cognitive deterioration in a range of group activities and discussions aimed at general enhancement of cognitive and social functioning (Table 2.2). The rationale for the use of a global method of cognitive stimulation, as opposed to a focus on specific functions, rests on the argument that cognitive functions are not used in isolation (Clare and Woods, 2004). The existing reviews of CS in people with mild to moderate dementia demonstrated consistent results of improvement in general cognition (Olazarán et al., 2010; Woods et al., 2012). The mechanisms and effects of CS are further detailed in other chapters of this book.

CT implies guided practice of a set of standard tasks designed to reflect particular cognitive functions, such as memory, attention, language, or executive function. CT may be offered through individual or group sessions. Usually a range of difficulty levels is available within a standardised set of tasks, to allow for selection of the level of difficulty that is most appropriate for a given individual (Clare and Woods, 2004).

The CR approach was developed mainly through work with younger brain-injured people, but is now increasingly being discussed in relation to chronic and progressive conditions, including dementia. CR was broadly defined as the use of any intervention strategy or technique which intends to enable clients or patients, and their families, to live with, manage, by-pass, reduce, or come to terms with deficits precipitated by injury to the brain (Wilson, 1997). CR was further defined as an individualised approach in which those affected by brain injury or disease, and their families, work together with healthcare professionals to identify personally relevant goals and devise strategies for addressing these (Wilson, 2002).

Cognitive training (CT)

Principles and mechanism of action

As mentioned above, CT involves guided practice on a set of standardised tasks designed to reflect particular cognitive functions. The intervention may be offered through individual or group sessions by professional therapists or facilitated by family members with the support of a therapist. Throughout the sessions, task difficulty is typically tailored and progressively adapted to the individual's performance level. Therapy can be provided with the traditional interpersonal approach as well as with specific computer platforms, or a combination of both.

The neuropsychological principles of CT are framed in the general principles of cognition-focused interventions (see non-pharmacological therapies: an expanding, versatile field for improving the quality of life of people with dementia and their caregivers and cognition-focused NPT). While progressive improvement in performance in trained tasks has been clearly demonstrated in people with mild dementia, the biological substrate or, in other words, the brain modifications accompanying that improvement have hardly been studied.

In one trial, 11 patients with mild to moderate AD received intense language training during five weeks. Before and after training, evoked potentials were recorded using scalp electrodes during a lexical decision task which required word/no-word discrimination. Stimuli included high and low-frequency words and no-words. After CT, a significant enhanced amplitude of the recognition potential (RP) to high-frequency words was observed. Since the initial RP did not differ from the RP observed in a matched group of cognitively healthy individuals, the results were interpreted in terms of intact functionality of left posterior linguistic networks, along with the possibility to increase plastically their activity after CT (Spironelli et al., 2013).

Clinical evidence from trials

The existing reviews of RCTs of CT have yielded conflicting results. The review by the International Non-Pharmacological Therapies Project (INPTP) concluded that CT has a positive effect on cognition, either using an individual or group format

(Olazarán et al., 2010). In contrast, the more recent Cochrane review obtained neutral results (Bahar-Fuchs et al., 2013). This discrepancy can be explained by two facts: different studies were included in both reviews, and computer-based CT was separately analysed in the INPTP review (yielding neutral results).

The INPTP did not include three neutral studies, which were included in the Cochrane review: a) the study of Neely et al. (2009), which was published beyond the time-limit of the INPTP search and implemented sessions only once a week, b) the study of Galante et al. (2007), which implemented a computer-based intervention and was therefore separately analysed in the INPTP review, and c) the study of Koltai et al. (2001), which implemented weekly sessions and was considered a multi-component intervention by the INPTP experts because coping and use of external memory aids were added to memory training.

In addition, there were two positive studies included in the INPTP review, which were not included in the Cochrane review: the study of Zarit et al. (1982), and the study of Günther et al. (1991). Both studies were excluded from the Cochrane review because participant inclusion criteria were not met. Definition of patients in Günther's and Zarit's studies were, respectively, 'elderly patients with abnormalities of cognition, memory and affect of organic causation' and 'demented persons'.

Practical conclusions

Clearly, there are insufficient data to establish a firm indication of CT in dementia. Several factors may be influencing the lack of consistent results, in contrast to those obtained by Cognitive Stimulation Therapy (CST) programmes: a) the need of highly individualised sessions, which may differ across studies; b) a possible dose-dependent effect (e.g. more effect with more frequent sessions), and c) the implementation of 'active' conditions (e.g. conditions providing similar amount of social attention in comparison to that provided to participants in the experimental group) rather than usual care in the control group in most RCTs of CT.

Nevertheless, there is also some concern regarding face validity of CT in dementia. The benefit of training of specific cognitive functions will hardly be generalised to other functions in a brain with diffuse damage. This view is supported by the studies of CT in healthy people, which demonstrate lack of transfer of effect, even to closely related cognitive areas (Owen et al., 2010). Highly individualised training, or facilitation of capacities which are personally relevant, may be certainly opportune in people with dementia, but that would be a CR approach.

Cognitive rehabilitation

Principles and mechanism of action

The already discussed neuropsychological principles of cognition-focused interventions (see non-pharmacological therapies: an expanding, versatile field for improving the quality of life of people with dementia and their caregivers and cognition-focused NPT) also apply for CR. CR programmes involve people with cognitive impairment and their families identifying personally relevant goals and devising strategies for addressing these. Hence, the emphasis is not on enhancing performance on cognitive tasks as such, but on improving functioning in the everyday context. CR targets everyday situations, and since there is no implicit assumption that changes implemented in one setting would necessarily generalise to another, it tends to be used in real-world settings (Bahar-Fuchs et al., 2013).

According to the utilised methods and techniques, two types of approaches may be distinguished in CR. The restorative approach uses methods that elicit the best possible performance of the subject's capacities. Typical examples of those methods are space retrieval, reinforcement at codification and retrieval, and vanishing cues. In contrast, the compensatory approach utilises prosthetic methods and techniques, such as environmental modifications and external aids.

Procedural tasks can best be trained using a stepwise approach, with the therapist modelling each step and providing verbal cues to guide the patient, while verbal instructions, spaced retrieval, and asking patients not to guess are most suitable for the acquisition of nonprocedural tasks. Vanishing cues are effective in steadily reducing the amount of help needed from the therapist and can be used in all types of tasks. Verbal facilitation and spaced retrieval are indicated in mild dementia, while modelling and the stepwise approach are indicated in advanced dementia. Training intensity and duration should be tailored to the needs of the individual patient and preferably take place in a familiar environment to facilitate acquisition (de Werd et al., 2013).

The biological substrate and mechanisms of CR in dementia have barely been investigated. In one RCT of CR in mild dementia (Clare et al., 2010), a subset of 19 participants underwent fMRI pre-treatment and post-treatment, while they learned and recognised unfamiliar face-name pairs. A decrease in brain function was observed in the right fusiform, parahippocampal, temporoparietal, and frontal regions in the control group, whereas patients who received CR showed an increase or remained stable in the MRI parameters. Interestingly, the fMRI differences were not observed during encoding, but only during the recognition phase of learning test, suggesting partial restoration of function in frontal brain areas (van Paasschen et al., 2013).

Clinical evidence from trials

The body of observational and controlled trials demonstrates that interventions based on errorless learning principles, which are targeted at specific everyday memory problems produce improvements in significant activities of daily living. Learning gains are usually maintained over prolonged periods of time, with or without refreshing sessions. Positive effects are mostly studied and obtained in the early stages of dementia (de Werd et al., 2013), but there are also reports of improving in procedural tasks in people with advanced dementia (Camp et al., 1997).

Sitzer et al. (2006) reviewed five non-RCT and 12 RCTs of heterogeneous interventions, which were classified on the basis of use of either compensatory or restorative approach. Overall effect sizes of (Cohen's) $d = 0.54$ and $d = 0.36$ were obtained, respectively, for restorative and compensatory approach. However, when only high quality trials were analysed, the effect sizes were 0.12 and 0.15, respectively.

There are two RCTs of CR in dementia. The Cognitive rehabilitation and cognitive-behavioural treatment for early dementia in Alzheimer's Disease (CORDIAL) was a well-powered RCT, which implemented CR and cognitive-behavioural therapy (CBT) in 201 people with mild dementia (mean Mini-Mental State Examination [MMSE] score of 25, standard deviation [SD] = 2) due to AD (Kurz et al., 2012). The intervention consisted of 12 weekly, one-hour sessions, which were organised in four thematic modules: external memory aids, identification of memory-related problems and ways of coping, reminiscence, and validation and structuring the day. The control condition was usual care. Conventional measures of cognition, functional autonomy, depression, neuropsychiatric symptoms, and caregiver burden were conducted before and after the intervention. Surprisingly, despite the fact that feasibility, treatment adherence, and carer commitment were excellent, no positive effect could be demonstrated. In fact, a mild worsening of caregiver burden was detected immediately post-intervention, although not at nine-month follow-up assessment.

In another RCT, 69 patients with mild AD (mean MMSE 23, SD = 3) were randomised to receive one of the following three conditions; CR, relaxation therapy, or usual care. The CR programme consisted of eight weekly sessions, focused on personally relevant goals. Although benefits were not demonstrated in conventional measures of cognition, functional autonomy, anxiety and depression, and memory awareness, benefits were demonstrated in a scale that evaluated performance in previously selected goals. Examples of therapy goals included; remembering details of jobs to be done around the house and learning to use a mobile phone (Clare et al., 2010; van Paasschen et al., 2013).

Practical conclusions

Based on different techniques, which should be used according to dementia severity, CR may improve predefined, personally relevant, therapy objectives. However, thorough assessment and high level of expertise on the part of the therapist are required, as well as collaboration from the person with dementia and their family.

Discussion

Pattern and predictors of response

The available trials and reviews of cognition-focused NPT in dementia demonstrate a pattern of specific response of targeted operations, which is consistent with a universal pattern of specific response to psychosocial and biological interventions in all human conditions. According to this pattern of response, CS should be preferable when general improvement in cognition is pursued, while CR will be indicated when more specific aims are desired.

A crucial question when choosing a therapy for the individual patient is the predictability of the response. This issue may be critical when facing older people, who frequently do not present well-defined processes, and are therefore amenable to different types of treatment. In fact, a high inter-individual variability of response is usually observed in older people, ranging from high resistance to unexpectedly high rate of response. Several factors have been proposed to explain this variability, including among others cognitive reserve and insight level. Surprisingly, most trials of NPT in dementia did not address the possible predictors of response. This may be explained by the typically small sample size, which prevents sub-analyses, but also by the absence of theoretically driven hypotheses.

Two RCTs of CS demonstrated more effect in patients with low education (Breuil *et al.*, 1994; Olazarán et al., 2004) and those results were interpreted in terms of cognitive reserve; given a similar level of clinical symptoms, AD could be more advanced in more educated people and thus could limit their learning ability (Olazarán et al., 2004). That interpretation was tested *ad hoc* and confirmed in a recent trial of CT enrolling 86 people with mild to moderate dementia AD. Patients with lower cognitive reserve benefited more than those with high cognitive reserve from CR on a measure of general cognition. Cognitive reserve was defined on the basis of education, working activity, and leisure time (Mondini et al., 2016).

Awareness of cognitive deficit may also predict the response to cognition-focused NPT. In a retrospective analysis of two RCTs of multi-component intervention programmes in mild to moderate AD, Fernández-Calvo et al. (2015) reported that patients in the experimental group with awareness of deficits showed positive effects on cognitive, functional, affective, and behavioural measures in comparison with patients in the waiting list group, while patients without awareness showed improvements in noncognitive symptoms only. Awareness of cognitive deficit may be needed for patient collaboration in therapy, but it could also be a surrogate marker of increased brain damage.

Several other factors may influence response to cognition-focused NPT, including biological factors (dementia aetiology, comorbidity, medications), premorbid psychological factors (IQ, personality traits), and clinical factors (cognitive performance, depressive and anxious symptoms, severity of behavioural disturbances) (Binetti et al., 2013). Clearly, large RCTs are needed to prospectively address the influence of those potential predictors and hence select the most suitable and efficient therapy for every person with dementia.

'Active ingredients'

A long-debated question in the field of CS of people with dementia is whether or not there are some 'active ingredients' which should be tapped to magnify and spread the effect of therapy all over the cerebral functions, and hence optimise the efficiency of the programmes. The above-described pattern of specific response to cognitive interventions goes against the existence of that type of intervention components. As previously discussed in this chapter, the rationale for the use of CS, as opposed to focusing on specific functions, rests on the argument that cognitive functions are not used in isolation. Instead, their operation requires a sophisticated integration with other functions such as attention, language, problem solving and so on. Possibly, the 'active ingredients' of CS and other cognition-focused NPT are those elements which elicit the relatively preserved capacities, reinforcing them and facilitating the use of other less preserved related capacities. This view of 'active ingredients' is supported from the biological perspective, since the relatively preserved neural systems have more synaptic connections than the damaged systems.

Consequently, it is preferable to tap into as many of those relatively preserved capacities as possible in order to achieve the maximal improvement in general cognition. If improvement in one particular function is desired, the relatively preserved capacities should also be utilised, in a context that facilitates the temporal relation between the preserved and the targeted function (e.g. conducting motor actions during verbal encoding and retrieval).

'Active ingredients' will therefore depend on the profile of damaged and preserved functions, which will mostly depend on dementia aetiology, but may also be modified by variation in lesion topography within the same aetiology, and by the individual background. Differences in the profile of damaged and preserved functions in patients receiving the same intervention may be in part responsible of the inter-individual variability of response.

Somehow related with the 'active ingredients' discussion, it remains to be clarified to what extent the benefits of cognition-focused interventions in dementia derive from social attention and interaction. In other words, these interventions might be beneficial just because they provide more opportunity for activities and social interaction that, due to consequences and stigma of dementia, are traditionally neglected. The available reviews and meta-analyses indicate that, when such interventions are tested against active control conditions, the magnitude of effect is lower than when the comparison group receives usual care (Sitzer et al., 2006; Olazarán et al., 2010). In fact, lack of active control groups in most RCTs of CS may have been decisive in reaching positive results in the meta-analyses. Conversely, the use of active control conditions in most RCTs of CT could explain the neutral results.

In a desirable and foreseeable context of progressive improvement in social attention and care for people with dementia, NPT are continuously challenged to find and offer relevant benefits for the affected people and the society. Non-pharmacological therapies are called to develop interventions for those aspects of dementias that produce special suffering and are not adequately covered, e.g. anxiety, depression, aggression, motor hyperactivity, and vocalisations.

What is the future of cognition-focused NPT in dementia?

While general recommendation for treatment could be established regarding CS, the reviews of CT and CR were not conclusive, due to very few trials (CR) or inconsistent results (CR). Supported by its cost-efficacy (Knapp et al., 2006) CS programmes should be universally offered across communities and institutions. Making such programmes accessible and feasible for people with physical disabilities or hard-to-reach populations is complex and may require involvement of local healthcare services. Well-designed e-health platforms and their implementation in homes and aged-care facilities could be an area worth developing.

Several issues remain critical and should be addressed in future research to consolidate cognition-focused NPT as first-line treatment for people with dementia. Important research is already being conducted to understand the time-course of CS benefits and the proper methods for the maintenance of effects (see the following chapters of this book). However, long-term trials should continue to address the effects of CS in noncognitive areas (functional autonomy, mood, behaviour) and also address the potential disease-modifying effects of the CS (i.e. effects beyond symptomatic improvement).

It also remains to be investigated how to balance frequency and intensity of various intervention components in the long term – particularly the elements targeted at stimulating advanced cognitive function. One RCT (Muñiz et al., 2015 which reports three-year results of the initial one year Olazarán et al., 2004 study) showed improved activities of daily living performance sustained during three years of the intervention. Unexpectedly, cognition improved after the first year, but fell below usual care control group performance after the third year.

The development of replicable, cost-effective CR programmes is a real challenge. To attain clinically meaningful treatment effects, it may be essential to use highly individualised interventions, focusing on a limited number of personally relevant needs and using the relatively preserved capacities. Treatment should be provided in real-life settings over a sufficiently long period so that acquired strategies can attain a sufficient degree of automatisation. Also, persistence in the day-to-day context should be ensured by regular follow-up visits or booster sessions. Since personally relevant goals can be achieved in multiple ways, ability-based assessments should be complemented by patient-centred outcome measures (Clare et al., 2010; Kurz et al., 2012).

Clearly, the global improvement of care of people with dementia is calling for an effort of imagination and methodological improvement on the part of NPT. In a context of optimal social care, interventions must be highly individualised, which raises the challenge of developing replicable interventions, with predictable results. Desirably, CR programmes will be developed, which will be available to citizens and will replace many of the current CT programmes.

Functional neuroimaging studies have demonstrated reallocation of neural resources after CT and CR in people with dementia, thus supporting neuroplasticity and intervention effect (van Os et al., 2015). However, neuroimaging studies are expensive and not always comfortable for the patient, raising concerns about its priority. In our view, clinical and personally relevant outcomes remain the gold standard for measuring the effects of NPT. Consequently, neuroimaging and other biological measurements should be regarded as less important than, and always accompanied by, clinical measurements to evaluate intervention effects and to gain insight into the clinical relevance of the observed neurobiological changes (Clare et al., 2009).

How control groups should be is another issue, particularly taking into account the desirability of carrying out long-term trials. Recently, a move forward from active control conditions to control conditions, which match treatment groups in terms of improvement expectation, has been suggested (Boot et al., 2013). However, it does not seem possible to separate expectations of cognitive improvement from cognitive effect itself, since expectations are elicited and modified not only before, but also during therapy. Rather than designing sophisticated control conditions, we believe that long-term studies recruiting large samples of well-defined patients (e.g. patients defined by clinical characteristics and AD biomarkers which are expected to have cognitive deterioration at a predictable pace) should be enough to demonstrate the general effects of cognitive interventions, even if usual care or historical control groups are utilised.

Beyond the cognition-focused NPT considered here, new approaches deserve consideration and further investigation. Recently, a trial compared mindfulness, CS, muscle relaxation, and usual care. After two years of intervention, benefits in a measure of general cognition were high for mindfulness, moderate for relaxation, and small for CS (Quintana-Hernández et al., 2016). While sharing the same objective, (improvement in general cognition) mindfulness and CS utilise quite different approaches; tapping into different cognitive functions. Clearly, emerging and traditional NPT should be tested directly against one another to compare their effects on general cognition, as well as the possible differences of effect in specific cognitive functions. Independence and similar motivation of therapists involved in the different experimental groups will be crucial for the validity of these future trials.

As different drugs with different mechanisms of actions are usually combined to treat complex conditions, a possible additive effect from other types of NPT to cognition-focused NPT should be investigated. It is well known that AD is accompanied by increase in cortisol levels, due to enhancement of the hypothalamus-hypophysis-adrenal axis. Physical exercise, possibly inhibiting that hyperactivation, may decrease cortisol levels, increase BDNF, and promote neuronal regeneration, providing biological substrate for the neural changes promoted by cognition-focused NPT (Adlard and Cotman, 2004). Promising results were recently reported from a trial of physical exercise, diet, CT, and vascular risk monitoring in older people who were at risk of dementia due to limited or slightly low cognitive performance (Ngandu et al., 2015).

In recent years, a reduction of dementia incidence was described, possibly due to a better control of some vascular risk factors, but also suggesting the beneficial effect of a stimulating environment and intellectual activities (Doblhammer et al., 2015; Satizabal et al., 2016). Although this appears encouraging, a progressive increase of dementia prevalence is expected over the next decades, given the continuous ageing of populations, the improvement in the treatment of old-age comorbidities, and the progressive advances in dementia care. The desired biological treatments will hopefully stabilise the disease at the initial clinical stages, but the number of old people with mild to moderate dementia will continue to grow, in most cases with a pathological substrate of combined or even not well-defined dementia. In this context, highly individualised, cognition-focused NPT will remain fully justified to improve relevant symptoms and disabilities of people with dementia and to alleviate the burden of their caregivers.

References

Adlard, P.A. and Cotman, C.W. (2004). Voluntary exercise protects against stress-induced decreases in brain-derived neurotrophic factor protein expression. *Neuroscience* 124(4), pp. 985–992.

Akanuma, K., Meguro, K., Meguro, M. et al. (2011). Improved social interaction and increased anterior cingulate metabolism after group reminiscence with reality orientation approach for vascular dementia. *Psychiatry Research: Neuroimaging* 192(3), pp. 183–187.

Ames, D., Burns, A. and O'Brien, J. (2010). *Dementia*, 4th ed. London: Arnold.

Bäckman, L. (1996). Utilizing compensatory task conditions for episodic memory in Alzheimer's disease. *Acta Neurologica Scandinavica* 93(Suppl 165), pp. 109–113.

Baglio, F., Griffanti, L., Saibene, F.L. et al. (2015). Multistimulation group therapy in Alzheimer's disease promotes changes in brain functioning. *Neurorehabilitation and Neural Repair* 29(1), pp. 13–24.

Bahar-Fuchs, A., Clare, L. and Woods, B. (2013). Cognitive training and cognitive rehabilitation for mild to moderate Alzheimer's disease and vascular dementia. *Cochrane Database of Systematic Reviews* Issue 6. Art. No.: CD 003260.

Binetti, G., Moretti, D.V., Scalvini, C. et al. (2013). Predictors of comprehensive stimulation program efficacy in patients with cognitive impairment: Clinical practice recommendations. *International Journal of Geriatric Psychiatry* 28(1), pp. 26–33.

Boot, W.R., Simons, D.J., Stothart, C. and Stutts, C. (2013). The pervasive problem with placebos in Psychology: Why active control groups are not sufficient to rule out placebo effects. *Perspectives on Psychological Science* 8(4), pp. 445–454.

Boyle, P.A., Wilson, R.S., Yu, L. et al. (2013). Much of late life cognitive decline is not due to common neurodegenerative pathologies. *Annals of Neurology* 74(3), pp. 478–489.

Breuil, V., De Rotrou, J., Forette, F. et al. (1994). Cognitive stimulation of patients with dementia: Preliminary results. *International Journal of Geriatric Psychiatry* 9, pp. 211–217.

Camp, C.J., Judge, K.S., Bye, C. et al. (1997). An intergenerational program for persons with dementia using Montessori methods. *Gerontologist* 37(5), pp. 688–692.

Clare, L., Linden, D.E., Woods, R.T. et al. (2010). Goal-oriented cognitive rehabilitation for people with early-stage Alzheimer disease: A single-blind randomized controlled trial of clinical efficacy. *American Journal of Geriatric Psychiatry* 18(10), pp. 928–939.

Clare, L., van Paasschen, J., Evans, S.J. et al. (2009). Goal-oriented cognitive rehabilitation for an individual with mild cognitive impairment: Behavioural and neuroimaging outcomes. *Neurocase: The Neural Basis of Cognition* 15(4), pp. 318–331.

Clare, L. and Woods, R.T. (2004). Cognitive training and cognitive rehabilitation for people with early-stage Alzheimer's disease: A review. *Neuropsychological Rehabilitation* 14, pp. 385–401.

Clare, L., Woods, R.T., Moniz-Cook, E.D., Orrell, M., & Spector, A. (2003). *Cognitive rehabilitation and cognitive training for early-stage Alzheimer's disease and vascular dementia.* Cochrane Database Syst Rev 4: CD003260.

de Werd, M.M., Boelen, D., Rikkert, M.G. and Kessels, R.P. (2013). Errorless learning of everyday tasks in people with dementia. *Clinical Interventions in Aging* 8, pp. 1177–1190.

Doblhammer, G., Fink, A., Zylla, S. and Willekens, F. (2015). Compression or expansion of dementia in Germany? An observational study of short-term trends in incidence and death rates of dementia between 2006/07 and 2009/10 based on German health insurance data. *Alzheimers Research and Therapy* 7(1), p. 66.

Fernández-Calvo, B., Contador, I., Ramos, F. et al. (2015). Effect of unawareness on rehabilitation outcome in a randomised controlled trial of multicomponent intervention for patients with mild Alzheimer's disease. *Neuropsychological Rehabilitation* 25(3), pp. 448–477.

Förster, S., Buschert, V.C., Buchholz, H.G. et al. (2011). Effects of a 6-month cognitive intervention program on brain metabolism in amnestic mild cognitive impairment and mild Alzheimer's disease. *Journal of Alzheimer's Disease* 25(4), pp. 695–706.

Foster, P.P., Rosenblatt, K.P. and Kuljiš, R.O. (2011). Exercise-induced cognitive plasticity, implications for mild cognitive impairment and Alzheimer's disease. *Frontiers in Neurology* 2(28).

Galante, E., Venturini, G. and Fiaccadori, C. (2007). Computer-based cognitive intervention for dementia: Preliminary results of a randomized clinical trial. *Giornale Italiano di Medicina del Lavoro ed Ergonomia* 29(3 Suppl B), pp. B26–B32.

Gidicsin, C.M., Maye, J.E., Locascio, J.J. et al. (2015). Cognitive activity relates to cognitive performance but not to Alzheimer disease biomarkers. *Neurology* 85(1), pp. 48–55.

Günther, V., Fuchs, D., Schett, P. et al. (1991). Kognitives training bei organischem psychosyndrom [Cognitive training in psycho-organic syndromes]. *Deutsche Medizinische Wochenschrift* 116(22), pp. 846–851.

Hosseini, S.M., Kramer, J.H. and Kesler, S.R. (2014). Neural correlates of cognitive intervention in persons at risk of developing Alzheimer's disease. *Frontiers in Aging Neuroscience* 6(231).

Iturria-Medina, Y., Sotero, R.C., Toussaint, P.J., Mateos-Pérez, J.M., Evans, A.C. and Alzheimer's Disease Neuroimaging Initiative. (2016). Early role of vascular dysregulation on late-onset Alzheimer's disease based on multifactorial data-driven analysis. *Nature Communications* 7(11934).

Katzman, R., Aronson, M., Fuld, P. et al. (1989). Development of dementing illnesses in an 80-year-old volunteer cohort. *Annals of Neurology* 25(4), pp. 317–324.

Kawas, C.H., Kim, R.C., Sonnen, J.A. et al. (2015). Multiple pathologies are common and related to dementia in the oldest-old: The 90+ Study. *Neurology* 85(6), pp. 535–542.

Knapp, M., Thorgrimsen, L., Patel, A. et al. (2006). Cognitive Stimulation Therapy for people with dementia: Cost-effectiveness analysis. *British Journal of Psychiatry* 188(June), pp. 574–580.

Koltai, D.C., Welsh-Bohmer, K.A. and Smechel, D.E. . (2001). Influence of anosognosia on treatment outcome among dementia patients. *Neuropsychological Rehabilitation* 11(3–4), pp. 455–475.

Kurz, A., Thöne-Otto, A., Cramer, B. et al. (2012). CORDIAL (cognitive rehabilitation and cognitive-behavioral treatment for early dementia in Alzheimer's disease): A multicenter, randomized, controlled trial. *Alzheimer's Disease and Associated Disorders* 26(3), pp. 246–253.

McDaniel, M.A. and Einstein, G.O. (2011). The neuropsychology of prospective memory in normal aging: A componential approach. *Neuropsychologia* 49(8), pp. 2147–2155.

Mondini, S., Madella, I., Zangrossi, A. et al. (2016). Cognitive reserve in dementia: Implications for cognitive training. *Frontiers in Aging and Neuroscience* 8(84).

Muñiz, R., Massegú, C., Reisberg, B. et al. (2015). Cognitive-motor intervention in Alzheimer's disease: Long-term results from the Maria Wolff Trial. *Journal of Alzheimer's Disease* 45, pp. 295–304.

Neely, A.S., Vikstrom, S. and Josephsson, S. (2009). Collaborative memory intervention in dementia: Caregiver participation matters. *Neuropsychological Rehabilitation* 19(5), pp. 696–715.

Ngandu, T., Lehtisalo, J., Solomon, A. et al. (2015). A 2 year multidomain intervention of diet, exercise, cognitive training, and vascular risk monitoring versus control to prevent cognitive decline in at-risk elderly people (FINGER): A randomised controlled trial. *Lancet* 385(9984), pp. 2255–2263.

OECD. 2014. Dementia prevalence. In OECD/European Union, Health at a Glance: Europe 2014 [Online]. OECD Publishing: Paris. Available at: http://dx.doi.org/10.1787/health_glance_eur-2014-18-en. Published December 3, 2014. Accessed 6 February 2017.

Olazarán, J., Muñiz, R., Reisberg, B. et al. (2004). Benefits of cognitive-motor intervention in MCI and mild to moderate Alzheimer disease. *Neurology* 63(12), pp. 2348–2353.

Olazarán, J., Reisberg, B., Clare, L. et al. (2010). Nonpharmacological therapies in Alzheimer's disease: A systematic review of efficacy. *Dementia and Geriatric Cognitive Disorders* 30(2), pp. 161–178.

Owen, A.M., Hampshire, A., Grahn, J.A. et al. (2010). Putting brain training to the test. *Nature* 465(7299), pp. 775–778.

Pouryamout, L., Dams, J., Wasem, J. et al. (2012). Economic evaluation of treatment options in patients with Alzheimer's disease: A systematic review of cost-effectiveness analyses. *Drugs* 72(6), pp. 789–802.

Prince, M., Bryce, R., Albanese, E. et al. (2013). The global prevalence of dementia: A systematic review and metaanalysis. *Alzheimer's & Dementia: The Journal of the Alzheimer's Association* 9(1), pp. 63–75.

Quintana-Hernández, D.J., Miró-Barrachina, M.T., Ibáñez-Fernández, I.J. et al. (2016). Mindfulness in the maintenance of cognitive capacities in Alzheimer's disease: A randomized clinical trial. *Journal of Alzheimer's Disease* 50(1), pp. 217–232.

Satizabal, C.L., Beiser, A.S., Chouraki, V. et al. (2016). Incidence of dementia over three decades in the Framingham Heart Study. *New England Journal of Medicine* 374(6), pp. 523–532.

Sitzer, D.I., Twamley, E.W. and Jeste, D.V. (2006). Cognitive training in Alzheimer's disease: A meta-analysis of the literature. *Acta Psychiatrica Scandinavica* 114(2), pp. 75–90.

Spironelli, C., Bergamaschi, S., Mondini, S. et al. (2013). Functional plasticity in Alzheimer's disease: Effect of cognitive training on language-related ERP components. *Neuropsychologia* 51(8), pp. 1638–1648.

Stern, Y. (2002). What is cognitive reserve? Theory and research application of the reserve concept. *Journal of the International Neuropsychological Society* 8(3), pp. 448–460.

Taulbee, L.R. and Folsom, J.C. (1966). Reality orientation for geriatric patients. *Hospital and Community Psychiatry* 17, pp. 133–135.

van Os, Y., de Vugt, M.E. and van Boxtel, M. (2015). Cognitive interventions in older persons: Do they change the functioning of the brain? *Biomed Research International* 2015(438908).

van Paasschen, J., Clare, L., Yuen, K.S. et al. (2013). Cognitive rehabilitation changes memory-related brain activity in people with Alzheimer disease. *Neurorehabilitation and Neural Repair* 27(5), pp. 448–459.

Vemuri, P., Fields, J., Peter, J. and Klöppel, S. (2016a). Cognitive interventions in Alzheimer's and Parkinson's diseases: Emerging mechanisms and role of imaging. *Current Opinions in Neurology* 29(4), pp. 405–411.

Vemuri, P., Lesnick, T.G., Przybelski, S.A. et al. (2016b). Effect of intellectual enrichment on AD biomarker trajectories: Longitudinal imaging study. *Neurology* 86(12), pp. 1128–1135.

Wilson, B.A. (1997). Cognitive rehabilitation: How it is and how it might be. *Journal of the International Neuropsychological Society* 3(5), pp. 487–496.

Wilson, B.A. (2002). Towards a comprehensive model of cognitive rehabilitation. *Neuropsychological Rehabilitation* 12(2), pp. 97–110.

Wolf, S.A., Kronenberg, G., Lehmann, K. et al. (2006). Cognitive and physical activity differently modulate disease progression in the amyloid precursor protein [APP]-23 model of Alzheimer's disease. *Biological Psychiatry* 60(12), pp. 1314–1323.

Woods, B., Aguirre, E., Spector, A.E. and Orrell, M. (2012). Cognitive stimulation to improve cognitive functioning in people with dementia. *Cochrane Database of Systematic Reviews* 2(CD005562).

Yang, H., Leaver, A.M., Siddarth, P. et al. (2016). Neurochemical and neuroanatomical plasticity following memory training and yoga interventions in older adults with mild cognitive impairment. *Frontiers in Aging Neuroscience* 8(277).

Zarit, S.H., Zarit, J.M. and Reever, K.E. (1982). Memory training for severe memory loss: Effects on senile dementia patients and their caregivers. *Gerontologist* 22(4), pp. 373–377.

Part II

The CST research findings

Chapter 3

CST

Development process

Bob Woods

Background

Cognitive Stimulation Therapy (CST) for dementia is now an accepted and increasingly implemented approach in the UK and across the world, as this book clearly indicates. However, readers may be surprised to learn that it has taken 60 years, with some considerable ups and downs along the way, to reach this point. This chapter will discuss the steps leading to the development of CST, and highlight some of the lessons learned.

Taking a historical perspective, cognitive stimulation for people with dementia, operationalised as CST, owes its development in the mid 1990s to the intersection of two distinct domains of knowledge and practice. The first domain reflected a growing interest in 'positive approaches to dementia care' (Holden and Woods, 1995). These approaches, including amongst others Reality Orientation (RO) and reminiscence therapy (RT), represented a rejection of the therapeutic nihilism which had for so long surrounded people with dementia. It was argued that psychological approaches could make a positive difference, when embedded in a value-system that recognised the human value of the person with dementia and the person's individuality, offering respect and dignity. These approaches were democratic, in that they did not require special qualifications or degrees to deliver them.

The second domain was methodological. This was a time when the first convincing evidence was emerging that pharmacological therapies could make a difference to cognitive function in people with Alzheimer's disease. Results from double-blind randomised controlled trials (RCTs) of a drug called 'tacrine' were boosting hopes that a treatment for Alzheimer's would soon be available. Indeed, licenced acetylcholinesterase inhibitors, such as donepezil, were just around the corner. Increasingly advocates of 'positive approaches' were challenged as to whether these psychological therapies could stand up to the same rigorous form of evaluation as was the accepted standard for pharmacological approaches.

By happy accident, the author, a clinical psychologist who is one of the UK pioneers of positive approaches to dementia, and Martin Orrell, an old-age psychiatrist with a particular interest in a psychological understanding of dementia, both had academic appointments at University College London (UCL) around this time, although employed in different areas of the National Health Service (NHS) in London and in different departments at UCL. They had previously worked closely, clinically as well as on research, at the Bethlem and Maudsley Hospitals in South London, where Orrell undertook his training as a psychiatrist and the author was the principal clinical psychologist for the older people's mental health service. A call for research proposals evaluating psychological therapies (not specifically for dementia) provided the impetus for a first (unsuccessful) proposal to carry out an evaluation of therapy groups (using positive approaches) for people with dementia, modelled on the methods used in a drug trial.

The collaboration on this unsuccessful proposal led to the publication of an editorial entitled 'Tacrine and psychological therapies in dementia: no contest?' (Orrell and Woods, 1996). This brief paper in retrospect may be seen as a manifesto for the body of work which has developed in subsequent decades, much of it documented in this volume. Orrell and Woods argued that it was premature to write off psychological therapies as a serious competitor to drugs in the treatment of dementia. They highlighted the low quality of the methodology used in studies of psychological approaches, with small sample sizes and poorly defined interventions (often without a sound theoretical underpinning), in comparison with the relatively large numbers and well-defined formulations used in drug trials. They called for standard and sensitive instruments to be used as outcome measures, to evaluate a range of areas, including quality of life (QoL) as well as cognitive function, selecting these from amongst those used in drug studies, for the purposes of comparability. They called for funding bodies to encourage large-scale well-designed studies, with researchers collaborating on multi-centre trials, and the evaluation including a cost-benefit analysis, recognising that psychological therapies are not necessarily a cheap option.

Thanks largely to the persistence of Martin Orrell, a year after the publication of this 'manifesto', funding had been obtained for 12 months for the development of a 'psychological therapy package' for dementia from the regional NHS research funder (North Thames NHS). Further grants followed over the next three years from the same funder and a local NHS organisation to support an RCT of this approach. Two talented and dedicated students, Aimee Spector and Lene Thorgrimsen, joined the team around this time to undertake their PhD studies on the programme, and they were instrumental in shaping how the programme developed. This early work will be described later in this chapter, after elaborating on the development of positive approaches and the methodology domain introduced above.

The development of positive approaches

Twenty years before the programme of work on CST began, Woods and Britton (1977) reviewed 'Psychological approaches to the treatment of the elderly'. Despite the generic title, the focus was on approaches which might prevent decline in the '10% of the elderly population suffering from mild mental deterioration and organic psycho-syndromes'. The approaches reviewed included stimulation and activity programmes, milieu treatment, behavioural approaches, and RO. The earliest study noted was carried out in a geriatric ward in the UK in 1958 (Cosin et al., 1958). The study concluded that deterioration was not inevitable, and that to have an effect programmes needed to be of sufficient intensity and engage the person in activity, as opposed to simply being exposed to increased stimulation. Addressing the person's motivation to participate and recognising the potential for negative effects and dissatisfaction were seen as important, but across all the approaches the need for changes in staff attitudes appeared paramount. Attitudes needed to be consistent and enabling, offering the person the opportunity to reach their potential level of function, and recognising that, however limited, some learning could be possible. While recognising the potential of behavioural approaches to be tailored to the individual and able to target specific areas of difficulty, the growing body of work on RO was evident, and this was the approach that went on to receive most research attention in the following decade.

RO was developed in the United States in the 1950s at the Veterans Administration (VA) Hospital in Topeka, Kansas, as an 'aide-centred activity programme for elderly patients'. Dr James Folsom was instrumental in its development, and the programme followed him to the VA Hospital at Tuscaloosa, Alabama. As described by Taulbee and Folsom (1966, p. 133) its effects were dramatic:

> In our geriatric unit we have 180 psychiatric, medically infirm patients, most of whom are ambulatory. They were sent to the unit because they were confused, disoriented, and lost to themselves and their families . . . When they arrived they all were frightened, unhappy and uncomfortable people, but their look of hopelessness soon changed to hopefulness when we told them their names, where they were and what date and day of the week it was. Thus we launched our unit program of reality orientation.

By 1969, the American Psychiatric Association (APA) had published a brief guide to the approach entitled 'Reality Orientation: a technique to rehabilitate elderly and brain-damaged patients with a moderate to severe degree of disorientation' (Stephens, 1969), and, building on the experience of over 10 years of training staff from all over the United States and further afield, the team at Tuscaloosa published a practical guide in 1978 (Drummond et al., 1978).

The approach as originally described comprised three components:

- 24-hour RO (or 'informal RO') involved staff in presenting information related to orientation in each interaction with the person, providing a commentary on events and reminding the person of time and place and people. These interactions were reinforced by environmental modifications, with signs, clocks, calendars, and noticeboards to assist the person remain aware of their surroundings.

- RO classes (or RO groups) were intended to be small group sessions, with perhaps five or six people with dementia and one or two staff. The session would commence with introductions around a RO board, discussing current information and orientation, such as the day, the place, news, and forthcoming events. This would be followed by a variety of other activities to enhance social interaction and learning, tailored to the abilities and interests of the group. Groups would meet as far as possible daily, for between 30 minutes and an hour. The groups aimed to help the person know what is happening, to communicate, and to experience success in activities, by offering activities geared to their level of ability.
- 'Attitude therapy' encouraged staff to be consistent in their attitudes towards particular patients or residents, with attitudes chosen to be a good fit with the person's personality, varying from active friendliness through no demand and matter-of-fact to kind firmness. This aspect of the original approach is the least well-documented, and does not appear to have been implemented widely.

By 1975, RO was being trialled in the UK, and the very first controlled trial of the approach was undertaken at Warley Hospital, Essex (Brook et al., 1975). The results of this study were published in the British Journal of Psychiatry and showed some positive indications on a behaviour rating scale, completed by nursing staff blind as to whether patients were attending RO sessions daily for 30 minutes, or were simply being taken to sit in the room where RO sessions took place, but without any activities. Eighteen patients took part in the study, over a four-month period, with nine attending RO sessions and nine in the control condition.

The following 10 years saw a rapid increase in the use of RO across the UK. Una Holden, working in Leeds, adapted the approach to fit better with the UK culture and context. In the VA Hospitals, group sessions were based on a classroom model, with a staff member as the instructor or teacher, and the focus on the whiteboard containing the orientation information. In Leeds, the RO sessions were held in a simulated pub, emphasising a social environment, and although a RO board would be used, there would be many other tangible props, photographs, and other materials to engage interest and attention. Elsewhere, the social atmosphere would be encouraged through meeting in a comfortable sitting room, with tea and other refreshments a central feature. Further UK controlled trials were published (Holden and Sinebruchow, 1978 [Leeds]; Woods, 1979 [Newcastle]; Johnson et al., 1981 [Dundee]; Hanley et al., 1981 [Edinburgh]; Merchant and Saxby, 1980 [Plymouth]), together with a similar number of studies from the United States, so that when in 1982 the first edition of 'Reality Orientation: psychological approaches to the 'confused' elderly' was published (Holden and Woods, 1982), there was a wealth of material on research and practice on RO and other approaches, filling over

300 pages. The book served as a practical manual as well as a research overview, and training materials were produced, with workshops and training courses on RO proving popular. A second edition of the book, updated and revised, appeared just six years later (Holden and Woods, 1988), reflecting the growth of the field, with international interest evident from Europe, Australia, and Japan.

However, in retrospect, the popularity of RO had peaked by the late 1980s, with widespread concern that its application was falling short of the aspirations of its pioneers. It seemed that some of those using it had focused on the name 'reality orientation' and had not gone beyond this to a broader understanding of what should be involved. The emphasis became on orientating the person, by correcting them, setting up a system of 'reality confrontation', which was never envisaged as a general communication strategy. The values of respect, dignity, individuality, and choice that Holden and Woods (1982) had seen as underpinning the approach in practice were too often disregarded. Even the most tangible indicator of the RO approach in practice, the orientation board at the centre of the ward or care setting, gave witness to the lack of consistent implementation of the approach. It appeared that every care setting for people with dementia in the UK now had a RO board, but that virtually every one of them had not been updated with the current date or other information.

Concerns were expressed regarding the value of orientating the person to his/her current environment when in so many instances it appeared to be an environment with little to commend it as a place to live or spend time. The challenge was to enrich the environment, to make it less institutional and clinical, less dominated by routine and the needs of the institution, so that it would be more homely and offering a much more extensive range of choices and activities. 'Does it matter whether it's Tuesday or Wednesday' was a question frequently asked in relation to RO's supposed relentless pursuit of correct and complete orientation. The answer, perhaps, was that it might make little difference in many care homes and wards, where each day might seem the same, but for a person living at home attending a day centre on Tuesdays and having a regular visit from a good friend on a Wednesday, it would be a different matter. Other concerns related to the power-imbalance that was seen to be inherent in RO. The person with dementia might have constructed their own reality, but the reality as perceived by the staff would always be seen as the 'correct' reality, again leading to reality confrontation, and the potential for distress in all its forms.

Case-reports such as reported by Dietch et al. (1989) powerfully illustrated the insensitive application of RO, exemplifying the way in which staff might impose their view on a person with dementia, in the guise of RO, through not seeking to see the world through the eyes of the person with dementia. Similar examples had been reported earlier by Gubrium and Ksander (1975) and Buckholdt and Gubrium (1983), of RO applied in a mechanical, depersonalised fashion. Such reports led to the APA (1997) in its practice guidelines for dementia concluding:

> The slight improvements observed with some of these treatments (cognition-oriented approaches) have not lasted beyond the treatment sessions and thus do not appear to warrant the risk of adverse effects.
>
> (APA, 1997)

The demise of RO is apparent in the change of title for the third edition of the Holden and Woods RO text-book, which in 1995 completely dropped RO from its title 'Positive approaches to dementia care', as well as embracing the change of language around the use of the terms 'confused' and 'dementia'. Much of the content of the book remained, albeit updated, as these authors had always viewed RO as part of an integrated, individualised approach, based on careful assessment and care-planning. In particular, while some in the field had seen reminiscence and validation therapy approaches as being in opposition to RO, these aspects had always been incorporated within the understanding of potentially effective communication strategies. As RO diminished in its influence, these other approaches came more to the fore.

Reminiscence approaches became widely used, with a broad range of memory triggers, such as photographs of previous decades, music and audio recordings, facsimiles of newspapers from the past and so on becoming commercially available. Many care settings developed collections of memorabilia, relating to particular phases of life or occupations that could become a tangible focus for a reminiscence session. Reminiscence rooms were created, furnished in the style from when the person with dementia would have been much younger. RO saw reminiscence as a valuable aid to communication, a bridge to the present. Reminiscence approaches sought to maintain the continuity of the person's identity, and to assist social interaction through the sharing of memories and experiences.

Validation therapy was developed in the United States by a social worker, Naomi Feil (e.g. Feil, 1993), in part from dissatisfaction with the over-confrontational application of RO that she observed. Whereas RO appeared to focus on facts – the day, the date, the place etc. – the validation approach acknowledged, and tried to validate, the emotions behind the communication of the person with dementia. For example, the person might talk about their mother, as if she were still alive. The validation approach would not seek to 'correct' the person, but would recognise the person's need to talk about their mother, perhaps as an expression of an attachment need, a desire for the safety and security a mother represented, when as a child we felt vulnerable or insecure. Simply saying 'tell me about your mother – do you have a picture of her?' opens up the communication of feelings rather than of facts about whether she is alive or dead. This communication strategy of 'acknowledge the feelings expressed, ignore the content' was recommended as part of the basic RO approach by Holden and Woods (1982), but was clearly over-shadowed in practice.

Kitwood's seminal work began to appear in the years before the publication of the third edition of the book (e.g. Kitwood, 1990), assisting in articulating more powerfully a strong emphasis on the need for person-centred values to underpin any psychological approach. Holden and Woods (1982) had emphasised the importance of dignity, respect, choice, individuality, and treating the person as an adult, but Kitwood's formulation of personhood and its significance enabled these messages to influence practice more directly.

Thus, by 1995, positive approaches had emerged post-RO to continue to have an influence on practitioners who had a sense of hope in their work with people with dementia, who felt that, in small ways, it was possible to make a difference. These approaches empowered staff, in providing a structure and framework to guide communication and activity.

Developing methodology for evaluating psychological approaches to dementia

Reflecting on the steps that followed from the Orrell and Woods (1996) manifesto, they can now be seen as fitting well with the widely accepted framework, developed by the Medical Research Council (MRC) (2008), for the evaluation of complex interventions. The framework includes four phases:

- Development
- Feasibility/piloting
- Evaluation
- Implementation

In the development of a complex intervention, such as a psychological approach to dementia, these phases are not seen as a linear progression, as might be the case in drug development, where laboratory tests lead to initial trials in humans, followed by full-scale effectiveness trials to licenced use in medical practice. With complex interventions, there are interactions between phases and there may be a need for example to carry out further development work on the basis of feasibility and piloting. Woods and Russell (2014) suggest that all the stages are important, and that adequate development and piloting work is needed to produce stronger interventions.

Thus, although Orrell and Woods envisaged from the outset setting up an RCT of a psychological approach to dementia, considerable preliminary work needed to be undertaken. Development work typically includes identifying and systematically reviewing the evidence base to establish what is already known. Understanding and developing the theory underlying the approach is also important to answer questions such as: Why would this approach make a difference? What difference exactly would it make – what are the areas on which the evaluation should focus?

Assessing the feasibility both of the intervention and proposed evaluation procedures is essential. Piloting the intervention on a small scale allows it to be refined so that a clear and full description of it can be drawn up, resulting in an intervention 'manual'. This will enable others to know exactly what the intervention comprised, and allow replication. Piloting, and if necessary, validating outcome measures, is important, especially where consideration of the theoretical basis of the intervention and the expected outcomes suggests that existing measures would not suffice. Preliminary work in feasibility and pilot studies also allows issues relating to recruitment of study sites and participants to be considered. For example, defining the appropriate inclusion and exclusion criteria, and answering questions such as; how difficult will it be to find sufficient participants, and what is the rate of likely loss of participants from the study? Often the feasibility study gives an indication of the potential size of any benefits, which can assist in calculating how many participants will be required in the full study for it to be highly probable that an effect, if it is present, has not been missed.

The development of CST

The first step in developing what was to become CST was to carry out systematic reviews of what was known already regarding the effects of psychological approaches for people with dementia. It was anticipated that there would be a number of studies of RO to review. Holden and Woods (1995) had identified 21 controlled studies of RO and cognitive approaches, including in total 677 patients with dementia (averaging 32 per study).

Systematic reviews published by the Cochrane Collaboration are viewed internationally as the authoritative source for evidence-based practice in medicine and healthcare. They are carried out to a rigorous protocol, and are peer-reviewed to assure their quality. It was decided to carry out Cochrane reviews for RO and RT in the first instance, both published in 1998 – other authors were working on a Cochrane review on validation therapy first published in 1999 (Neal and Barton-Wright, 2009).

The review of RT (Spector et al., 1998) found very little evidence from RCTs, with much of the (broadly encouraging) evidence in support coming from descriptive or observational studies. The RO review (Spector et al., 2000) identified 43 studies, but only eight of these met the criteria for inclusion as *randomised* controlled trials of RO sessions. A meta-analysis, combining comparable data across studies, was possible for six of the studies, with 125 participants. This analysis indicated that there were significant benefits on cognitive function and on behaviour associated with RO. The results for a number of the individual studies were not statistically significant, but pooling the data, which showed a similar trend across studies, revealed an effect not apparent in small-scale studies. The results were strongly influenced by a French study, with 56 participants (Breuil et al., 1994), which had shown a significant effect on cognition. They described their approach as 'cognitive stimulation' and their programme was much more informed by a neuropsychological understanding of dementia. It aimed to capitalise on preserved skills, such as implicit memory, and mental imagery was used to stimulate encoding, consolidation, and retrieval of information. Typical activities included word association, object naming, and categorising, and it was considered that there was sufficient similarity with other RO programmes to include it in the review.

In designing the intervention, a broader range of literature than had been included in the meta-analysis was used to identify what appeared to be the components of successful approaches (Spector et al., 2001). A total of 28 studies, including studies on reminiscence and validation, provided enough details on activities used in their interventions, and these were then used to develop the first CST programme.

The decision was taken to initially develop a group-based programme, in view of the apparent effectiveness of RO sessions. Twenty-four hour RO was seen as potentially more difficult to 'package' or to monitor its implementation. Five principles were followed in designing the programme, with a view to ensuring the values-base underpinning it was explicit, and in line with Kitwood's conception of person-centred care (Spector et al., 2001):

1 Experiential learning using all five senses to promote cognitive stimulation and memory processes.
2 Focused psychological interventions relevant to the difficulties of everyday living.
3 Acknowledgment of the emotional lives and enhancement of the cognitive skills of people with dementia.
4 Implicit learning (familiarity and 'intuition'), rather than explicit 'teaching'. Extensive rehearsal and consolidation of essential information about themselves and their world.
5 The reciprocal, psychological process (involving cognitive and emotional states) in which people with dementia and those who care for them learn more about each other's capabilities and vulnerabilities.

A 15-session programme was designed with four phases:

1 The senses e.g. sounds and music
2 Remembering the past e.g. childhood
3 People and objects e.g. cookery, famous faces
4 Everyday practical issues e.g. money

Sessions were planned to last 45 minutes, commencing with a 10-minute opening phase where the group was to be welcomed, the 'theme song' sung, current information discussed around a board, and tea and biscuits consumed. This was to be followed by a 25-minute session focusing on the main activity of the day, with the session ending with 10 minutes of consolidation where the discussion and ideas could be summarised, the theme song sung again, and farewells said.

Feasibility and piloting

Having developed the initial CST programme, its feasibility needed to be evaluated in practice. Accordingly, it was piloted in one day centre and three care homes, with 35 participants being randomly allocated to either attend the CST sessions or to receive treatment as usual. The decision not to have the control group receive an alternative intervention was based on several considerations. Firstly, the Cochrane review of RO did not suggest that the type of control group (active versus treatment as usual) made any difference to outcomes. Secondly, achieving a plausible, credible active control group is quite challenging. Thirdly, the ultimate research question is whether adding a psychological intervention to usual care makes a difference. An implication of this decision is that the subsequent RCT could not be 'double-blind' as in a drug trial. Inevitably, the participants and group leaders will be aware that they are taking part in the intervention being trialled. However, by ensuring those carrying out the assessments and outcome evaluations are blinded to group membership, it is possible for such trials to be conducted on a single-blind basis, and to reduce the bias that would potentially result if assessors knew which participants had received the intervention. This single-blinding was implemented in the full RCT (Spector et al., 2003) which is detailed in Chapter 4.

Criteria for inclusion and exclusion were piloted, based on pragmatic considerations. It was decided that all participants should meet diagnostic criteria for dementia, but it was recognised that in care homes it would be difficult to establish the specific type of dementia (e.g. Alzheimer's or vascular). Other criteria were set to ensure that those included were not prevented from taking an active part in the group through uncorrected sensory or communication difficulties or through serious illness or distress.

A range of outcome measures were incorporated, notably the MMSE and ADAS-Cog, as had been used in virtually all the drug trials to assess cognitive change. Measures of depression and anxiety and behaviour and communication rated by staff members were also included, as these were thought to be aspects that could be influenced by participation in the group sessions. Relatives of those attending the group sessions at the day centre were also invited to complete scales relating to their own levels of stress, as a previous study (Greene et al., 1983) had shown an impact on carers from their relative attending RO sessions at a day unit.

Recruitment was possible from both the day centre and the care homes. More participants were randomised to the intervention group to ensure there were sufficient numbers in each setting to run a viable group (6 in the day centre, 5 in each of the care homes). Attrition between baseline and the assessment after the end of the sessions was comparable in treatment and control groups, being 23% overall. Over half the losses were due to ill health or the person moving away.

Following the feasibility study, the content of all the sessions was reviewed, and a number of changes made (documented in Spector et al., 2001). A session focusing on the senses in isolation proved difficult for many, and so this session was dropped, and an emphasis on multi-sensory stimulation added throughout. Throughout it was noted that discussion needed to be enabled by specific prompts or activities, and these were incorporated throughout the programme. It was also clear that provision needed to be made for different levels of ability between groups, and so for the modified programme most sessions have two levels of activity, to offer a choice of ability level. However, this is not prescriptive, and a 'mix and match' approach can be used across the levels as preferred. The final programme comprised 14 sessions, to be delivered twice a week over a seven-week period, and forms the basis of the Making a Difference CST Manual (Spector et al., 2006).

The outcome measures worked well and appeared acceptable. However, while measures of mood and behaviour could tap into reduced problems, there was no measure of QoL or well-being included. The QoL-AD, a 13-item self-report quality of life measure for people with dementia had just become available (Logsdon et al., 1999) and it was decided to include this in the outcome measures in the main trial. The research team undertook additional work on this measure to ensure its validity in the UK context (Thorgrimsen et al., 2003).

The results from the feasibility/pilot study were used to calculate what sample size would be required in the full trial. This analysis suggested that a sample size of 64 in each group would be needed to ensure that a difference of two points on the MMSE would be detected, using a 5% significance level, with 80% probability. The full trial then aimed to achieve a sample size of 128 or greater.

The evaluation of CST

Once the changes to the intervention programme and assessment measures had been made, arising from the learning gained in the feasibility study, all was set for an RCT of the new intervention, named Cognitive Stimulation Therapy. The name acknowledged the influence of the work of Breuil et al. (1994) and sought to leave behind some of the negative perceptions associated with RO, while incorporating all that had been learned from the research on RO and other positive approaches.

The multi-centre single-blind randomised controlled trial (Spector et al., 2003) is described fully in Chapter 4 of this volume. The RCT recruited 201 people with dementia from 18 care homes and 5 day centres. Three points from the RCT are especially relevant here:

- There were improvements on the QoL-AD for those receiving CST, as well as on the cognitive measures. This was an important finding, as a change of a few points on a cognitive measure such as the MMSE may not translate into a meaningful difference in the person's life, whereas improvement in the person's own report of their quality of life suggests the approach is having a broader, and arguably more meaningful, effect.

- On some outcome measures there were differences between centres in the size of the effect. This may be one reason why small studies produce discrepant results – perhaps because of the make-up of a group, or the effects of a negative institutional environment, results are not entirely consistent from group to group, and hence a large-scale study is needed to detect the underlying effect.
- The Spector et al. (2003) report of the RCT provided a first response to the question raised in Orrell and Woods's (1996) manifesto: could psychological approaches have just as much effect as the acetylcholinesterase inhibitor medications becoming available? A comparison table takes published figures from the drug studies and compares them with the CST results for the cognitive measure, the ADAS-Cog, and so the comparison is not completely like for like – there may have been differences in the participants included in the different studies, and different time-scales of effect. However, it was evident that CST appeared to be just as effective (if not more so) as the then available medications in producing a significant improvement in ADAS-Cog scores.

Conclusion

The story of the development of CST does not end, of course, with the first RCT, important and landscape-changing as that turned out to be. This chapter has not addressed the implementation phase of the MRC Framework, and the issues arising in taking CST from an approach with evidence of effect in a RCT to a widely implemented approach in health and social care are addressed in Chapter 6.

In developing the approach, its eventual implementation was considered in terms of frequency and length of sessions, relating to what would be feasible in real-life practice outside a research setting. One hour, twice a week, was more likely to be achievable than daily groups, for example. The involvement of staff from the care home or day centre as co-facilitators of the groups also ensured that this was an approach that would not need higher degrees or specific professional qualifications in order to deliver it. The cost-effectiveness of the approach was established early on, using data from the RCT (Knapp et al., 2006). Implementation has also involved working on the adaptation of the programme for different cultures and language groups (see Chapters 10–16). Further development work has been necessary, of course, in relation to maintenance sessions (Chapter 4) and individual cognitive stimulation (Chapter 5).

It is also important that the evidence base does not come from just one study or one research group. The Cochrane review of RO was later replaced by a review of cognitive stimulation, which by 2012 was able to conclude that: 'There was consistent evidence from multiple trials that cognitive stimulation programmes benefit cognition in people with mild to moderate dementia over and above any medication effects' (Woods et al., 2012), with studies from a number of countries adding to the evidence base. Implementation of CST was also aided by its recommendation in the NICE-SCIE guidelines on the management of dementia, reflecting best practice in health and social care in the UK:

> People with mild/moderate dementia of all types should be given the opportunity to participate in a structured group cognitive stimulation programme . . . provided by workers with training and supervision . . . irrespective of any anti-dementia drug received.
>
> (NICE-SCIE, 2006)

Later it was included in the influential Royal College of Psychiatrists' Memory Services National Accreditation Programme (MSNAP). These are good examples of the evidence base providing a platform for implementation.

This chapter has traced CST back to its roots in RO. It is worth documenting how similar CST sessions are to the RO sessions described by Holden and Woods (1982). Indeed, the great majority of the session activities in both the CST and maintenance CST manuals (Aguirre et al., 2011) can be identified in Holden and Woods's chapter entitled '101 ideas for formal RO sessions', together of course with the opening introduction of names and current information around a board, and the importance of refreshments! It is this combination of cognitive and social domains which is the hallmark of cognitive stimulation. Arguably this combination produces stronger effects in each domain: laughter and having fun promotes cognitive function and achievement/success on a cognitive activity promotes self-esteem and well-being. The influence of the French cognitive stimulation programme (Breuil et al., 1994) is also interesting. According to Spector et al. (2001), the group in Paris were people recently diagnosed who wished to improve their cognitive function. They were quite different in attitude and phase of dementia and much younger (average age 77) than the care home/day centre populations included in Spector et al. (2001) and (2003) who had an average age of around 85. These differences led to the CST programme presenting cognitive tasks in a game-like manner wherever possible, and focusing on implicit memory, active engagement with materials, and the provision of retrieval cues to avoid the risk of overt failure, with its potential detriment to self-esteem. The lack of emphasis on specific neuropsychological mechanisms, that might be seen in some cognitive training programmes, leads to greater generalisability and the active engagement and encouragement in a social setting challenges the excess disability that too often accompanies dementia, and poses a real threat to personhood.

References

Aguirre, E., Spector, A., Streater, A., Hoe, J., Woods, B., and Orrell, M. (2011). *Making a Difference 2: An Evidence-based Group Programme to Offer Maintenance Cognitive Stimulation Therapy (CST) to People With Dementia*. London: Hawker.

American Psychiatric Association. (1997). Practice guideline for the treatment of patients with Alzheimer's disease and other dementias of late life. *American Journal of Psychiatry, 154*(5 Supplement), 1–39.

Breuil, V., Rotrou, J. D., Forette, F., Tortrat, D., Ganansia-Ganem, A., Frambourt, A. et al. (1994). Cognitive stimulation of patients with dementia: Preliminary results. *International Journal of Geriatric Psychiatry, 9*, 211–217.

Brook, P., Degun, G., and Mather, M. (1975). Reality orientation, a therapy for psychogeriatric patients: A controlled study. *British Journal of Psychiatry, 127*, 42–45.

Buckholdt, D. R., and Gubrium, J. F. (1983). Therapeutic pretence in reality orientation. *International Journal of Aging & Human Development, 16*, 167–181.

Cosin, L. Z., Mort, M., Post, F., Westropp, C., and Williams, M. (1958). Experimental treatment of persistent senile confusion. *International Journal of Social Psychiatry, 4*, 24–42.

Dietch, J. T., Hewett, L. J., and Jones, S. (1989). Adverse effects of reality orientation. *Journal of American Geriatrics Society, 37*, 974–976.

Drummond, L., Kirchhoff, L., and Scarbrough, D. R. (1978). A practical guide to reality orientation: A treatment approach for confusion and disorientation. *The Gerontologist, 18*(6), 568–573.

Feil, N. (1993). *The Validation Breakthrough: Simple Techniques for Communicating With People With "Alzheimer's Type Dementia"*. Baltimore: Health Professions Press.

Greene, J. G., Timbury, G. C., Smith, R., and Gardiner, M. (1983). Reality orientation with elderly patients in the community: An empirical evaluation. *Age & Ageing, 12*, 38–43.

Gubrium, J. F., and Ksander, M. (1975). On multiple realities and reality orientation. *Gerontologist, 15*, 142–145.

Hanley, I. G., McGuire, R. J., and Boyd, W. D. (1981). Reality orientation and dementia: A controlled trial of two approaches. *British Journal of Psychiatry, 138*, 10–14.

Holden, U. P., and Sinebruchow, A. (1978). Reality orientation therapy: A study investigating the value of this therapy in the rehabilitation of elderly people. *Age and Ageing*, 7(2), 83–90.

Holden, U. P., and Woods, R. T. (1982). *Reality Orientation: Psychological Approaches to the 'Confused' Elderly*. Edinburgh: Churchill Livingstone.

Holden, U. P., and Woods, R. T. (1988). *Reality Orientation: Psychological Approaches to the 'Confused' Elderly* (Second ed.). Edinburgh: Churchill Livingstone.

Holden, U. P., and Woods, R. T. (1995). *Positive Approaches to Dementia Care*. Edinburgh: Churchill Livingstone (3rd revised edition of 'Reality Orientation': Psychological approaches to the 'confused' elderly').

Johnson, C. H., McLaren, S. M., and McPherson, F. M. (1981). The comparative effectiveness of three versions of 'classroom' reality orientation. *Age and Ageing, 10*(1), 33–35.

Kitwood, T. (1990). The dialectics of dementia: With particular reference to Alzheimer's disease. *Ageing & Society, 10*, 177–196.

Knapp, M., Spector, A., Thorgrimsen, L., Woods, R. T., and Orrell, M. (2006). Cognitive Stimulation Therapy for people with dementia: Cost effectiveness analysis. *British Journal of Psychiatry, 188*, 574–580.

Logsdon, R., Gibbons, L. E., McCurry, S. M., and Teri, L. (1999). Quality of life in Alzheimer's disease: Patient and caregiver reports. *Journal of Mental Health & Aging, 5*, 21–32.

Medical Research Council. (2008). *Developing and Evaluating Complex Interventions: New Guidance*. London: MRC.

Merchant, M., and Saxby, P. (1980). Reality orientation – A way forward. *Nursing Times*, 77(33), 1442–1445.

Neal, M., and Barton-Wright, P. (2009). Validation therapy for dementia (Cochrane review). *The Cochrane Library*, Issue 2. Chichester: Wiley.

NICE-SCIE. (2006). *Dementia: Supporting People With Dementia and Their Carers in Health and Social Care: Clinical Guideline 42*. London: National Institute for Health and Clinical Excellence.

Orrell, M., and Woods, R. T. (1996). Tacrine and psychological therapies in dementia: No contest? *International Journal of Geriatric Psychiatry, 11*, 189–192.

Spector, A., Orrell, M., Davies, S., and Woods, B. (2001). Can reality orientation be rehabilitated? Developing and piloting of an evidence-based programme of cognition-based therapies for people with dementia. *Neuropsychological Rehabilitation, 11*(3/4), 377–397.

Spector, A., Orrell, M., Davies, S., and Woods, R. T. (1998). Reminiscence therapy for dementia: A review of the evidence of effectiveness (Cochrane Review). *The Cochrane Library*, Issue 3. Oxford: Update Software.

Spector, A., Thorgrimsen, L., Woods, B., Royan, L., Davies, S., Butterworth, M., and Orrell, M. (2003). Efficacy of an evidence-based Cognitive Stimulation Therapy programme for people with dementia: Randomised controlled trial. *British Journal of Psychiatry, 183*, 248–254.

Spector, A., Thorgrimsen, L., Woods, R. T., and Orrell, M. (2006). *Making a Difference*. London: Hawker.

Spector, A., Woods, B., Davies, S., and Orrell, M. W. (2000). Reality orientation for dementia: A systematic review of the evidence of effectiveness from randomized controlled trials. *The Gerontologist, 40*(2), 206–212.

Stephens, L. P. (1969). *Reality Orientation*. Washington, DC: American Psychiatric Association Hospital and Community Psychiatric Service.

Taulbee, L. R., and Folsom, J. C. (1966). Reality orientation for geriatric patients. *Hospital & Community Psychiatry, 17*, 133–135.

Thorgrimsen, L., Selwood, A., Spector, A., Royan, L., de-Madariaga-Lopez, M., Woods, R. T., and Orrell, M. (2003). Whose quality of life is it anyway? The validity and reliability of the Quality of Life – Alzheimer's Disease (QoL-AD) Scale. *Alzheimer Disease and Associated Disorders, 17*(4), 201–208.

Woods, B., Aguirre, E., Spector, A. E., and Orrell, M. (2012). Cognitive stimulation to improve cognitive functioning in people with dementia. *Cochrane Database Systematic Reviews, 2*.

Woods, B., and Russell, I. (2014). Randomisation and chance-based designs in social care research. *NIHR School for Social Care Research Methods Review 17*. London: NIHR SSCR.

Woods, R. T. (1979). Reality orientation and staff attention: A controlled study. *British Journal of Psychiatry, 134*, 502–507.

Woods, R. T., and Britton, P. G. (1977). Psychological approaches to the treatment of the elderly. *Age & Ageing, 6*, 104–112.

Chapter 4

Group cognitive stimulation therapy

Clinical trials

Martin Orrell and Lene Thorgrimsen Forrester

Introduction

Psychological interventions for dementia, such as Reality Orientation (RO; Brook et al., 1975), have been in use for more half a century (Taulbee and Folsom, 1966). However, despite their longevity, their effects remained controversial and studies were either small, of poor methodological quality, or both (Orrell and Woods, 1996). A Cochrane review found that RO was associated with significant improvements in both cognition and behaviour, but also identified the need for large, well-designed, multi-centre trials (Spector et al., 1998, 2000). The results of the Cochrane review were used to develop a programme of evidence-based therapy focused on cognitive stimulation (Spector et al., 2001).

The Cognitive Stimulation Therapy (CST) programme developed consists of 14 sessions, lasting 45 minutes, held twice weekly, over seven weeks. It was designed using the theoretical concepts of RO and cognitive stimulation, largely building on a trial by Breuil et al. (1994), which was identified through the systematic reviews as having the most significant results (Spector et al., 1998, 2000). CST includes topics such as using money, word games, and faces and scenes, and an RO board to prompt and create continuity, displaying both personal and orientation information such as the group name chosen by participants. Each session begins with a gentle, noncognitive warm-up activity such as a softball game, and then moves to a main themed activity. Reminiscence as a natural process is a feature of CST, but there is also additional focus on the current day. Multisensory stimulation is incorporated as much as possible, and sessions encourage the use of information processing rather than factual knowledge, avoiding potential failure experiences with regards to memory impairments. The key principles of CST are described in Chapter 1. A range of ideas for each session enables the facilitator to pitch activities to the group's cognitive capabilities and interests (see Spector et al., 2006 for detailed descriptions of the programme).

CST feasibility and pilot study

The investigation of CST began with a feasibility and pilot study conducted in three care homes and one day centre in the Greater London area. The study indicated people with dementia participating in the programme experienced improvements in cognition and depression when compared to usual care control participants in the same centres (Spector et al., 2001). Based on these findings, the effects of CST groups on cognition, mood, functioning, and quality of life (QoL) for people with dementia were investigated in a larger scale, single-blind, multi-centre, randomised controlled trial (RCT; See Spector et al., 2003 for a detailed report).

The first clinical trial of CST

Methods

A total of 201 people with dementia took part in the RCT within 18 residential homes and five day centres in the Greater London area, making a total of 23 groups. The inclusion criteria all participants met for the study were as follows:

1. Diagnostic and Statistical Manual of Mental Disorders Fourth Edition (DSM – IV) criteria for dementia (American Psychiatric Association, [APA] 1994),
2. Score of between 10 and 24 on the Mini-Mental State Examination (MMSE; Folstein et al., 1975),
3. Some ability to communicate and understand communication as measured by the Clifton Assessment Procedures for the Elderly-Behaviour Rating Scale (CAPE-BRS) (Pattie and Gilleard, 1979),
4. Able to see and hear well enough to participate in the group and make use of most of the material in the programme,
5. No major physical illness, learning disability, or other disability that could affect participation.

These criteria have been widely used in subsequent investigation and evaluation of CST-based approaches, and are referred to as the Spector et al. (2003) standardised criteria for psychological treatment of people with dementia.

Participants were randomly allocated either into CST treatment groups (n = 115) or treatment as usual (TAU) control groups (n = 86). The appropriate multi-centre and local research ethics committees granted ethical approval, and written informed consent was obtained from all participants. Based on the results from the pilot study, the estimated required sample size to achieve 80% power to detect a difference of two points on the MMSE was 64 in each group, assuming common standard deviation to be 4.0, and using a two-group t-test with a 0.05 (two-tailed) significance level. The characteristics of the participants are outlined in Table 4.1.

Results

The trial flowchart is shown in Figure 4.1, which illustrates that 97 participants in the CST treatment group and 70 controls were assessed at follow-up. Mean group attendance was 11.6 sessions (range 2–14) and 89% of people attended seven or more sessions.

Table 4.1 Characteristics and mean scale scores of participants at baseline

Characteristics	*Treatment (SD)*	*TAU control (SD)*	*All (SD)*
Number	115	86	201
Mean age	85.7 (6.2)	84.7 (7.9)	85.3 (7.0)
Female	96 (84.3%)	62 (72.1%)	158 (78.6%)
MMSE	14.2 (3.9)	14.8 (3.8)	14.4 (3.8)
ADAS-Cog	27.4 (7.2)	26.8 (7.9)	27.0 (7.5)
CDR	1.4 (0.5)	1.4 (0.5)	1.4 (0.5)
QoL-AD	33.2 (5.9)	33.3 (5.7)	33.3 (5.8)
Cornell	5.2 (5.0)	6.9 (4.7)	5.5 (4.9)
RAID	8.4 (8.0)	10.1 (8.5)	9.1 (8.2)
CAPE-BRS	11.3 (4.7)	11.5 (5.1)	11.4 (4.8)
Holden	11.1 (5.9)	9.9 (5.5)	10.6 (5.7)

Key:
MMSE: Mini-Mental State Examination (Folstein et al., 1975)
ADAS-Cog: Alzheimer's Disease Assessment Scale – Cognition (Rosen et al., 1984)
QoL-AD: Quality of Life – Alzheimer's Disease scale (Logsdon et al., 1999)
Cornell: Cornell Scale for Depression in Dementia (Alexopoulos et al., 1988)
RAID: Rating Anxiety in Dementia (Shankar et al., 1999)
CAPE-BRS: Clifton Assessment Procedures for the Elderly-Behaviour Rating Scale (Pattie and Gilleard, 1979)
Holden: Holden Communication Scale (Holden and Woods, 1995)

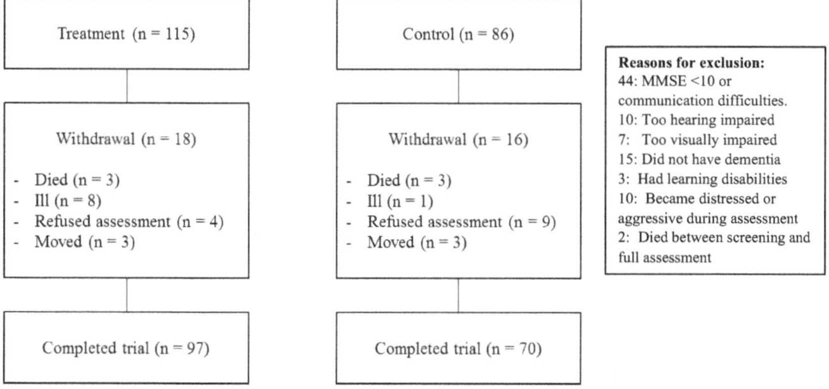

Figure 4.1 Profile of trial and attrition

Table 4.2 Change from baseline in measures of efficacy at follow up: intention to treat analysis

Measure	*Mean change from baseline (SD)*		*Mean group difference (SE), [95% CI]*	*ANCOVA: between-group difference*	*ANCOVA: other significant differences*
	Treatment	*TAU Control*			
MMSE[1]	+0.9 (3.5)	–0.4 (3.5)	+1.14 (0.09) [0.57, 2.27]	F = 4.14 p = 0.044	None
ADAS–Cog[2]	+1.9 (6.2)	–0.3 (5.5)	+2.37 (0.87) [0.64, 4.09]	F = 6.18 p = 0.014	C: p = 0.006
No with >/= 0 pts improvement	58 (50%)	32 (37%)			
No with >/= 4 pts improvement	34 (30%)	11 (13%)			
QoL–AD[2]	+1.3 (5.1)	–0.8 (5.6)	+1.64 (0.78) [0.09, 3.18]	F = 4.95 p = 0.028	G: p = 0.010
Holden	+0.2 (6.1)	–3.2 (6.3)	+2.3 (0.93) [–0.45, 4.15]	F = 2.92 p = 0.090	C: p = 0.009 G: p = 0.001
CAPE–BRS	–0.2 (6.1)	–0.7 (5.5)	+0.40 (0.65) [–0.9, 1.69]	F = 0.58 p = 0.449	C: p < 0.001 G: p = 0.001
RAID	–0.5 (10.2)	–0.7 (10.3)	–1.30 (1.10) [–3.48, 0.87]	p = 0.200	C: p < 0.001
Cornell	0 (6.2)	–0.5 (7.0)	+0.12 (0.72) [–1.56, 1.31]	p = 0.648	C: p < 0.001

Key:
1 = Primary outcome measure CI = Confidence interval SE = Standard error
2 = Secondary outcome measure F = F value + = Change in positive direction
C = Difference between centres G = Difference between genders – = Change in negative direction

The findings of the RCT are displayed in Table 4.2 and indicate that people with dementia who completed CST treatment groups performed significantly higher with regards to cognitive functioning measured by MMSE (Folstein et al., 1975) and the Alzheimer's Disease Assessment Scale-Cognition (ADAS-Cog; Rosen et al., 1984) in comparison to the TAU group, with confidence intervals for the differences between groups being above zero for all both measures. There was a trend towards an improvement on the Holden Communication Scale (Holden and Woods, 1995) for participants in the treatment group (p = 0.09). No difference was detected between the groups in terms of functional ability measured by the Clifton Assessment Procedures for the Elderly-Behaviour Rating Scale (CAPE-BRS; Pattie and Gilleard, 1979), nor for scores on the Rating Anxiety in Dementia (RAID; Shankar et al., 1999) scale or the Cornell Scale for Depression in Dementia (Alexopoulos et al., 1988). Centre emerged as a significant covariate in relation to ADAS-Cog, Holden Communication Scale, Cornell, and RAID scales, and CAPE-BRS score.

Self-rated QoL measured by the Quality of Life-Alzheimer's Disease scale (QoL-AD; Logsdon et al., 1999), was rated higher by people from the CST groups than those in the TAU group, with confidence intervals above zero for the difference between groups. QoL scores for women in the treatment group improved more than those for men, whereas QoL for men in the control group deteriorated significantly more than it did for women.

Reflection on the outcomes from the original trial of CST

The significant improvements found in the RCT on cognitive functioning and QoL are consistent with findings of earlier studies (Woods, 1979; Breuil et al., 1994). Moreover, since the first trial, further research has showed that CST can make a significant impact on particular language skills including naming, word-finding, and comprehension (Spector et al., 2010). From interviewing people with dementia, carers, and staff about their experiences of CST sessions, key themes including positive experiences of being in the groups due to a supportive and non-threatening environment, as well as improvements in mood, confidence, and concentration have emerged (see Chapter 8 and Spector et al., 2011).

In terms of cognition, the overall change indicated improvement in a number of areas. With the exception of explicit rehearsal in place orientation, which is directly questioned, there was no obvious reason why participation in groups should have had a direct practice effect on any other cognitive tasks, such as word recall or recognition. This suggests that generalised cognitive benefits resulted from inclusion in the programme. Some authors (Zanetti et al., 1995) have identified that behavioural outcome measures are often not sensitive enough to detect the functional impact of cognitive stimulation programmes. There were positive trends in communication, which were not shown empirically in earlier RO trials. Communication is a factor that is likely to deteriorate in individuals moving into residential care, and the small group context was probably novel for many of the participants, perhaps exercising long unused communication skills. It is not known why women reacted more favourably to the programme. However, being in the minority in most groups could have created discomfort for male participants, making them less inclined to fully participate.

There was a significant variation between centres from baseline to follow-up on measures of cognition, behaviour, mood, and communication. Experiences from the research team suggested that some centres appeared more institutionalised, and in these the staff-patient relationships were poorer and so functioning was not optimised. Thus, it may be the case that the effects of groups were not strong enough to combat the effects of a negative environment overall. Moreover, in some centres with a better quality of social environment, perhaps having a local programme of activities available as part of regular care, residents might have been functioning near their optimum, leaving little scope for improvement. Groups including people at different stages of dementia were sometimes difficult to run, as people with milder dementia could become irritated by those with more severe cognitive impairment, and observing their confusion might have been off-putting and hence detrimental to the group process. As such, pitching the sessions at an appropriate level appears to be an important consideration. Outside the context of a research trial, groups can be selected through clinical judgement, with a consideration of how people would mix.

Comparisons of outcomes with medication

In order to perform comparisons with anti-dementia medication (e.g. acetylcholinesterase inhibitors), number-needed-to-treat (NNT) analyses were performed identically to trials of three acetylcholinesterase inhibitors: tacrine, rivastigmine, and donepezil (Livingston and Katona, 2000). Calculations were also included for galantamine, using the results from another trial (Wilcock et al., 2000). These comparisons show that for small improvements, or no deterioration, the programme was not quite as effective as rivastigmine, donepezil, and galantamine. For greater improvements (four or more points), CST did as well as galantamine or tacrine and substantially better than rivastigmine, or the lower dosage of donepezil (5 mg). Only the higher dosage of donepezil (10 mg) had a smaller NNT. These results are particularly interesting considering that the drug programmes lasted for 24 weeks, 26 weeks, or 30 weeks compared with only seven weeks of CST. However, since these drug studies applied only to Alzheimer's Disease (AD), and since drug therapy and psychological therapy are different forms of treatment, some caution is required when interpreting these comparisons.

Mechanisms of change

There are a number of possible mechanisms of change relevant to the improvement found for people with dementia completing the CST groups. The learning environment during sessions was designed to be optimal for the impairments found in this group, for example focusing on implicit memory and integrating reminiscence and multi-sensory stimulation throughout the programme. Stimulation in the group could improve cognition and might make participants feel more able to communicate. The groups could also serve to work against the experience of 'excess disability' due to the 'malignant social psychology' of a negative social environment (Kitwood, 1997) by improving self-esteem through social stimulation and encouragement. Finally, groups positively reinforced questioning, thinking, and interacting with other people, objects, and the environment. This effect might have extended beyond the groups, with people communicating more effectively and responding more to the environment and to others.

It is possible that the social interaction provided by the groups could have been of benefit in the centres which provided some activities as part of normal care. However, our Cochrane Review of RO (Spector et al., 1998) found that in RCTs, social groups appeared to be of no benefit to cognition. This suggests that the results are because of the specific effects of CST rather than the non-specific effects of attention or social interaction.

Limitations and challenges

There were a number of limitations with the RCT. For example, the randomisation procedure involved drawing numbers from a hat to allocate people to trial arm, but ideally the generation of the allocation sequence, enrolment into the trial and allocation to group should be separate and performed by people independent of the research trial. In later studies (Orrell et al., 2014, described later in this chapter), this was improved upon by using remote randomisation through the North Wales Organisation for Randomised Trials in Health and Social Care (NWORTH) Clinical Trials Unit, and enhanced procedures to ensure researcher performing assessments were blind to intervention or TAU allocation.

Another limitation was that differences in control conditions between centres meant that the 'control group' was not homogeneous, although 'usual activities' generally meant doing nothing. Lastly, in contrast to the results on the primary and secondary outcome measures which were rated directly with the participants, none of the scales rated by staff (e.g. mood, communication, behaviour) showed significant improvements for the CST group. Staff perceptions about the therapy groups might have introduced bias into the ratings of the scales. Centres appeared to vary to which degree they were open to participating in the study, or perceived it to be threatening in terms of challenge or implying criticism of their established activities. Efforts were made to engage local members of staff acting as co-therapists, and these staff members were not involved in completion of the rating scales. However, it is likely the staff completing the rating scales would have had good awareness of the trial and group allocation, which might have influenced their ratings.

Historically, early guidelines cautioned against the use of cognitive stimulation programmes because of the possibility of adverse reactions such as frustration (APA, 1994). However, this RCT showed that cognitive improvements were associated with benefits to QoL rather than deterioration, and was the first study to show improvements in QoL of people with dementia participating in such a programme.

The short follow-up period (eight weeks) did not inform the potential longer-term implications of delivering CST to older people with dementia. The CST groups were delivered by trained researchers in this study. It would be less expensive to deliver CST by training care home staff, or home care workers, but we do not know whether this would generate different outcomes from those observed. Most participants had mild to moderate dementia and often had some hearing and vision difficulties, and it is difficult to generalise to other groups from the present results. Centres with fewer than eight eligible participants had to be excluded, although there is no reason to believe that this has biased the findings.

Long-term impact of CST

Over the past decade, there has been much interest in the potential for mental exercises and activities to maintain and improve cognitive function for people with dementia (Orrell et al., 2012). However, research has found that interventions utilising specific cognitive tasks only induced improvements in the domains trained, and the effects tend not to generalise to general cognitive functioning (Owen et al., 2010). As outlined in this chapter, there is good evidence for the benefits of CST for people with dementia, and this method of implicitly enhancing cognitive functioning utilising a comprehensive set of methods has now superseded more generic approaches such as reminiscence therapy and RO (Orrell et al., 2012). Following the initial trial, group-based CST has become widely used and is now a well-established, evidence-based and cost-effective approach (Orrell et al., 2012). A recent Cochrane review showed that CST improved both cognition and QoL, and concluded that the benefits of CST enhanced those of medication, and that it was effective whether or not acetylcholinesterase inhibitors (ACHEIs) were prescribed (Woods et al., 2012). The 2011 World Alzheimer report concluded 'there is strong evidence to support cognitive stimulation programmes and these interventions should therefore be routinely offered' (Prince *et al.*, 2011). However, despite this evidence, little was known about the impact of CST beyond the original eight weeks, demonstrating the need for more research to look at potential longer-term outcomes of CST (Orrell et al., 2014).

Maintenance CST (MCST) pilot

A pilot study of MCST was conducted, which continued for an additional 16 weekly sessions beyond the standard seven-week, 14-session programme. Thirty-five people with dementia were included, and the once weekly MCST sessions ran in two residential homes for the additional 16 weeks. Two treatment as usual control care homes did not receive the MCST intervention. Using repeated measures ANOVAS, there was a continuous, significant improvement in cognitive function (MMSE) for those receiving MCST (CST plus MCST sessions) compared to CST alone, or no treatment (p = 0.012). There were no effects on QoL, behaviour, or communication following maintenance sessions. The initial cognitive improvements following CST were only sustained at follow-up when followed by the programme of MCST sessions. As such, the MCST programme found a sustained significant improvement in cognitive function compared with CST alone (Orrell et al., 2005).

The Cochrane Review of CST found no link between duration or frequency of the programme and degree of improvement (Woods et al., 2012). Some studies have continued cognitive stimulation for six months or more (Buschert et al., 2011; Requena et al., 2006), but there is little evidence about how far potential benefits may continue after sessions end (Orrell et al., 2014). The Cochrane Review suggested that after the sessions finished, the effects on cognition were evident for three months at most (Woods et al., 2012), and another study found no continuing effects at 10 months (Chapman et al., 2004). On this basis, a trial was conducted which aimed to evaluate the effectiveness of maintenance CST in improving cognition and QoL in people with dementia who had completed the standard CST programme (Aguirre et al., 2010). In addition, a sub-study focused on the effects of MCST on people with dementia taking ACHEIs.

Development of the MCST programme

The MCST programme was based on the theory of cognitive stimulation as applied to the original CST programme (Spector et al., 2003, 2006), and its development was guided by the Medical Research Council (MRC) framework for complex interventions (Craig et al., 2008; MRC, 2000). The intervention was developed based on a mixed methods approach, using evidence obtained from: (1) the Cochrane review of cognitive stimulation for dementia (Woods et al., 2012), (2) a consultation with key stakeholders using a Delphi Consensus Process (including an expert consensus conference), (3) focus groups with the target population and, (4) a Delphi survey. These techniques were used to complete the theoretical, preclinical, and phase I modelling described in the MRC framework. It was feasible and effective to use a systematic development process to produce successive modifications of the draft MCST manual. Close involvement of users and carers ensured that the manual was well tailored to the preferences and abilities of people with dementia.

The final MCST programme and manual includes themed sessions (e.g. current affairs, my life, word games) and adheres to the consistent structure which characterises the original CST programme, including an orientation-based activity, refreshments, and a group song with which to begin.

MCST trial

Methods

The MCST trial was a single-blind, multi-centre, pragmatic RCT comparing (1) MCST groups after completing standard CST versus (2) CST followed by TAU (Aguirre et al., 2012). There were no modifications in design or eligibility criteria from the study protocol of the original CST trial (Spector et al., 2003). Potential centres were screened for eligibility to determine whether there were sufficient numbers of potential participants with dementia, and participants all met the Spector et al. (2003) standardised criteria for psychological treatment of people with dementia (see 'The first clinical trial of CST' in this chapter). Most had either AD or vascular dementia and mild (45%) to moderate (55%) dementia on the Clinical Dementia Rating (CDR) scale (Hughes et al., 1992).

All trial participants completed seven weeks of CST (Spector et al., 2003) comprising 14 twice-weekly 45-minute sessions according to the CST manual (Spector et al., 2006). Approximately half of the participants were from nine care homes, and half were from nine community services within London, Essex, and Bedfordshire. The community centres included four voluntary sector specialist dementia day centres and five centres based in local Community Mental Health Teams (CMHTs) for older people. The nine care homes included five provided by social services, one by the private sector, and three from voluntary organisations.

Upon completion of seven weeks of CST, participants were randomised within each centre to either the 24-week MCST programme (Aguirre et al., 2011) or the treatment as usual (TAU) control group. TAU varied across the 18 centres, but other activities were generally available to both groups.

Randomisation and blinding

The NWORTH Clinical Trials Unit remotely randomised participants in equal proportions between groups after stratifying for centre (community service or care home), whether ACHEI was prescribed, and previous CST group. The random allocation sequence was computer-generated and in the ratio of 1:1. Researchers who were blind to allocation conducted initial and subsequent interviews, usually in care homes or participants' own homes.

Delivery and training

Each group had two facilitators, one from the research team and one staff member from the participating care home or community service. All facilitators had at least one year of experience in dementia care, and had attended the one-day CST training course.

Outcomes and assessments

Participants were interviewed at baseline, before randomisation, at three months (intermediate end-point), and after six months (primary end-point). The primary outcome measures were the ADAS-Cog (Rosen et al., 1984) and QoL-AD (Logsdon et al., 2002), as described above. Secondary outcomes were:

1 MMSE (Folstein et al., 1975),
2 Dementia Quality of Life scale (DemQoL; Smith et al., 2005) covering five domains of quality of life using self-reporting and rating by family carer or staff member as proxy,

3 Neuropsychiatric Inventory (NPI; Cummings et al., 1994), which assesses 10 behaviours commonly occurring in dementia and,
4 Alzheimer's Disease Cooperative Study-Activities of Daily Living (ADCS-ADL; Galasko et al., 1997), assessing functional capacity over the range of dementia severity.

Sample size

Based on the Cochrane Review, an estimated effect size MCST of 0.39 on the ADAS-Cog was calculated, with power of 80% when using 5% significance level and estimating attrition at 15% between baseline and six months. This required a sample size of 230 participants randomised at baseline and an estimated 195 at follow up. It was estimated that 60 participants with Alzheimer's disease were taking AChEIs, which provided sufficient numbers for the maintenance CST/AChEIs sub-study to estimate effect size and the feasibility of a full-scale trial.

Trial results

Two hundred and seventy-two people with dementia started CST groups and were considered for the trial. Two hundred and thirty-six were available for randomisation after the CST groups finished. Of these, 218 participants (92% of 236; 96% of those still alive) were followed up at three months, and 199 (84% of 236; 89% of those still alive) at six months, with a similar withdrawal rate in both arms of the trial (Figure 4.2).

Of the 236 participants, 123 were allocated to the MCST group and 113 to TAU. The groups were similar at baseline as randomisation avoided imbalances. The mean age was 83 years and most participants were white and female (Tables 4.3 and 4.4). On average, participants allocated to the MCST groups attended 18 of the 24 available sessions.

At the six-month primary end-point, the MCST group had significantly higher scores than the TAU group on self-rated QoL-AD (first primary outcome) (mean difference 1.78; 95% CI 0.00 to 3.60; $p = 0.03$). There were no significant differences on ADAS-Cog (second primary outcome), nor secondary outcomes at six months.

At three months, there were no significant differences on either primary outcome. For secondary outcomes, participants in the MCST group had significantly better scores than controls on proxy ratings of QoL (QoL-AD and DEMQOL) and daily activities. The mean difference on the proxy QoL-AD was 1.53 (95% CI 0.35 to 2.71; $p = 0.01$), and for the proxy DEMQOL it was 3.24 (95% CI 0.24 to 6.24; $p = 0.03$). The difference on the ADCS-ADL was 2.64 (95% CI 0.04 to 5.24; $p = 0.04$).

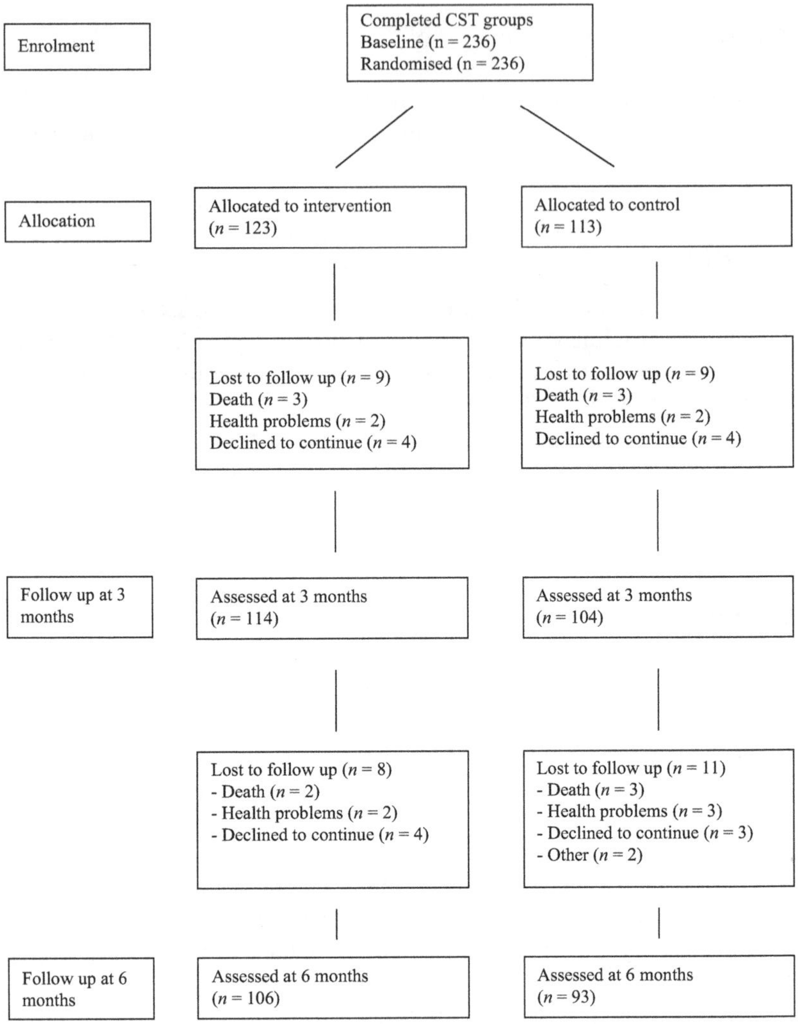

Figure 4.2 Consort flowchart of participants' progress

Table 4.3 Baseline characteristics of participants in MCST trial

Participants before start of CST groups	272
Total lost from the beginning of CST groups	36
Reason for withdrawal	
Did not like CST groups and wanted to withdraw	17 (49%)
Health issues	15 (40%)
Difficulties with group time or other participants	2 (6%)
Moved to a different care home	2 (6%)
Participants after completion of CST groups	236

Table 4.4 Baseline characteristics of participants by allocated group

Characteristics	*Intervention (n = 123)*	*TAU Control (n = 113)*
	Number (%)	*Number (%)*
Female	80 (65%)	70 (62%)
Ethnicity (white)	111 (90%)	104 (92%)
Marital status (widow)	54 (44%)	57 (50%)
Dementia diagnosis (AD)	38 (31%)	35 (31%)
On AChEIs	42 (34%)	34 (30%)
In care home	51 (41%)	50 (44%)
	Mean (SD)	**Mean (SD)**
Age (years)	82.7 (7.9)	83.5 (7.2)
ADAS-Cog	31.1 (14.6)	33.2 (13.0)
QoL-AD	36.1 (4.8)	36.5 (5.7)
MMSE	17.8 (5.6)	17.8 (5.4)
DEMQOL	94.8 (10.9)	95.1 (11.7)
NPI	13.8 (12.9)	11.3 (9.1)
ADCS-ADL	42.7 (17.2)	41.5 (18.1)
Proxy QoL-AD	33.7 (5.9)	33.3 (4.9)
Proxy DEMQOL	102.2 (13.5)	102.2 (11.2)

Key:
AChEIs – Acetylcholinesterase Inhibitors
ADAS-Cog – Alzheimer's Disease Assessment Scale–Cognitive Subscale
QoL-AD – Quality of Life in Alzheimer's Disease scale
MMSE – Mini-Mental State Examination
DEMQOL – Dementia Quality of Life scale
NPI – Neuropsychiatric Inventory
ADCS-ADL – Alzheimer's Disease Cooperative Study-Activities of Daily Living scale

Quality of delivery

To measure the quality of delivery of MCST, the researchers rated a range of factors related to the successful running of the groups, including manager's attitude, centre atmosphere, co-facilitator input, group atmosphere, and average number of sessions attended by participants after each session. Centres were divided into low quality and high quality based on this information. Eight of the nine community centres were considered 'high quality' sites, compared to only six of the nine care homes. The quality indicator was incorporated into the model of analysis with primary outcome results, with baseline score, centre type, age, and allocation as a fixed effect, with a random effect of centre nested within the interaction of quality and type. The analysis showed that both centre type and quality of MCST provision were not significant in the model using either

QoL-AD or ADAS-Cog, and as such, the differences among the centres could not be explained by amount of sessions attended or quality of MCST provision.

With regards to the sub-study exploring MCST with participants in receipt of AChEIs, there were no significant results in relation to the primary outcomes. Table 4.4 shows observed means and standard deviations (SD) at baseline. The means and SDs at the three and six-month follow-ups were adjusted for the factors and covariates in the fitted model, including the treatment group by AChEIs interaction term. The follow-up means were standardised to a common baseline mean value. The significance levels reported below are for the interaction term. Only MMSE at both three and six months follow-up showed significant interactions.

There was evidence that AChEIs and MCST had a synergistic effect. The results show that starting from a mean baseline MMSE of 17.8, there was the smallest decrease to 17.25 (95% CI 14.63 to 19.87, $p = 0.03$) at the six-month follow-up in those taking AChEIs and receiving MCST. The largest decrease occurred in those taking AChEIs who did not receive MCST, where the mean was 14.62 (95% CI 11.81 to 17.43, $p = 0.03$). There were no other significant differences between groups on any other outcome measures. Between baseline and second follow up, 92% of participants had no changes to their to AChEI status, three participants stopped taking them (1 TAU/2 MCST), and 11 started with the medication (4 TAU/7MCST).

There were no differences between the groups (intervention and TAU) in the number of reported adverse events or severity. In the intervention group there were five deaths and four withdrawals due to health issues. In the usual care group there were six deaths and five withdrawals due to health issues. All events were judged as unrelated to trial treatment or assessment contacts by the study trial coordinator and Principal Investigator.

Reflections on the MCST trial

The trial found that after the initial CST programme, a further 24-week course of weekly MCST improves QoL at six-month follow up, but confers no additional benefit to cognition. At six months, it was only participants who reported improved QoL (a small standardised difference of 0.35), whereas at three months only the proxy respondents (carers/care staff) noted the improvement (a small standardised difference of 0.30). Participants in the intervention group also improved in their activities of daily living at three months (a very small standardised difference of 0.15). There were no significant differences in other outcomes at either three or six months.

The sub-study results demonstrate that MCST may provide people on AChEI medication with cognitive benefits, which is in line with other studies combining AChEIs and cognitive stimulation, and the Cochrane review (Woods et al., 2012), which concluded that the effect of cognitive stimulation on cognition is over and above the effects of medication alone. The relevance in terms of clinically significant change is less clear. A mean decrease of one point versus four points on the MMSE scale may make a big difference for some people with dementia. The difference might translate into economic benefits since a difference of one point in the MMSE score may be associated with substantial reductions in the costs of caring for people with dementia (Jonsson et al., 1999). Participating in the CST programme prior to MCST baseline resulted in mean improvements of 4.4 points on the ADAS-Cog and 2.7 points on the MMSE (Aguirre et al., 2012). Since dementia is associated with progressive cognitive decline, there may be limited potential for further cognitive improvement with the maintenance programme. This means that at six-month follow-up both groups were likely to have declined from the assessment carried out after the CST groups finished, and so significant differences in cognition were only likely to be found if the usual care (CST only) group had declined more than the maintenance group.

QoL was found to have improved at six-month follow-up, which in chronic conditions may be more important than disease-specific outcomes, and is a key outcome that interventions for dementia should target. Benefits to cognition alone may not be sufficient to justify an extensive programme of intervention unless they are accompanied by other benefits such as QoL (Woods et al., 2006). Two recent systematic reviews highlighted that there are few well-designed studies on the effectiveness of either pharmacological (Cooper et al., 2012a) or psychosocial (Cooper et al., 2012b) interventions on QoL. Similar to other follow up studies, we found that individual changes in QoL were apparent for nearly three-quarters of our sample (Selwood et al., 2005; Lyketsos, 2003; Missotten et al., 2007). In contrast to the Cochrane review of cognitive stimulation, the MCST study found that activities of daily living improved at three-month follow-up. However, previous research suggests that there may be a correlation between proxy-rated QoL and activities of daily living (Selwood et al., 2005). It might be that the effects of the intervention on proxy-rated QoL were linked with the effects on activities of daily living. At six-month follow-up these proxy-rated domains showed no difference. However, for the person with dementia, a temporary improvement in QoL, cognition, or activities of daily living may be considered worthwhile.

Strengths and limitations

As participants came from nine care homes and nine community services across London, Essex, and Bedfordshire, this pragmatic trial is likely to be generalisable in many respects. Since participants were almost all white and women, it is hard to say how far CST is useful for other ethnic or cultural groups. However, the CST and MCST programmes are being adapted and used internationally (see Chapters 10–16). Although great care was taken to blind researchers to allocated treatment, the care staff, and family carers who provided proxy ratings for four measures (ADCS-ADL, NPI, QoL-AD and DEMQOL) could not be blinded, and this means there is a risk of detection bias. Notably, these measures provided three of the four significant findings. Compared to the original CST study, this trial had more diversity in dementia severity due to a much higher proportion recruited from the community (50% vs. 15%). This resulted in the standard deviations of the cognitive measures being much higher than in the original trial of CST making it harder to find a significant effect size.

This was the first rigorous trial of MCST. The results are encouraging, but not conclusive and suggest that further trials are needed, and it is important for other groups to evaluate MCST. Future research could look in more depth at the optimum frequency and duration of CST groups. For example, to continue to provide CST twice a week (rather than once weekly) for a six-month period. Another option would be to repeat the standard seven-week CST programme after a break. However, this option could be disruptive to the groups, and would not mirror the standard approach used in drug interventions, which are given without interruption rather than as a short course.

Conclusions

Weekly MCST over 24 weeks provides some potential benefit beyond the basic CST programme, and may offer short- and long-term benefits to QoL, and may in combination with AChEI medication also have longer-term benefits to cognition (Orrell et al., 2014). Pharmacological and psychosocial interventions may potentially work better together than either alone. Considering the positive impact of CST upon the lives of people of dementia as described in this chapter, investigating the long-term implications of CST in order to maximise these benefits seems of utmost importance. Following the first rigorous trial of MCST, others are encouraged to implement and evaluate this novel extension in other populations in other contexts with other staff.

References

Aguirre, E., Hoare, Z., Streater, A., Spector, A., Woods, B. and Orrell, M. (2012). Cognitive Stimulation Therapy (CST) for people with dementia – Who benefits most? *International Journal of Geriatric Psychiatry*, doi:10.1002/gps.3823.

Aguirre, E., Spector, A., Hoe, J., Knapp, M., Woods, B. and Orrell, M. (2010). Maintenance Cognitive Stimulation Therapy (CST) for dementia: A single-blind, multi-centre, randomised controlled trial of Maintenance CST vs. CST for dementia. *Trials*, 11(46).

Aguirre, E., Spector, A., Hoe, J., Streater, A., Woods, R. T. and Orrell, M. (2011). Development of an evidence- based extended programme of maintenance Cognitive Stimulation Therapy (CST) for people with dementia. *Non-pharmacological Therapies in Dementia Journal*, 1, 198–215.

Alexopoulos, G. S., Abrams, R. C., Young, R. C. and Shamoian, C. A. (1988). Cornell Scale for depression in dementia. *Biological Psychiatry*, 23, 271–284.

American Psychiatric Association. (1994). *Diagnostic and statistical manual of mental health disorders*. 4th ed. Washington, DC, APA.

Breuil, V., De Rotrou, J., Forette, F., Tortrat, D., Ganansia-Ganem, A., Frambourt, A., Moulin, F. and Boller, F. (1994). Cognitive stimulation of patients with dementia: Preliminary results. *International Journal of Geriatric Psychiatry*, 9, 211–217.

Brook, P., Degun, G. and Mather, M. (1975) Reality orientation, a therapy for psychogeriatric patients: A controlled study. *British Journal of Psychiatry*, 127, 42–45.

Buschert, V. C., Friese, U., Teipel, S. J., Schneider, P., Merensky, W. and Rujescu, D. (2011). Effects of a newly developed cognitive intervention in amnestic mild cognitive impairment and mild Alzheimer's disease: A pilot study. *Journal of Alzheimer's Disease*, 25, 679–694.

Chapman, S. B., Weiner, M. F., Rackley, A., Hynan, L. S. and Zientz, J. (2004). Effects of cognitive-communication stimulation for Alzheimer's disease patients treated with donepezil. *Journal of Speech, Language & Hearing Research*, 47, 1149–1163.

Cooper, C., Mukadam, M., Katona, C., Lyketsos, C., Ames, D. and Livingston, G. (2012a). Systematic review of the effectiveness of non-pharmacological interventions to improve quality of life of people with dementia. *International Psychogeriatrics*, doi:10.1017/S1041610211002614.

Cooper, C., Mukadam, N., Katona, C., Lyketsos, C. G., Blazer, D. and Livingston, G. (2012b). Systematic review of the effectiveness of pharmacologic interventions to improve quality of life and well-being in people with dementia. *American Journal of Geriatric Psychiatry*, PMID: 22245881.

Craig, P., Dieppe, P., MacIntyre, S., Mitchie, S., Nazareth, I. and Petticrew, M. (2008). Developing and evaluating complex interventions: The new Medical Research Council guidance. *BMJ*, 337, a1655.

Cummings, L., Mega, M., Gray, K., Rosenberg-Thompson, S., Carusi, D. A. and Gornbein, J. (1994). The neuropsychiatric inventory: Comprehensive assessment of psychopathology in dementia. *Neurology*, 44, 2308–2314.

Folstein, M. F., Folstein, S. E. and McHugh, P. R. (1975). Mini mental state: A practical method for grading the cognitive state of patients for the clinician. *Journal of Psychiatry Research*, 12, 189–198.

Galasko, D., Bennet, D., Sano, M., Ernesto, C., Thomas, R. and Ferris, S. (1997). An inventory to assess activities of daily living for clinical trials in Alzheimer's disease: The Alzheimer Disease Cooperative Study. *Alzheimer Disease & Associated Disorders*, 11, S33–39.

Holden, U. P. and Woods, R. T. (1995). *Positive approaches to dementia care*. 3rd ed. Edinburgh, Churchill-Livingstone.

Hughes, C., Berg, L., Danziger, W., Coben, L. A. and Martin, R. L. (1992). A new clinical scale for the staging of dementia. *British Journal of Psychiatry*, 140, 566–572.

Jonsson, L., Lindgren, P., Wimo, A., Jonsson, B. and Winblad, B. (1999). *Costs of Mini Mental State Examination-related cognitive impairment. Pharmacoeconomics*, 16, 409–416.

Kitwood, T. (1997). *Dementia reconsidered*. The Open University, UK.

Livingston, G. and Katona, C. (2000). How useful are cholinesterase inhibitors in the treatment of Alzheimer's disease? A number needed to treat analysis. *International Journal of Geriatric Psychiatry*, 15, 203–207.

Logsdon, R.G., Gibbons, L.E., McCurry, S.M.Teri, L. (1999). *Quality of life in Alzheimer's Disease: Patient and caregiver reports. Journal of Mental Health and Aging*, 5(1), 21–32.

Logsdon, R. G., Gibbons, L. E., McCurry, S. M. and Teri, L. (2002). Assessing quality of life in older adults with cognitive impairment. *Psychosomatic Medicine*, 64, 510–519.

Lyketsos, C. G., Gonzales-Salvador, T., Chin, J., Baker, A., Black, B. and Rabins, P. (2003). A follow-up study of change in quality of life among persons with dementia residing in a long-term care facility. *International Journal of Geriatric Psychiatry*, 18, 275–281.

Medical Research Council. (2000). *A framework for development and evaluation of RCTs for complex interventions to improve health*. London, MRC.

Missotten, P., Ylieff, M., Di Notte, D., Paquay De Lepeleire, J. and Fontaine, O. (2007). Quality of life in dementia: A 2-year follow-up study. *International Journal of Geriatric Psychiatry*, 22, 1201–1207.

Orrell, M., Aguirre, E., Spector, A., Hoare, Z., Streater, A., Woods, B., Streater, A., Donovan, H., Hoe, J. and Russell, I. (2014). Maintenance Cognitive Stimulation Therapy (CST) for dementia: A single-blind, multi-centre, randomised controlled trial of Maintenance CST vs. CST for dementia. *British Journal of Psychiatry*, 204, 454–461.

Orrell, M., Spector, A., Thorgrimsen, L. and Woods, B. (2005). A pilot study examining the effectiveness of Maintenance Cognitive Stimulation Therapy (Maintenance CST) for people with dementia. *International Journal of Geriatric Psychiatry*, 446–451.

Orrell, M. and Woods, B. (1996). Tacrine and psychological therapies in dementia – No contest? Editorial comment. *International Journal of Geriatric Psychiatry*, 11, 189–192.

Orrell, M., Woods, B. and Spector, A. (2012). Should we use Cognitive Stimulation Therapy to improve cognitive function in people with dementia? *BMJ*, 344, e633, doi:10.1136/bmj.e633.

Owen, A. M., Hampshire, A., Grahn, J. A., Stenton, R., Dajani, S., Burns, A. S., Howard, R. J. and Ballard, C. G. (2010). Putting brain training to the test. *Nature*, 465, 775–778.

Pattie, A. H. and Gilleard, C. J. (1979). *Clifton Assessment Procedures for the Elderly (CAPE)*. Sevenoaks, Hodder and Stoughton.

Prince, M., Bryce, R. and Ferri, C. (2011). *World Alzheimer report: The benefits of early diagnosis and intervention*. London, Alzheimer's Disease International, p. 49, www.alz.co.uk/worldreport2011.

Requena, C., Maestu, F., Campo, P., Fernandez, A. and Ortiz, T. (2006). Effects of cholinergic drugs and cognitive training on dementia: 2-year follow up. *Dementia and Geriatric Cognitive Disorders*, 22, 339–345.

Rosen, W. G., Mohs, R. C. and Davis, K. L. (1984). A new rating scale for Alzheimer's disease. *American Journal of Psychiatry*, 141, 1356–1364.

Selwood, A., Thorgrimsen, L. and Orrell, M. (2005). Quality of life in dementia – A one-year follow-up study. *Internal Journal of Geriatric Psychiatry*, 20, 232–237.

Shankar, K., Walker, M., Frost, D. and Orrell, M. W. (1999). The development of a valid and reliable scale for anxiety in dementia. *Aging & Mental Health*, 3, 39–49.

Smith, S. C., Lamping, D. L., Banerjee, S., Harwood, R., Foley, B. and Knapp, M. (2005). Measurement of health-related quality of life for people with dementia: Development of a new instrument (DEMQOL) and an evaluation of current methodology. *Health Technology Assessment*, 9(10).

Spector, A., Davies, S., Woods, B. and Orrell, M. (2001). Can reality orientation be rehabilitated? Development and piloting of an evidence-based programme of cognition-based therapies for people with dementia. *Neuropsychological Rehabilitation*, 11, 377–397.

Spector, A., Gardner, C. and Orrell, M. (2011). The impact of Cognitive Stimulation Therapy groups on people with dementia: Views from participants, their carers and group facilitators. *Ageing & Mental Health*, 15(8), 945–949.

Spector, A., Orrell, M., Davies, S. and Woods, B. (1998). Reality Orientation for dementia: A review of the evidence for its effectiveness. *The Cochrane Library*, Issue 4. Oxford, Update Software.

Spector, A., Orrell, M., Davies, S. and Woods, B. (2000). Reality orientation for dementia: A systematic review of the evidence of effectiveness from randomised controlled trials. *Gerontologist*, 40(2), 206–212.

Spector, A., Orrell, M., Davies, S. and Woods, B. (2001). Can reality orientation be rehabilitated? Development and piloting of an evidence-based programme of cognition-based therapies for people with dementia. *Neuropsychological Rehabilitation*, 11(3/4), 377–397.

Spector, A., Orrell, M. and Woods, B. (2010). Cognitive Stimulation Therapy (CST): Effects on different areas of cognitive function for people with dementia. *International Journal of Geriatric Psychiatry*, 25(12), 1253–1258.

Spector, A., Thorgrimsen, L., Woods, B. and Orrell, M. (2000). Reality orientation for dementia: A systematic review of the evidence of effectiveness from randomised controlled trials. *The Gerontologist*, 40, 206–212.

Spector, A., Thorgrimsen, L., Woods, B., Royan, L., Davies, S. and Orrell, M. (2003). Efficacy of an evidence-based Cognitive Stimulation Therapy programme for people with dementia: Randomised controlled trial. *British Journal of Psychiatry*, 183, 248–254.

Taulbee, L. R. and Folsom, J. C. (1996). Reality Orientation for geriatric patients. *Hospital and Community Psychiatry*, 17, 133–135.

Wilcock, G. K., Lilienfeld, S. and Gaens, E. (2000). Efficacy and safety of galantamine in patients with mild to moderate Alzheimer's disease: Multicentre randomised controlled trial. *BMJ*, 321, 1445–1449.

Woods, B., Aguirre, E., Spector, A. and Orrell, M. (2012). Cognitive stimulation to improve cognitive functioning in people with dementia. *Cochrane Database of Systematic Review*, Issue 2. Art. No.: CD005562. doi:10.1002/14651858.CD005562.pub2.

Woods, B., Thorgrimsen, L., Spector, A., Royan, L. and Orrell, M. (2006). Improved quality of life and Cognitive Stimulation Therapy in dementia. *Aging and Mental Health*, 10, 219–226.

Woods, R. T. (1979). Reality orientation and staff attention: A controlled study. *British Journal of Psychiatry*, 134, 502–507.

Zanetti, O., Frisoni, G. B., De Leo, D., Buono, M. D., Bianchetti, A. and Trabucci, M. (1995). Reality orientation therapy in Alzheimer's disease: Useful or not? A controlled study. *Alzheimer's Disease and Associated Disorders*, 9, 132–138.

Chapter 5

Individual cognitive stimulation therapy (iCST)

Lauren A. Yates

Rationale for the development of iCST

The body of evidence demonstrating the short- and long-term benefits of group Cognitive Stimulation Therapy (CST) for people with dementia is substantial (Woods et al., 2012). As a result, its popularity continues to grow. In the UK, CST has been integrated into routine practice, with a reported 66% of memory services offering groups (MSNAP, 2014), and over 20 countries are part of the International CST Centre, established at University College London (UCL). Although the availability of CST is increasing, the intervention may not be accessible to certain individuals (Orrell et al., 2012), for example:

- Those with mobility or health issues which make getting to groups difficult,
- Those living in remote geographical areas,
- Those living in areas in which local services do not offer CST, or have waiting lists for groups,
- Those who would prefer not to take part in group activities,
- Those with sensory impairments or problems with communication who may find a group environment challenging,
- Those who have completed a CST programme, but would like to continue participating in similar activities.

In recognition of the need to provide other avenues by which people could access CST and its benefits, a home-based, carer-delivered, one-to-one version of the intervention was developed.

Development of iCST (Yates et al., 2015a)

In line with the previous body of CST research (Spector et al., 2003; Orrell et al., 2014), the development and evaluation of iCST followed the Medical Research Council (MRC) framework (Craig et al., 2008). Figure 5.1 shows the research activities conducted within each phase of the iCST trial in the context of this framework.

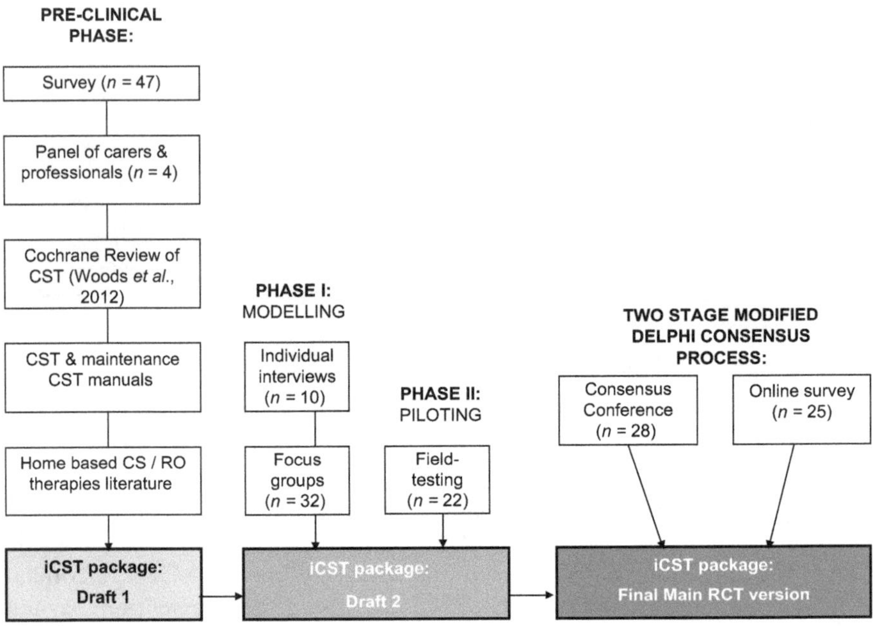

Figure 5.1 Development of iCST intervention within MRC framework

The iCST programme and materials were progressively refined according to feedback from key stakeholders (carers and people with dementia, healthcare professionals) and experts in the field. The development phase activities were reported in detail in journal articles (Yates et al., 2015a; Yates et al., 2015b; Yates et al., 2016).

Pre-clinical phase of development

Prior to designing the iCST programme and drafting the materials, people with dementia, carers and care staff were consulted on the feasibility of the idea of iCST. In addition, the research team reviewed existing literature on group CST, including the CST (Spector et al., 2006) and maintenance CST (mCST) manuals, (Aguirre et al., 2011) and one to one programmes of Cognitive Stimulation (CS) and Reality Orientation (RO) (*Moniz-Cook et al.*, 1998; Quayhagen and Quayhagen, 2001; Onder et al., 2005). This evidence was also examined by a small group of carers and healthcare professionals, who gave advice about how the group CST materials and the individual approaches identified could be adapted to best effect (see Box 5.1).

Box 5.1 Views of consultees

- iCST will be useful and should be a priority for research.
- iCST could help to bring the person and carer closer together, provide those unable to get out of the house an opportunity to take part in CST, and could be an alternative for those unable to take anti-dementia medication.
- Sessions should not be too long, around 30 minutes.
- Manual for family carers should be more concise than group manuals, and free of 'academic' terminology.
- Manual should be visually appealing with a simple and clear layout.
- Dyadic nature of the intervention should be emphasised.
- Varied activities to cater for the abilities of the person with dementia

Phase I modelling: focus groups and interviews (Yates et al., 2015b)

The first drafts of the iCST manuals and activity workbooks (sessions 1–12), and prototype toolkit items were presented to 24 carers and 28 people with dementia for appraisal in a series of 10 interviews and six focus groups (including three groups of people with dementia, two groups of carers, and one collaborative group of carers and their relative with dementia). Participants were recruited from a variety of settings, including voluntary and local authority organisations and memory services. Second drafts of the iCST materials were created based on the data collected from the groups, interviews, and field-testing phase (see Box 5.2).

Box 5.2 Data from interviews and focus groups

Views on mentally stimulating activities

> May I just say I believe that we are all crying out for help and stimulation but we can't, haven't so much got ideas in our own head as we hope other people can encourage us.
>
> (Person with dementia, focus group)

Feasibility of iCST

> The idea of activities (in the home) is good, people with dementia just need assistance with it.
>
> (Person with dementia, focus group)

You know, there's a physical side of it and a mental side of it, I don't know how many carers would be able to follow this programme consistently for 25 weeks.

(Family carer, focus group)

My reaction was that I could see more benefits in this approach, but I find it difficult to identify who actually would give the programme because I think anyone from the family, it probably wouldn't work because it's too formal and you'd need a lot of co-operation from the person who you have given it to.

(Family carer, focus group)

Dad felt at first that it was going to be treating him like a child [. . .] but I think once it comes to doing the manual, he'll realise it can be quite fun [. . .] It mustn't become a bore, a chore. It's got to be fun. Dad's got to enjoy it.

(Family carer, interview)

I can imagine saying to him 'come on we'll have a game of skittles' and he'd say 'oh I don't feel up to it at the moment'. There's all those factors to consider really so then, by the time you come to do it on that day, something else has gone on and it hasn't happened. So I think the flexibility here is important.

(Family carer, focus group)

iCST materials

Well it was plain speaking, it wasn't fancy words [. . .] It was straightforward so you couldn't mess about you know, you wouldn't make a mistake reading it would you? I found it good.

(Family carer, interview)

I like the attractive cover. It gives one the impression it's going to be interesting.

(Family carer, interview)

Phase II piloting (Yates et al., 2016)

The data from the focus groups and interviews were limited as participants had not tried the programme, and as such they could only discuss the programme 'in theory'. Additionally, only the materials for the first 12 sessions were available for appraisal at this stage. As a result, and in line with the MRC framework, a field-testing phase was conducted. Given the limited time available for field-testing, the programme was not tested in full (75 sessions over 25 weeks) by any one dyad (carer and person with dementia pair), and instead

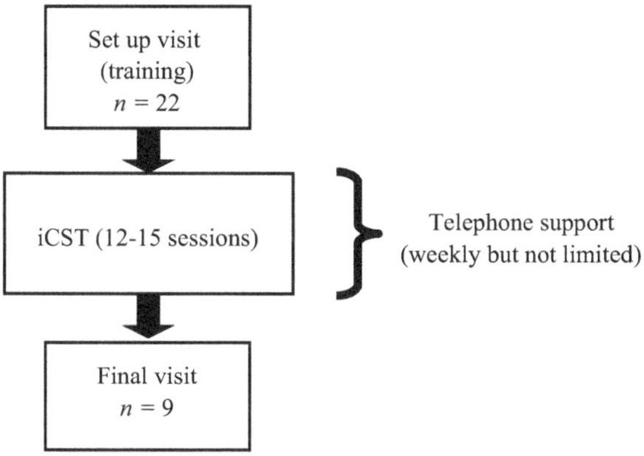

Figure 5.2 Procedure of the field-testing phase

it was split into six sections, with each dyad being allocated 12–15 sessions to complete (see Figure 5.2).

The sample was predominantly made up of family carers ($n = 16$), but in response to data from Phase I indicating iCST may be suitable, or even best delivered by a professional carer, paid carers were also recruited from a home care agency ($n = 6$). Dyads received training and support from a researcher comprising of a home visit to familiarise participants with iCST and the programme materials, and weekly telephone calls. Collection of qualitative and quantitative data was embedded into the telephone support contacts and visits. In addition, dyads completed 'monitoring progress' forms which gathered data about each activity, including quantitative ratings of enjoyment, interest, communication, and level of difficulty.

All data gathered were taken into account regardless of whether a complete set (set-up questionnaires, telephone support questionnaires, and final visit questionnaires) was obtained. The loss to follow-up rate in this phase was high, with only nine dyads available for the final follow-up visit. Despite this, dyads were generally able to participate in iCST together with minimal support from the research team. Most dyads were not able to do three sessions per week as recommended in the protocol with lack of time, illness, and motivation acting as barriers to delivery.

Two-stage modified Delphi consensus process (Yates et al., 2015a)

A modified Delphi process consisting of two rounds (an online survey and a conference) was conducted to achieve consensus on themes that participants had been unable to reach agreement on in the focus groups, interviews, and field-testing. Twenty-five participants completed the online survey, and 28 participants subsequently attended the conference. Sixteen participants took part in both rounds (57%). The sample included academics, healthcare professionals, researchers, and carers (family and paid home carers).

iCST intervention

Features of the programme

A key feature of the group CST sessions is their consistent structure (Figure 5.3) which is designed to support memory and learning. The 'introduction' and 'closing' elements of group sessions were omitted, as these were seen as 'too formal' in the context of delivery by a family member or friend. However, iCST sessions include the discussion of orientation information (e.g. date, time, weather), current affairs, and a themed activity which feature in the group CST programme.

Lasting around 20–30 minutes, iCST sessions are shorter than group CST sessions. A study of home-based cognitive stimulation (CS) by Onder et al. (2005) suggested this duration was feasible. It is unclear whether there is an optimum 'dose' of CST. However, given that group participants receive 90 minutes of CST per week and experience benefits, the research team reasoned that participating in iCST sessions for an equal amount of time may have a similar effect. Each CST (14 sessions) and maintenance CST (24 sessions) session (38 in total) was split to create two iCST sessions, with the exception of the final session, resulting in a 75-session programme delivered over 25 weeks.

Content of the iCST sessions

Although the group CST and maintenance CST programmes are manualised, activity resources are not provided for either as sessions are delivered by healthcare staff who are often allocated time and a budget to source materials. By contrast, informal carers may not be able to provide their own resources, or may be inconvenienced in doing so (e.g. time, cost), therefore iCST resources

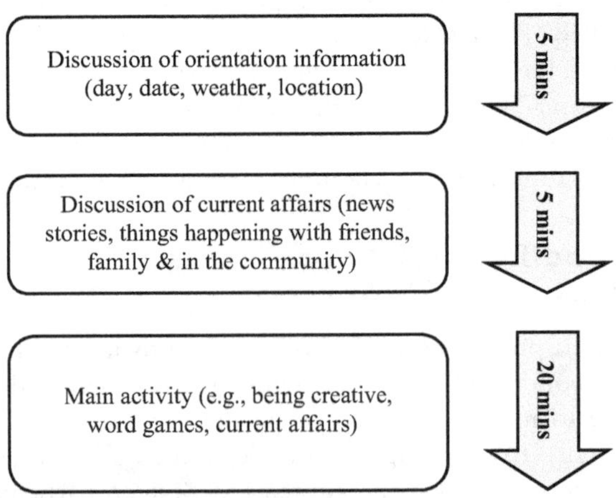

Figure 5.3 Structure of iCST sessions

Table 5.1 iCST session themes

iCST Session themes	
My life	Thinking cards
Current affairs	Visual clips discussion
Food	Art discussion
Being creative	Faces/scenes
Number games	Word games
Quiz games	Slogans
Sounds	Association words discussion
Physical games	Orientation
Categorising objects	Using money
Household treasures	Childhood
Useful tips	

were developed. It is important to note that people taking part in iCST are not restricted to using only the materials provided in the manual (see Box 5.3).

The iCST session themes (Table 5.1) and many of the suggested activities that appear in the iCST manual were taken directly from the group CST manuals (Spector et al., 2006; Aguirre et al., 2011). The research group also had access to a bank of resources that had been created by researchers who facilitated groups in the maintenance CST trial (Orrell et al., 2014). Activities were reviewed and included in the iCST programme if they could be easily adapted for a one-to-one session, and if they had generally been received well by groups in the trial.

A choice of activities is suggested for each session. These suggestions are graded by difficulty so the programme can be tailored to the person's abilities. Level A activities are typically more discussion based than level B activities, which tend to be more cognitively demanding. Box 5.3 provides tips on how to tailor iCST activities effectively.

iCST key principles

The guiding principles of CST and maintenance CST were adapted to create the 15 key principles of iCST (see Table 5.2). Principles specific to a group environment were omitted, and some academic terminology was rephrased in accordance with feedback from consultation with carers who felt that the manual should be easy to understand.

The person with dementia and their carer are encouraged to take part in the activities together, allowing the person to practice their cognitive skills and maximise their potential. Along with the feeling of 'togetherness', iCST encourages the carer and person with dementia to have fun and to see the time spent doing the activities as quality time together. A key goal of the sessions is to stimulate discussion, which can improve the language skills of the person with dementia.

Box 5.3 Tailoring activities effectively

- Include materials that have personal significance where possible to maximise engagement. For example, in a 'childhood session' the person delivering the session could prepare a selection of the person with dementia's photographs and some from their own collection as well as generic photos of a particular childhood scene or era.
- Pay attention to the level of challenge to which the person typically responds well. Are they the sort of person who enjoys completing tasks with ease? Do they become disheartened if they find activities difficult? Or do they relish a challenge? Choose level A or level B, or source additional materials accordingly.
- It's not necessary to stick to the same level of difficulty throughout the programme. Mix and match, according to which activity appeals to the person.
- Offer the person a choice of activities and themes each time you do a session together.
- Find ways to incorporate the person's interests into sessions where possible, e.g. when choosing a news topic to discuss.
- Try a range of session themes, but if there are any the person would prefer not to do, substitute these for themes the person enjoys.
- Use multi-media such as music and video clips where possible.

Table 5.2 iCST key principles

iCST Key Principles	
1	Mental stimulation
2	Develop new ideas, thoughts, and associations
3	Use orientation in a sensitive manner
4	Focus on opinions, rather than facts
5	Use reminiscence
6	Provide triggers to help memory
7	Stimulate learning and communication
8	Stimulate language and discussion
9	Stimulate everyday planning ability
10	Use a person-centred approach
11	Offer choice of activities
12	Enjoyment and fun
13	Maximise potential
14	Spend quality time together
15	Strengthen the caregiving relationship

Exploring the effectiveness of iCST: main trial

Design

A multi-centre, single-blind, clinical randomised controlled trial (RCT) of iCST over 25 weeks vs. treatment as usual (TAU) was conducted (Orgeta et al., 2015). All dyads recruited began by completing a baseline assessment.

Subsequently, they were randomly allocated into either the treatment group (completing three, 30 minute sessions of iCST per week for 25 weeks) or control group (receiving TAU for 25 weeks). Primary and secondary outcome measures were completed at three time points; baseline (BL) prior to randomisation; first follow-up 13 weeks after baseline (FU1); and second follow-up 26 weeks after baseline (FU2) (Figure 5.4).

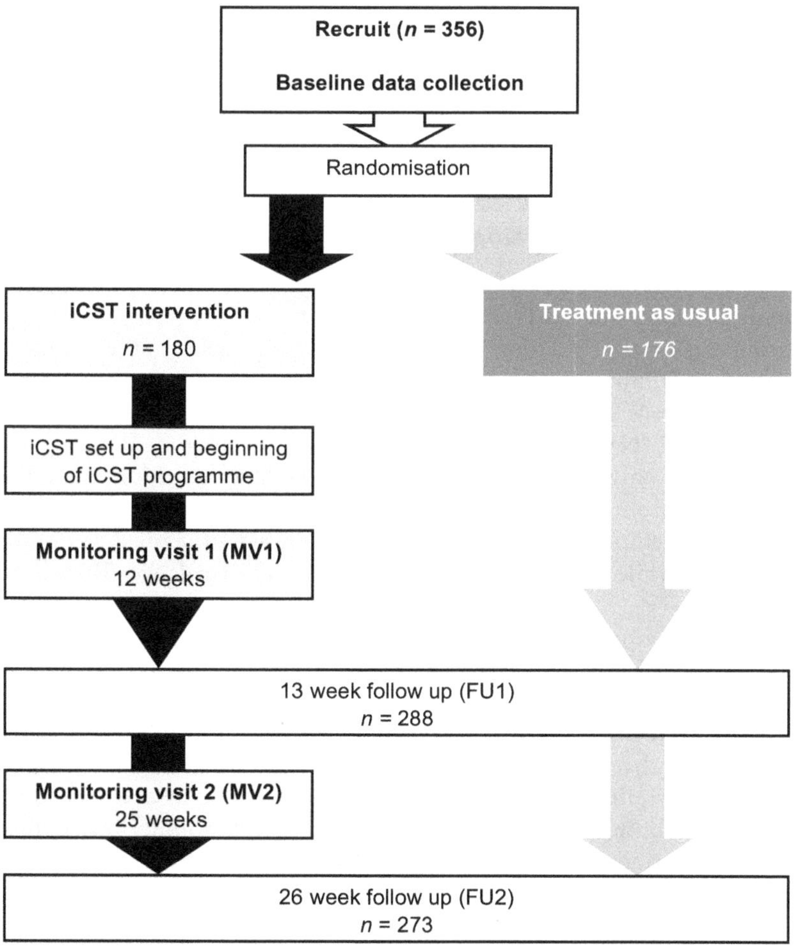

Figure 5.4 Design of the iCST trial

Sample

The trial was run from eight University and National Health Service (NHS) sites across the UK, including; London, Bangor, Hull, Manchester, Norfolk and Suffolk, Devon, Lincolnshire, and Dorset. Recruitment to the trial took place in a variety of community settings, including community mental health teams for older people (OPCMHTs), memory clinics, outpatient clinics, day centres, and voluntary sector organisations such as the Alzheimer's Society. In total, 356 dyads enrolled in the trial, with 273 completing FU2.

Inclusion criteria

Participants referred to the trial were screened for eligibility using the Spector et al. (2003) standardised criteria for psychological treatment of people with dementia (see Chapter 4 for full inclusion criteria). Additional criteria included living in the community and having regular contact with an informal carer. An 'informal carer' was defined as an unpaid carer in regular contact with the person with dementia who could deliver the programme, and act as an informant for the assessments at BL, FU1, and FU2. Many of the carers were relatives (e.g. spouses or children), or were close friends of the person.

Randomisation and blinding

Participants were randomised on a 1:1 ratio into either the iCST intervention group or TAU. In order to ensure participants were evenly distributed between the groups, they were stratified by centre and whether they were taking anti-cholinesterase inhibitors. The web-based randomisation service was managed by a Clinical Trials Unit in the UK (North Wales Organisation for Randomised Trials in Health [NWORTH]). A dynamic, adaptive randomisation algorithm was selected to ensure balance overall, within each stratification variable and within each stratum.

Using this method, participants can be randomised sequentially, minimising selection bias while maintaining an acceptable level of balance (Russell et al., 2011).

Due to the nature of the iCST intervention, it was not possible to blind dyads to their allocation. However, treatment allocation was not disclosed to the researchers conducting the assessments at FU1 and FU2. Blinded assessors recorded their impression of the allocation of each dyad and their confidence in that prediction at FU1 and FU2. Based on this data, the integrity of blinding was examined retrospectively to test whether inadvertent loss of blinding resulted in bias, and to adjust for any bias detected. The trial statisticians remained blind to allocation while performing the main analyses. Unblind adherence data was analysed after the main analyses were complete.

iCST package and training

Carers received the iCST manual which provided guidance and session plans, an activity workbook containing resources for activities suggested in the session plans, and a toolkit including a set of boules, playing cards, dominoes, magnifying card, sound activity CDs, coloured pencils, and world and UK maps. Carers were trained in their homes by a researcher. In most cases both the carer and the person with dementia were present during the session. Training was standardised and designed to be interactive, including a role-play exercise, clips of the maintenance CST training DVD, 'Making a Difference 2' (Aguirre et al., 2011), and the opportunity to complete the first session with support from the researcher.

Support and measures of adherence

Adherence to the iCST programme was measured throughout dyads' participation. A carer's diary was provided in which carers were required to record which sessions had been completed, when, assessments of the person's response to each session, and comments about their experience of each session.

Researchers provided dyads with regular support via telephone throughout their participation in the trial. Calls were semi-structured according to a standardised telephone support questionnaire; however, the carer was also invited to discuss their experience of the programme, or request advice from the researcher.

Monitoring visits were scheduled for 12 and 25 weeks, prior to the FU1 and FU2 assessments. The purpose of the visits was to collect the carer diaries and complete a brief questionnaire with the carer requiring them to reflect on their success with the programme, and discuss the dyad's experience of the programme, problem solving any issues if necessary. The researcher recorded their impressions of the visit using the researcher monitoring questionnaire. Any additional visits (e.g. additional training) or carer-initiated contacts were classified as 'out of protocol' and recorded.

Treatment as usual (TAU)

Dyads randomised into the TAU arm did not receive any additional intervention for the duration of their participation. The services and treatments accessed by control group dyads varied between and within centres, and changed over time. As expected, a large proportion of the people with dementia involved in the trial were on cholinesterase inhibitor medication. The services and treatments available to the control were also expected to be accessible to the intervention group; therefore the trial evaluated the additional effects of iCST.

Assessment procedure

Assessments took place at dyads' homes. In most cases one researcher conducted the visit, interviewing both the carer and the person with dementia. The person with dementia and the carer were interviewed separately whenever possible.

Assessment visits usually lasted around one and a half to two hours. Cognition, quality of life, mood, and quality of the caregiving relationship were assessed in the person with dementia's interview. Carers were interviewed about their health and well-being, as well as behavioural and psychological symptoms, functional status, and quality of life of the person with dementia (see Table 5.3). Socio-demographic data for the dyad and service use were also collected from the carer.

Consent

People with dementia recruited into the trial were in the mild to moderate stages of dementia, and able to give informed consent to participate. Consent was regarded as a continuing process rather than a one-off decision, thus willingness to participate was checked during the assessments. The terms of the Mental Capacity Act (Department of Health, 2005) were followed in instances where the person with dementia's level of impairment increased to the extent that they were no longer able to provide informed consent.

Outcome measures

The key outcomes of interest for people with dementia were cognition and quality of life, and quality of life for the carer. Table 5.3 shows all primary and secondary outcomes assessed in the trial.

Table 5.3 Outcome measures

Person with dementia	*Person with dementia proxy*	*Carer*
****Alzheimer's Disease Assessment Scale (ADAS-Cog) (Rosen et al., 1984)**	DEMQoL Proxy	****Short Form 12 (SF-12) (Ware, Kosinski, and Keller, 1996)**
****Quality of Life – Alzheimer's Disease Scale (QoL-AD) (Logsdon et al., 1999)**	Neuropsychiatric Inventory (NPI) (Cummings et al., 1994)	Hospital Anxiety and Depression Scale (HADS) (Zigmond and Snaith, 1983)
Mini-Mental State Examination (MMSE) (Folstein et al., 1983)	Bristol Activities of Daily Living Scale (BADLS) (Bucks et al., 2001)	European Quality of Life-5 Dimensions (EQ-5D) (Brooks et al., 2013)
Dementia Quality of Life Scale (DEMQoL) (Smith et al., 2005)	Client Service Receipt Inventory (CSRI) (Beecham and Knapp, 2001)	Resilience Scale-14 (RS-14) (Wagnild, 2009)
Geriatric Depression Scale (GDS) (Sheikh and Yesavage, 1986)		Client Service Receipt Inventory (CSRI) (Beecham and Knapp, 2001)
Quality of the Caregiving Relationship Scale (QCPR) (Spruytte et al., 2002)		Quality of the Caregiving Relationship Scale (QCPR) (Spruytte et al., 2002)

****indicates primary outcomes. Person with dementia proxy measures were completed by the carer**

Analyses

An intention-to-treat (ITT) analysis was carried out including available data. Sample size calculations were based on the numbers estimated to be available at the study primary end-point (FU2) 26 weeks after randomisation into the iCST intervention group, or TAU control.

Analysis of covariance (ANCOVA) was performed for each of the measures. The 26-week primary end-point of the study (FU2) was the dependent variable, and the centre was used as the random factor in the model. Marital status, living status, gender of the participant, use of anti-dementia medication, and treatment allocation (iCST or TAU) were the fixed factors. Age, baseline outcome score, and dyadic relationship were fitted covariates in the model. A similar model was fitted for the carer primary outcome including baseline measurement, age of carer, and relationship with the person with dementia as covariates. Fitted fixed factors were sex and marital status, and site was a random factor. The same models were applied to outcomes at the shorter-term 13-week follow up (FU1) and for all secondary outcomes. The number of iCST sessions was also factored into the model of the main analysis as a continuous variable to determine whether number of sessions completed was associated with the outcomes.

Results

Outcomes for people with dementia

The analyses demonstrated no significant difference between the iCST and TAU groups at either FU1 (MD = 0.29, 95% CI -1.10–1.68, $p = 0.68$) or FU2 (MD = -0.55,95% CI -2.00–0.90, $p = 0.45$) for cognition measured by the ADAS-Cog. Nor did the groups differ significantly on the primary measure of QoL (QoL-AD) at FU1 (MD = -0.14, 95% CI -1.12–0.84, $p = 0.78$) or FU2 (MD = -0.02, 95% CI -1.04–1.00, $p= 0.97$).

Improvements in the quality of the caregiving relationship (QCPR) from the person's perspective were found at FU2, with a mean difference of 1.77 (95% CI 0.26–3.28, $p = 0.02$) between the groups. Amongst the remaining secondary outcomes, there was no evidence that people with dementia allocated to iCST experienced improvements in activities of daily living (ADLs), or behavioural, psychological, or depressive symptoms.

Outcomes for carers

No significant differences in the primary carer outcome (SF-12) were detected between the iCST and TAU groups at either FU1 or FU2. However, at FU2, EQ-5D scores were significantly better in the iCST group (MD = 0.06, 95% CI 0.01–0.10, $p = 0.014$). Resilience, anxiety, and depressive symptoms did not appear to be significantly impacted by iCST.

Adherence analysis

Adherence was monitored and factored into analysis in order to explore any potential dose relationship. A relatively large proportion of dyads (22%) did not complete any sessions. Fifty-one percent completed 30 or more sessions by FU2. For people with dementia, the total number of sessions completed at FU2 was significantly associated with improvements in the QCPR. For carers, completing a higher number of sessions was associated with a significant reduction in HADS score at FU2.

Commentary and reflections

Previously, CST (Spector et al., 2003) had only been delivered in a group setting by a member of staff or healthcare professional, thus the home-based, family carer-led format of iCST represents an innovation in CST-based approaches. Furthermore, this is the largest known piece of CST research to date.

iCST did not yield significant cognitive or QoL benefits for people with dementia as hypothesised. However, iCST appeared to enhance the quality of relationship between the person with dementia and their carer, from the person with dementia's perspective. When level of adherence to the programme (number of sessions completed) was factored into analyses, it emerged that people with dementia who participated in more sessions were much more likely to experience gains in the quality of the relationship with their carer at 26 weeks.

iCST may be useful to help carers and people with dementia actively improve the quality of their relationship. Improvements in the caregiving relationship may contribute to the QoL of the person with dementia and potentially result in reduced institutionalisation. These outcomes are valuable, thus the intervention manual and DVD have now been published (Yates et al., 2014) so that they are widely available for carers and people with dementia.

Reflecting on the results of the trial

The results of the trial are not consistent with previous studies of group short-term CST (Spector et al., 2003), longer-term maintenance CST pilot (Orrell et al., 2005), and one-to-one, home-based programme of reality orientation (RO)/cognitive stimulation (CS) (Moniz-Cook et al., 1998; Quayhagen and Quayhagen, 2001; Onder et al., 2005).

It is possible that shorter-term, more intense programmes of CS are more effective. Indeed, short-term CST (14 sessions over 7 weeks) consistently yields cognitive benefits (Woods et al., 2012), whereas longer-term maintenance CST (7 weeks of CST followed by 24 weekly sessions) does not appear to do so (Orrell et al., 2014).

Lack of cognitive benefits may reflect a 'ceiling effect' whereby participants were already functioning at their maximum level of cognitive performance at baseline, thus were not able to glean any significant improvement from the intervention. Indeed 70% of the sample had mild dementia (Clinical Dementia Rating Scale [CDR] score = 1; Morris, 1993). If this is the case, individuals may benefit if they were to participate in the intervention at a later stage in the progression of dementia. However, the evidence for group cognitive stimulation suggests that the effects of the intervention are similar regardless of the severity of dementia (Woods et al., 2012).

For some dyads, iCST activities may not have been mentally stimulating enough. This may account for cases in which the person did not engage in the sessions and subsequently failed to adhere to the programme, or dropped out of the trial completely. Moreover, the activities may have failed to provide enough stimulation to have an impact on cognition. Given the majority of the sample had mild dementia, this experience may have been common enough to contribute to the lack of significant result for this outcome.

In addition, in contrast to the findings of the trial, QoL benefits have been consistently associated with both short- and longer-term programmes of CST (Spector et al., 2003; Orrell et al., 2014; Woods et al., 2012). Woods and colleagues (2012) suggest that the QoL benefits associated with CST are likely to be mediated by improvements in cognition. Thus, the lack of significant cognitive change experienced by iCST participants may account for the findings on QoL outcomes.

Adherence to the intervention

Adherence to iCST was much lower than expected. On average, dyads completed just less than half (31.68) of the recommended number of sessions (75) over 25 weeks and 22% were not able to complete any sessions. Intention-to-treat (ITT) analyses are not sensitive to variations in receipt of an intervention, thus using all available data including that of dyads who received less or none of the planned intervention, may have under-powered the study against a potential significant result.

The patterns of adherence, and large variation in number of sessions completed between dyads (SD = 26.81) suggest that very few dyads participated in sessions consistently week to week. There may be a relationship between regular engagement and capacity to benefit from cognitive-stimulation-based interventions. For example, delivering the intervention intermittently, with long periods of 'rest' in between, or bouts of intense participation in sessions followed by inactivity may not be effective approaches. There is evidence to suggest that participating in group CST once, as opposed to twice weekly as recommended does not yield the cognitive or QoL benefits typically associated with the intervention (Cove et al., 2014). Thus, it is conceivable that 'dose' is similarly important with iCST.

Dyads were given flexibility to fit in sessions when possible, in response to development phase feedback from carers who emphasised the need for this approach. However, based on the adherence data, this pragmatic approach did not appear to be effective in ensuring dyads completed the recommended number of sessions. In terms of strategies to improve adherence, it seems unlikely that provision of more detailed and fixed schedules of delivery for iCST would have made an impact, particularly if the reasons for non-adherence in the main trial were related to practical issues such as lack of time or illness as described in the field-testing phase.

How can we explain the discrepancy between the impact of group CST and iCST?

The social setting and additional stimulation from participating in a group context may account for the difference in outcomes between iCST and group CST. When non-specific components of CST such as receiving social attention are controlled for, the intervention still has a significant impact on cognition and some neuropsychological symptoms including apathy and depression (Niu et al., 2010). However, they do appear to contribute to cognitive change (Woods et al., 2006). Being involved in a social setting may generate more stimulation through development and expression of new ideas, thoughts, and associations and use of language skills, owing not only to the input of the facilitator, but the group members who prompt responses from one another. In a one-to-one setting fewer, and crucially less diverse, ideas may be exchanged between two people, and the onus is on the carer to constantly encourage the person to discuss their opinions and respond to the stimuli presented as part of the activity. If the carer is not adept at this, or if there are challenges in communication between the dyad, the sessions may be missing a crucial component which may elicit benefits.

Suitability of the carer as an interventionist

The findings of the trial demonstrate that it is feasible for carers to deliver therapeutic interventions, and importantly that their involvement benefits them in terms of quality of life, but also extends to the quality of the caregiving relationship. As a result iCST could be considered a 'relationship-centred' approach, helping people with dementia and those around them actively manage how they live with dementia together. Still, taking on the role of interventionist may not suit all carers. In certain circumstances it might be preferable for the intervention to be delivered by healthcare professionals, befrienders, or paid carers. Certainly it seems this would be feasible given iCST was successfully field-tested by a small sample of paid carers in the development phase, and group CST is typically facilitated by healthcare professionals and/or care staff. Prospectively, delivery by a paid carer, befriender, or healthcare professional would offer several advantages in research and real-world settings:

- Paid carers or healthcare professionals may have dementia care skills and previous experience of interventions, which may enhance the quality of delivery, or fidelity to the principles and techniques of iCST.
- Professionals may be more likely to be able to deliver the intervention consistently as visits are often scheduled regularly.

- As carers highlighted in consultations during the development phase of the trial, interactions with a professional are more likely to be free from any relationship dynamics that may compromise successful engagement in sessions. For instance, some carers felt that an 'outsider' might elicit a more positive response from the person.
- In circumstances in which iCST would not be feasible for a family carer (e.g. lack of time, carer ill health or frailty, feeling burdened) it would be useful to have a professional available to deliver the sessions. Delivery by a professional would also suit people who do not have a family carer, or have family who live a long distance away, as is now common.
- Offering a structured intervention with demonstrated benefits is advantageous for healthcare services and care agencies. For healthcare services using iCST could demonstrate compliance with guidelines and recommendations on early, home-based interventions issued by the government and bodies such as the National Institute for Clinical Excellence (NICE). Use of interventions by paid staff from care agencies is not compulsory, but may set their services apart from others.

Further research and the future of iCST

Given that a major limitation of this study was low adherence, more work is needed to explore whether it can be improved. This may be achieved by enhancing methods of support or training, changing the format of delivery (e.g. via a paid carer/healthcare professional, on a computer platform), or identifying characteristics of dyads which might predict suitability and likelihood of benefit.

The iCST materials are currently only available in paper-based format. However, there may be benefit in adapting them for a computer-based platform. This would be convenient for people who have difficulty handling a manual, meaning that the materials can be re-used, and if on a computer tablet, the sessions could be done while out and about (e.g. in a café or at another person's home). A computer-based programme would also have the capacity to track or monitor progress, record adherence to sessions, and help users decide which level of activity (A or B) is most appropriate for them. On a computer-based platform there is more scope for sessions to include media (e.g. images, video clips, audio tracks) which could be easily accessed using the internet, and unlike the manual, which is restricted in terms of content, a large bank of activity materials could be made available and regularly updated. A computer platform would also have the facility for social interaction tools such as forums and online help, which could be useful for users to discuss their experiences of the programme, share materials and tips, as well as seek support. There is evidence to suggest that using computers can enhance participation in mentally stimulating activities and may be associated with maintenance of cognition (Almeida et al., 2012); thus delivering cognitive stimulation via computer could maximise or enhance the effects of the intervention.

References

Aguirre, E., Spector, A.E., Streater, A., Hoe, J., Woods, B., and Orrell, M. (2011). *Making a Difference 2: An Evidence Based Group Program to Offer Maintenance Cognitive Stimulation Therapy (CST) to People With Dementia.* London: Hawker Publications.

Almeida, O.P., Yeap, B.B., Alfonso, H., Hankey, G.J., Flicker, L., and Norman, P.E. (2012). Older men who use computers have lower risk of dementia. *PLoS ONE*, 7(8), pp. e44239.

Beecham, J., and Knapp, M. (2001). Costing psychiatric interventions. In G. Thornicroft (Ed.), *Measuring Mental Health Needs* (pp. 179–190). London: Gaskill.

Brooks, R., Rabin, R., and De Charro, F., eds. (2013). *The Measurement and Valuation of Health Status Using EQ-5D: A European Perspective: Evidence From the EuroQol BIOMED Research Programme.* Berlin: Springer Science & Business Media.

Bucks, R.S., Ashworth, D.L., Wilcock, G.K., and Siegfried, K. (1996). Assessment of activities of daily living in dementia: Development of the Bristol Activities of Daily Living Scale. *Age Ageing*, 25, pp. 113–120.

Cove, J.E. Jacobi, N., Donovan, H., Orrell, M., Stott, J., and Spector, A. (2014). Effectiveness of weekly Cognitive Stimulation Therapy (CST) for people with dementia and the additional impact of enhancing CST with a carer training programme. *Clinical Interventions in Aging*, 9, pp. 2143.

Craig, P., Dieppe, P., Macintyre, S., Michie, S., Nazareth, I., and Petticrew, M. (2008). Developing and evaluating complex interventions: The new Medical Research Council guidance. *BMJ*, pp. 337.

Cummings, J.L., Mega, M., Gray, K. et al. (1994). The neuropsychiatric inventory: Comprehensive assessment of psychopathology in dementia. *Neurology*, 44, pp. 2308–2314.

Department of Health. (2005). *Mental Capacity Act.* London: HMSO.

Folstein, M.F., Robins, L.N., and Helzer, J.E. (1983). The mini-mental state examination. *Arch Gen Psychiatry*, 40, p. 812.

Hodge, S., Hailey, E., and Orrell, M. (2014). *Memory Services National Accreditation Programme (MSNAP) Standards for Memory Services.* 4th ed. London: Royal College of Psychiatrists.

Logsdon, R.G., Gibbons, L.E., and McCurry, S.M. (1999). Quality of life in Alzheimer's disease: Patient and caregiver reports. *Journal of Mental Health and Aging*, 5, pp. 21–32.

Moniz-Cook, E., Agar, S., Gibson, G., Win, T., and Wang, M. (1998). A preliminary study of the effects of early intervention with people with dementia and their families in a memory clinic. *Aging & Mental Health*, 2(3), pp. 199–211.

Morris, J.C. (1993). The Clinical Dementia Rating (CDR): Current version and scoring rules. *Neurology*.

Niu, Y.X., Tan, J.P., Guan, J.Q., Zhang, Z.Q., and Wang, L.N. (2010). Cognitive stimulation therapy in the treatment of neuropsychiatric symptoms in Alzheimer's disease: A randomized controlled trial. *Clinical Rehabilitation.*

Onder, G., Zanetti, O., Giacobini, E. et al. (2005). Reality orientation therapy combined with cholinesterase inhibitors in Alzheimer's disease: Randomised controlled trial. *British Journal of Psychiatry*, 187, pp. 450–455.

Orgeta, V., Leung, P., Yates, L. et al. (2015). Individual Cognitive Stimulation Therapy for dementia (iCST): Effectiveness and cost-effectiveness pragmatic multicentre randomised trial. *Health Technology Assessment*, 19(64).

Orrell, M., Aguirre, E., Spector, A. et al. (2014). Maintenance Cognitive Stimulation Therapy for dementia: Single-blind, multicentre, pragmatic randomised controlled trial. *The British Journal of Psychiatry*, 204(6), pp. 454–461.

Orrell, M., Spector, A., Thorgrimsen, L., and Woods, B. (2005). A pilot study examining the effectiveness of maintenance Cognitive Stimulation Therapy (MCST) for people with dementia. *International Journal of Geriatric Psychiatry*, 20(5), pp. 446–451.

Orrell, M., Woods, B., and Spector, A. (2012). Should we use individual Cognitive Stimulation Therapy to improve cognitive function in people with dementia? *BMJ*, 344, pp. e633.

Quayhagen, M.P., and Quayhagen, M. (2001). Testing of a cognitive stimulation intervention for dementia caregiving dyads. *Neuropsychological Rehabilitation*, 11(3–4), pp. 319–332.

Rosen, W.G., Mohs, R.C., and Davis, K.L. (1984). A new rating scale for Alzheimer's disease. *American Journal of Psychiatry*, 141, pp. 1356–1364.

Russell, D., Hoare, Z.S., Whitaker, R., Whitaker, C.J., and Russell, I.T. (2011). Generalized method for adaptive randomization in clinical trials. *Stat Med*, 30(9), pp. 922–934.

Sheikh, J.I., and Yesavage, J.A. (1986). Geriatric Depression Scale (GDS): Recent evidence and development of a shorter version. In T.L. Brink (Ed.), *Clinical Gerontology: A Guide to Assessment and Intervention* (pp. 165–173). New York: The Haworth Press.

Smith, S.C., Lamping, D.L., Banerjee, S. et al. (2005). Measurement of health-related quality of life for people with dementia: Development of a new instrument (DEMQOL) and an evaluation of current methodology. *Health Technology Assessment*, 9, pp. 1–93.

Spector, A., Thorgrimsen, L., Woods, B., and Orrell, M. (2006). *Making a Difference: An Evidence-based Group Programme to Offer Cognitive Stimulation Therapy (CST) to People With Dementia*. London: Hawker Publications.

Spector, A., Thorgrimsen, L., Woods, B., Royan, L., Davies, S., Butterworth, M., and Orrell, M. (2003). Efficacy of an evidence-based Cognitive Stimulation Therapy programme for people with dementia. *British Journal of Psychiatry*, 183(3), pp. 248–254.

Spruytte, N., van Audenhove, C., Lammertyn, F., and Storms, G. (2002). The quality of the caregiving relationship in informal care for older adults with dementia and chronic psychiatric patients. *Psychology & Psychotherapy*, 75, pp. 295–311.

Wagnild, G.M. (2009). *Resilience Scale User's Guide for the US English Version of the Resilience Scale and the 14-item Resilience Scale (Version 3.08)*. Worden, MT: The Resilience Center PLLP.

Ware, J., Jr, Kosinski, M., and Keller, S.D. (1996). A 12-Item short-form health survey: Construction of scales and preliminary tests of reliability and validity. *Medical Care*, 34, pp. 220–233.

Woods, B., Aguirre, E., Spector, A.E., and Orrell, M. (2012). Cognitive stimulation to improve cognitive functioning in people with dementia. *Cochrane Database of Systematic Reviews*, 2.

Woods, B., Thorgrimsen, L., Spector, A., Royan, L., and Orrell, M. (2006). Improved quality of life and Cognitive Stimulation Therapy in dementia. *Aging and Mental Health*, 10(3), pp. 219–226.

Yates, L., Orrell, M., Leung, P., Spector, A., Woods, B., and Orgeta, V. (2014). *Making a Difference 3 Individual CST: A Manual for Carers*, volume 3. London: Hawker.

Yates, L.A., Leung, P., Orgeta, V., Spector, A., and Orrell, M. (2015a). The development of individual Cognitive Stimulation Therapy (iCST) for dementia. *Clinical Intervention Aging*, 10, pp. 95–104.

Yates, L.A., Orgeta, V., Leung, P., Spector, A., and Orrell, M. (2016). Field testing phase of the development of individual Cognitive Stimulation Therapy (iCST) for dementia. *BMC Health Services Research*, 16(233).

Yates, L.A., Orrell, M., Spector, A., and Orgeta, V. (2015b). Service users' involvement in the development of individual Cognitive Stimulation Therapy (iCST) for dementia: A qualitative study. *BMC Geriatrics*, 15(1), p. 1.

Zigmond, A.S., and Snaith, R.P. (1983). The hospital anxiety and depression scale. *Acta Psychiatrica Scandinavica*, 67(6), pp. 361–370.

Chapter 6

Cognitive stimulation therapy

Implementation in practice

Amy Streater

Introduction

The development, implementation, and evaluation of CST and MCST have adhered to the Medical Research Council (MRC) framework for the development and evaluation of complex interventions (Craig et al., 2008). Consequently, CST research has established a strong evidence base to support its use in routine practice (Spector, Orrell & Aguirre, 2011; Orrell et al., 2005; Orrell et al., 2014) for cognitive and quality of life (QoL) benefits for people with mild to moderate dementia. This has led to both programmes being widely used in a variety of healthcare settings in practice. However, less is known about the level of support required by staff members to deliver the programmes, and adaptations in practice are not consistently formally evaluated from a research perspective. Evaluation in this way is necessary due to the well-documented gap between research and practice (Grol and Grimshaw, 2003). This chapter describes a phase IV study (MRC framework) examining implementation and long-term follow up of CST.

Justification for the outreach support options

A previous pilot study investigated the implementation of CST after one-day training (Spector et al., 2011). One hundred and sixty-eight staff working with people with dementia who attended CST training were followed up by email/post with a questionnaire. The questionnaire asked whether the person had run CST groups, problems/barriers to running groups, and what extra support may be useful. In addition, staff completed outcome measures, including approaches to dementia (Lintern and Woods, 2001), learning transfer (Holton et al., 2000), and job satisfaction (Barkham et al., 1989). From the 76 respondents, a *t*-test was used to compare staff who had run CST to those who had not.

Staff who ran CST groups scored significantly higher on the three subscales of the brief Learning Transfer System Inventory (LTSI, Spector et al., 2011): learner characteristics, work environment, and ability/enabling. Approaches to dementia and job satisfaction did not change across the two groups. Those running the groups reported perceived barriers as lack of staff time and resources, not enough suitable people with dementia or a suitable room, transport difficulties, and lack of managerial support. These barriers were the same for those who did not run groups.

Even though 86% of survey respondents felt skilled enough to deliver the programme after receiving CST training, there was however, feedback to suggest that access to additional support may enhance delivery. Suggestions for methods of support included more support from other members of staff, regular and specialist supervision, an online forum, and additional training in other areas. Respondents also felt it would be helpful to have support and learning from colleagues, training in group facilitation, experience and understanding of running groups, and work flexibility. The authors recommended comparing the effectiveness of different training methods, as well as the impact on outcome measures for people with dementia. The outreach support options derived from this research for the following study included: email support, an online forum, and local supervision.

Exploring the implementation of CST with outreach support: main trial

Aims

This study (Streater et al., 2017) aimed to: (1) evaluate the effectiveness of outreach support options offered to staff, including an online forum, email support, and local supervision, and (2) determine the effects of outreach support on the implementation of CST and MCST in practice.

Design

The study was a multi-centre, single-blind, randomised controlled trial (RCT) of staff in receipt of CST training, or with previous experience of CST, who were then cluster randomised to outreach support comprising of an online forum, email support, and local supervision, or a usual CST control group. Participants were expected to deliver the CST and MCST programmes over the duration of the study. All participants completed a baseline, six, and 12-month assessments, as well as attendance and adherence records of group members after each session. The trial team consisted of senior members of clinical staff, a researcher, an administrator, and a local collaborator or principal investigator at each recruited site.

Sample

Staff members with varying levels of CST experience who worked with people with dementia were recruited across 63 dementia care settings. Participating Trusts included North East London Foundation Trust, Tees, Esk and Wear

Valleys NHS Trust, Worcestershire Health and Care NHS Trust, Kent and Medway NHS and Social Care Partnership Trust, and North Staffordshire Combined Healthcare NHS Trust. In addition, Olympuscare services, and voluntary organisations contributed to the research study. Staff members were either 'new' to CST, having never delivered the programme prior to their research involvement, had previously attended CST training, or were already using the CST 'Making a difference' manual (Spector et al., 2006). In total, 241 staff members enrolled in the study, and 140 completed the final follow up (Figure 6.1).

Inclusion criteria

Each staff member met the following inclusion criteria: (1) adequate written and spoken English, (2) ability to complete online assessment at three time points, (3) availability of two additional staff members to support the running of groups, (4) agreement from management to have time set aside to run groups,

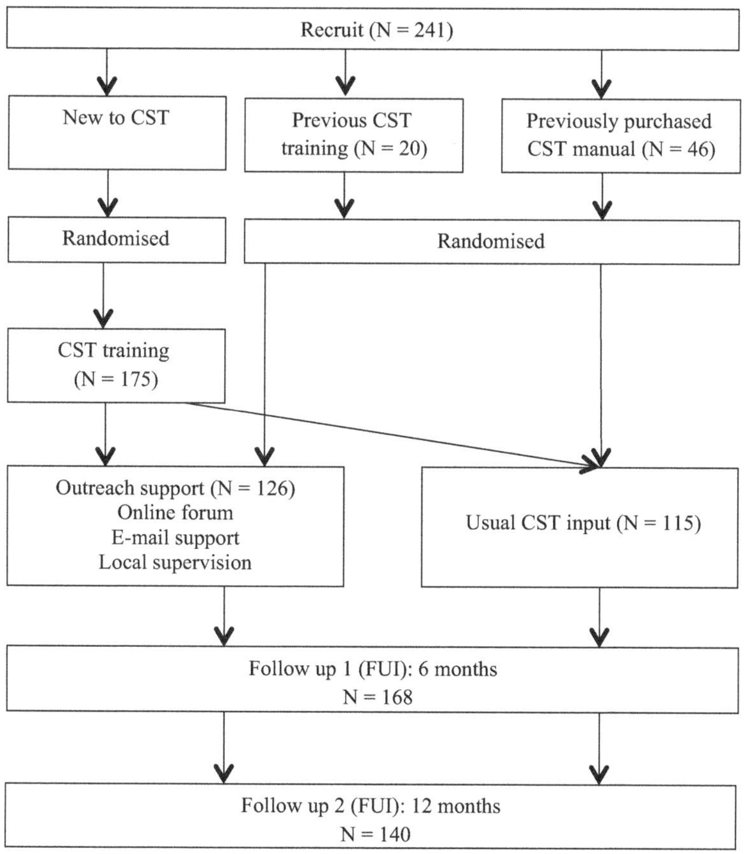

Figure 6.1 Design of the MCST implementation trial

and (5) able to identify 5–8 people with mild to moderate dementia to participate in the programmes.

Randomisation and masking

Randomisation occurred in clusters to avoid contamination within centres. For staff members in receipt of the CST training day, randomisation occurred prior to the day via a Clinical Trials Unit (North Wales Organisation for Randomised Trials in Health [NWORTH]). Randomisation of staff who had previously received CST training, or had the CST manual occurred on a day when there was a relatively equal pairing of participants across centres to avoid imbalance between the outreach support and usual CST control groups. Participants were allocated their identification number by an administrator and completed their questionnaires online, so the researcher was masked to the randomisation result.

Consent

Consent was provided electronically by each staff member at the point of the baseline assessment, either prior to the CST training day or date of randomisation. A paper consent form was also completed by each staff member either on the training day or completed and mailed back to the researcher. Consent was considered an ongoing process and the completion of the questionnaire at each time point was taken as an indicator of participants' agreement to continue in the study.

CST training and outreach support package

Staff members 'new' to CST received CST training delivered by Dr Aimee Spector or Dr Amy Streater. The training included: background to CST and evidence base, role-play, problem solving, and video clips of the MCST sessions. Each session theme was discussed with the attendees to help them consider what they could realistically deliver in practice. An evaluation form was completed at the end of each day by each participant to ensure the standardised delivery of the training day.

The outreach support options (online forum, local supervision, and email support) were made available as much as required for the duration of the participant's study involvement. Staff members created login details for the online forum. Once alerted to each registration, the researcher activated their username and checked that they had been randomised into the outreach support group. The purpose of the online forum was to provide an online community for the participants to discuss any issues or barriers they may be experiencing, or to let others know what was working well in practice. The email support was provided by the researcher and was available 24/7. For those 'new' to CST, supervision was provided by a clinical practitioner e.g. occupational therapist or psychologist in the local area, or if this was not possible the researcher took on this role. For those with previous CST experience, the participant was expected to identify their own local supervision, and if this did not happen this was recorded to reflect what was likely to currently be happening in practice. All outreach support options required active engagement from the staff members. Additionally, the researcher contacted those in receipt of outreach support in a monthly phone call to monitor each centre. Outreach support options were logged by the researcher and followed up when required.

Usual CST control group

Centres randomised to the usual CST control group did not receive any additional intervention. Randomised staff members were considered in the usual CST control group irrespective of their previous CST experience. Centres varied in the level of external support received, and this remained unaltered for the study to reflect the running of groups in practice. The administrator, with no experience of CST, contacted those not in receipt of outreach support in a monthly phone call to monitor each centre. It was expected that varying levels of support would also be seen in the intervention group, thus the trial evaluated the additional effects of the outreach support options made available through the study.

Assessment procedure

The assessment was completed online, or in paper form and then entered online by the researcher or administrator. The assessment was designed to be completed in approximately 45 minutes. In addition to socio-demographic data, approaches to dementia, barriers to change, learning transfer, controllability beliefs, dementia knowledge, job satisfaction, and sense of competence were measured.

Measures of attendance and adherence

Attendance and adherence to the programme were measured using an attendance and adherence booklet completed by each centre delivering the programme. Information collected included name of group, group song, facilitators, date, names of group members and their attendance, level of interest, communication, enjoyment, and mood on a five-point Likert scale (e.g. 1 = no interest to 5 = shows great interest). The attendance record sheet can be found in the Making a Difference 2 manual (Aguirre et al., 2011). The overall records allowed us to look at the primary outcome of average number of attendees recorded across the CST and MCST programmes. The attendance records were also used to rate the level of delivery of the programme in practice as: (1) 'low' use of CST – fewer than three people per session, (2) 'medium' use of CST – three to four group members per session, and (3) 'high' use of CST – five or more group members per session. 'High' use of CST, or successful implementation of the programme was considered five or more group members in accordance with the recommended group size in both CST manuals (Spector et al., 2006; Aguirre et al., 2011).

Secondary outcome measures

Secondary outcome measures included; Approaches to Dementia Questionnaire (ADQ; Lintern and Woods, 2001), Barriers to Change Questionnaire (BARCQ; Corrigan et al., 1992), Brief Learning Transfer System Inventory (Brief LTSI; Spector *et al.*, 2011), Controllability Beliefs Scale (CBS; Dagnan et al., 2004), Dementia Knowledge–20 (DK-20; Shanahan et al., 2013), Minnesota Satisfaction Questionnaire (MSQ; Weiss et al., 1967), and Sense of Competence in Dementia care Staff (SCIDS; Schepers et al., 2012). These measures were considered appropriate to determine change over time across the CST and MCST programmes.

Analyses

Primary outcome

An intention-to-treat (ITT) analysis was carried out. The sample size calculation was based on estimated numbers available at the study primary end-point (follow up 2, FU2) of 12 months after randomisation into the outreach support group, or usual CST control group. A Mann-Whitney U test was applied to the primary outcome of average number of attendees at seven of 14 weeks (after CST), and 31 weeks after the initial CST programme. All participants were included irrespective of CST experience prior to their research involvement. The average number of attendees was calculated for each centre (total number of sessions run multiplied by the average number of people at each session) assuming an intra-cluster correlation of $p < .05$.

Secondary outcomes

A one-way between-groups analysis of covariance (ANCOVA) was fitted and adjusted for baseline differences to compare the effectiveness of outreach support versus usual CST control. An ANCOVA was considered an appropriate method given there was an experimental and control group with repeated measures (baseline [BL], follow up 1 [FU1], FU2), and this method controls for the variability in pre-test scores (the covariate). Variances in the dependent variables, such as individual differences, were estimated by scores on covariates. By allowing for these adjustments, the covariates can be used as a control variable.

Results

The outreach support options were accessed 21 times, with 25 individual issues raised, mainly through the monthly follow-up telephone calls. These were split across eight categories: group participation, inclusion criteria, practicalities, delivery of the programme, group facilitation, after CST, activity theme, and general queries.

Six questions were raised under 'group participation' including; attendance, group size, and relationships amongst group members. Four questions related to suitability of group members and were grouped as 'inclusion criteria'. Two questions were considered 'group facilitation' as they were regarding staff availability. Four issues were raised in relation to sourcing materials and room availability and so were grouped as 'practicalities related to running groups'. Three queries, including the length and duration of the programme were raised under 'programme delivery'. Two questions regarding activity appropriateness came under 'activity theme', and two questions raised related to what to do after the programme and so were considered under the 'after CST' theme. Finally, there were two general queries about other cognitively stimulating activities and the use of a carer measure.

Information on additional support provided external to the research team was not collected. A series of focus groups was run with staff members who had gone on to deliver the MCST programme to gather general feedback on implementation, perceptions of the intervention, and practical considerations of delivering the programme (Box 6.1).

Perceived benefits of CST included: motivation of the staff member, opportunity to be involved in a group setting, support from other staff members, usability of the training manuals, and flexibility in the delivery of the session. Practical considerations highlighted by the focus groups were: the length of time of the MCST programme, lack of flexibility in introducing new group members, increased level of impairment for the person with dementia, transport difficulties, and outdated resources.

Primary outcome measure

Twenty-nine out of 63 (46%) centres ran the CST programme. Of the 29 centres that delivered the original programme, 20 centres (69%) initiated the MCST programme. A large number of centres did not run the CST programme; thus an independent sample *t*-test was not appropriate as the sample was not normally distributed ($W(69) = 0.817$, $p = < .001$). As an alternative, a Mann-Whitney U test was applied. There was no significant difference in the average number of attendees for the CST programme between the centres that received outreach support ($MD = 3.57$, $n = 38$), and usual CST control group ($MD = 0$, $n = 31$), $U = 571$, $z = -.231$, $p = 0.81$, $r = 0.03$. Similarly, fewer MCST groups were run and this was not normally distributed ($W(69) = 0.650$, $p < .001$). There was no significant difference in the average number of attendees to the MCST programme across outreach support ($MD = 0$, $n = 38$) and usual CST control ($MD = 0$, $n = 31$), $U = 586$, $z = -.043$, $p = 0.97$, $r = 0.05$.

Secondary outcome measures

Staff members' approaches to dementia were not significantly different between the outreach support group and usual CST control group at the primary endpoint at FU2 ($MD = 0.6$, 95% CI [-0.92, 2.13], $p = 0.44$). No significant

Box 6.1 Perceptions and considerations of MCST by staff members

Practical considerations of delivering the programme:

> Getting enough people in the first place to actually commit to that length of time.
>
> (Group 3)
>
> If we hadn't been doing the long programme we could have got other new people in and through the CST programme thus making the waiting list shorter.
>
> (Group 2)
>
> Couple . . . started to obviously be more impaired and it was a little tricky to try and keep the thing running when they were obviously struggling.
>
> (Group 3)
>
> If you can't provide transport for the older person then, unless they've got a really well motivated carer they are not going to get there.
>
> (Group 3)
>
> Outdated resources couldn't really use them . . . we couldn't reproduce those.
>
> (Group 2)

Perceived benefits of CST:

> Staff commitment, you need passion really to do it, you need a quiet room and an uninterrupted space.
>
> (Group 1)
>
> One chap said . . . it's not often you get the chance to be in a group.
>
> (Group 4)
>
> There was enough of us to give each other lots of support and learn as we went along'
>
> (Group 4)
>
> 'What's nice about the programme is that you have that element of structure and it's nice to have that guide of what you're doing.
>
> (Group 2)
>
> We let the group choose whatever they want to do and we just go with it.
>
> (Group 1)

differences were demonstrated across staff members in the outreach support or usual CST control group for job satisfaction (MD = 1.56, 95% CI [-16.62, 19.74], p= 0.87), controllability belief (MD = 0, 95% CI [-1.26, 1.26], p = 0.99), sense of competence (MD = 0.75, 95% CI [-2.59, 1.10], p = 0.43), learning transfer (MD = 1.08, 95% CI [-3.35, 1.19], p = 0.35), barriers to change (MD = 1.11, 95% CI [-6.28, 4.06], p = 0.67), or dementia knowledge (MD = 0.05, 95% CI [-0.62, 0.73], p = 0.88).

Commentary and reflections

Outreach support does not seem to impact on the average number of attendees to either the CST or MCST groups. However, since the study was based on an ITT model and the outreach support options were rarely accessed, there was no particular 'dosage' of outreach support that could be directly compared. It was also not feasible to collect generalised support from external staff members as this was happening on an ad hoc and informal basis and three Trusts had general clinical supervision already set up for their service prior to their study involvement. Consequently, additional support may be beneficial, but it was not possible to definitively determine this due to the naturalistic design of this study. Previous studies have used researchers to lead the delivery of both programmes with trained staff members co-facilitating the groups. Thus, recruiting staff members to deliver the programme, and then evaluating the impact this has on how the programme is run is a useful and necessary step forward in CST research.

The emphasis on the study being in line with phase IV of the MRC framework meant the study was kept as naturalistic as possible to reflect the dissemination and long-term follow up of CST. As a result, both staff with previous experience of CST as well as those staff members 'new' to the therapy were recruited into the study. This may have impacted on the number of times outreach support was accessed, as it might be expected that those familiar with the therapy were less likely to require the additional support. Even though outreach support did not impact on the average number of attendees to the CST or MCST programme, it demonstrated that irrespective of outreach support all groups were run at a 'medium' (3–4 group members) or 'high' (5+ group members) level. This is a positive finding as it supports the ease at which centres can independently implement the programmes in practice without the use of additional support.

There was no difference in staff outcome measures on the implementation of the programmes. Arguably, it is unsurprising that staff measures remained unchanged over the duration of both programmes because the outreach support was rarely accessed, and not all staff members went on to deliver either the CST or MCST programme in their workplace. Yet, the outcome measures allowed us to provide an overview of the demographics of the staff members enrolled in the research study. In retrospect, each staff member could have been required to deliver a certain number of sessions to take part in the study. This would have led to greater control in the delivery of the programmes, but would not have reflected the reality of running groups in practice.

At the time this research was conducted, there had been no studies looking at the impact of outreach support on the delivery of the CST and MCST. Although the findings of this trial indicated outreach support made no difference to delivery and adherence, a localised version of outreach support was investigated as a service evaluation (Streater et al., 2016a). This is reported later in this chapter (see service evaluation of CST in care homes).

Service evaluation of CST in care homes

Staff training in dementia care is inconsistent and varied in care homes (Care Quality Commission [CQC], 2014). To support the delivery of CST as a National Institute for Health and Care Excellence (NICE) recommended psychosocial intervention, it was recognised that staff required training and could potentially benefit from ongoing localised support. North East London Foundation Trust (NELFT) received funding from the London Borough of Redbridge to support the implementation of CST in care homes for people with dementia.

Aim

The service evaluation (Streater et al., 2016a) aimed to: (1) assess the effectiveness of outreach support options offered to staff members, and (2) determine the effects of outreach support on the implementation of CST and MCST in care home settings.

Design

This study was a service evaluation of care home staff in receipt of CST training and outreach support, that included an optional set-up visit, spot visits, and telephone support. Care home staff were required to deliver the CST and MCST programmes over a nine-month period. All staff members completed a questionnaire prior to receiving CST training and at six-month follow up.

Sample

The Redbridge Care Directory 2013 was used to identify care homes that offered care for people with dementia. Care home staff were 'new' to CST with no previous experience of the intervention. No randomisation occurred, and so all care homes were offered the outreach support options. Fourteen care homes enrolled in the service evaluation and 46 staff members completed the baseline assessment. Thirty-one staff members completed the six-month follow up.

Inclusion criteria

The following were required of staff at each participating care home: (1) a minimum of two participating staff members, who were willing to attend a training day, (2) adequate written and spoken English, (3) ability and willingness to complete the questionnaire at two time points, and (4) willingness to complete attendance records after each session.

Consent

Consent was received electronically by each staff member at the baseline assessment time point. Consent was considered an ongoing process and the completion of the questionnaire at both time points was considered an indicator of the participants' agreement to continue in the study.

Assessment procedure

The questionnaire was completed online or in paper format and then entered electronically into Surveymonkey. The measures included: approaches to dementia, dementia knowledge, sense of competence, and learning transfer. The questionnaire was completed prior to attending the training day and at six months. Attendance records were completed after each session.

CST training and outreach support package

The CST training day was delivered by Dr Amy Streater. The outreach support consisted of an optional set-up visit, spot visits, and telephone support. The additional support options were provided by two researchers familiar with the development, evaluation, and delivery of the CST and MCST programmes. Support involved assisting the care home staff to identify suitable residents to participate in the programmes, providing feedback to the staff members, helping with problem solving, and ongoing support.

Analyses

The number of programmes run was recorded, as well as whether CST was delivered to a low, medium, or high level (determined by the number of attendees). This was calculated in the same way as the main trial (see 'Exploring the implementation of CST with outreach support: main trial'). The staff outcome measures were compared using a paired sample *t*-test.

Results

Seven care homes successfully ran the CST programme, three care homes attempted to run the programme, and four care homes were unable to run the CST programme. Four care homes ran the programme twice weekly and three care homes ran the programme once weekly. Five of the seven care homes delivered CST to a 'high' level (Table 6.1). From the seven care homes that ran the CST programme, two care homes ran the full MCST programme, four care homes were part way through, and one care home was unable to run the MCST programme.

Table 6.1 Delivery and level of implementation for CST programme

CST implementation				
Delivery of CST	*Number of programmes*	*CST low*	*CST medium*	*CST high*
Yes n(%)	7(70)*	1(14)	1(14)	5(72)
Partially n(%)	3(30)	2(67)	1(33)	0(0)

(Adapted from Streater et al. 2016a)
*attendance records missing for one centre, entered in table as CST low

A paired sample *t*-test of staff outcome measures showed that there was a significant improvement in approaches to dementia (MD = 2.87, 95% CI [-5.18, -0.56], $p = 0.01$) and sense of competence (MD = 8.8, 95% CI [-11.53, -6.05], $p = 0.00$). Both learning transfer and dementia knowledge improved between baseline and follow up, but were not statistically significant.

Commentary and reflections

The service evaluation was a new approach to looking at the delivery of CST in care home settings. Every staff member enrolled in the study received CST training and could access the outreach support as much as required. This was a proactive form of outreach support as the researcher was in weekly contact with each care home. Arguably, this approach was more successful in comparison to the previously reported RCT of CST implementation and outreach support (see 'Exploring the implementation of CST with outreach support: main trial') as the localised support and more frequent contact allowed the researcher to support the running of the groups and provide feedback after sessions. Anecdotally, care home staff said they appreciated receiving feedback to enable them to improve the running of each session.

Amongst the staff outcome measures, improvements in sense of competence, and approaches to dementia could be attributed to the person-centred approach of CST and the provision of training that otherwise would be difficult to access for a member of staff working in a care home. The frequent contact with the researcher also encouraged proactive thinking and provided positive feedback that may have impacted on the staff members perceived sense of competence in their work role.

A limitation of the study design is the lack of a control group, which meant it was not possible to determine whether the change in staff outcome measures could have occurred over the nine-month timeframe regardless of the CST training and additional support. However, the primary intention of this piece of work was to increase the delivery of CST in Redbridge care homes and so this was not an option.

Exploring the implementation of CST in practice

Aim

This study (Streater et al., 2016b) aimed to evaluate the effectiveness of the programme in practice by gathering cognition and quality of life (QoL) measures with people with dementia prior to, during, and after the CST and MCST programmes.

Design

As an observational study, people with dementia who were in receipt of CST as part of their usual care were recruited into the trial and so no randomisation occurred. Participants were expected to remain in the trial for up to 12 months for there to be enough time to deliver both programmes and collect the outcome measures at baseline, and after the delivery of the CST and MCST programmes.

Sample

Eleven centres across five National Health Service (NHS) trusts, including NELFT, North Staffordshire Combined Healthcare NHS Trust, Nottinghamshire Healthcare NHS Foundation Trust, Kent and Medway NHS Trust, and South Staffordshire and Shropshire Healthcare participated in the observational study. The centres included memory clinics, day hospitals, Community Mental Health Teams (CMHTs), a day centre, and a care home. All people with dementia recruited into the study received CST and MCST as part of their usual care.

Inclusion criteria

All people with dementia met the following criteria: (1) a formal diagnosis of mild to moderate dementia according to the Clinical Dementia Rating (CDR) scale (Hughes et al., 1982), (2) adequate written and spoken English, (3) ability to have a 'meaningful' conversation, (4) good eyesight and hearing, (5) ability to remain in a group for 45 minutes, (6) no physical illness or disability that may impact on their participation, (7) no diagnosed learning disability, and (8) willingness to complete three assessments over the duration of the study. This is in line with previously conducted CST research (Aguirre et al., 2010). At baseline, 89 people with dementia entered the study and 56 people remained at follow up 2.

Consent

The Mental Capacity Act (Department of Health, 2005) was adhered to when people were entered into the study and this continued throughout their participation in the study. As the study included people with mild to moderate dementia, it was expected that each person would be able to give informed consent. The initial agreement to participate in the study was taken as an indication of preference for their future study involvement, but consent was considered an ongoing process and was confirmed at each follow up time point.

Assessment procedure

The interviews were carried out by the researcher, or a staff member trained in Good Clinical Practice (GCP) and in obtaining informed consent. Measures of cognition (Mini-Mental State Examination [MMSE]; Folstein et al., 1975) and QoL (Quality of Life-Alzheimer Disease [QoL-AD]; Logsdon et al., 1999) were collected pre and post-CST and post-MCST.

Analyses

A paired sample *t*-test was carried out on the full dataset. A separate analysis was then carried out to include participants that scored mild to moderate on the MMSE (10–24). This criteria was in line with previously conducted CST research (Spector et al., 2003; Aguirre et al., 2010; Orrell et al., 2014).

Results

The original analysis demonstrated no significant difference in cognition at follow up 1 (MD = 0.37, 95% CI-1.13. 0.39, $p = 0.17$), or follow up 2 (MD = 0.02, 95% CI -0.80, 0.76, $p = 0.48$). Similarly, there was no significant difference in QoL at follow up 1 (MD = 0.88, 95% CI -0.64, 2.40, $p = 0.13$) or follow up 2 (MD = 0.39, 95% CI -2.21, 1.43, $p = 0.34$) (Table 6.2).

Notably, there was a difference in the level of cognition for people with dementia entering the programme compared to previous CST research (Spector et al., 2003, Orrell et al., 2014). When people with dementia that scored over 24 on the MMSE were excluded from the analysis, improvements in cognition were significant after CST at follow up 1 (MD = 0.99, 95% CI -1.92, -0.04, $p = 0.02$), but not at follow up 2 (MD = 0.25, 95% CI -1.28, 0.78, $p = 0.32$). QoL improved over the duration of the programme but there was no statistically significant difference between groups at follow up 1 (MD = 1.39, 95% CI -0.45, 3.23, $p = 0.68$), or follow up 2 (MD = 1.00, 95% CI -3.28, 1.28, $p = 0.19$).

Commentary and reflections

Both CST and MCST are easily delivered group programmes for people with dementia. Although the programmes are now widely used, less is known about the effect of the programmes on people with dementia who receive them as part of usual practice.

It is important to note that the people with dementia with a score of 18–30 were included in this study compared to previous trials of CST which included

Table 6.2 Results of people with dementia outcome measures. Overall analysis and sub-analysis of participants scoring <25 according to the MMSE

Measure	*Follow up time points*	*n*	*Mean (SD)*	*Mean difference (95% CI)*	*Interaction p (1-tailed)*
MMSE	Baseline	67	21.45 (4.70)	−0.37 [-1.13, 0.39]	0.17
	FU1	67	21.82 (4.88)		
	Baseline	56	21.48 (4.94)	−0.02 [-.80, 0.76]	0.48
	FU2	56	21.50 (5.66)		
MMSE (< 25 MMSE)	Baseline	47	19.12 (3.48)	−0.99 [-1.92, -0.04]	0.02
	FU1	47	20.11 (4.56)		
	Baseline	40	19.30 (4.04)	−0.25 [-1.28, 0.78]	0.32
	FU2	40	19.55 (5.34)		
QoL-AD	Baseline	66	36.53 (7.32)	0.88 [-.64, 2.40]	0.13
	FU1	66	35.65 (8.37)		
	Baseline	56	36.34 (7.64)	−0.39 [-2.21, 1.43]	0.34
	FU2	56	36.73 (5.30)		
QoL-AD (< 25 MMSE)	Baseline	46	35.74 (7.54)	1.39 [-0.45, 3.23]	0.68
	FU1	46	34.35 (9.35)		
	Baseline	40	35.25 (7.70)	−1.00 [-3.28, 1.28]	0.19
	FU2	40	36.25 (5.64)		

(Adapted from Streater et al. 2016b)
**FU1 – follow up 1, FU2 – follow up 2*

participants scoring between 10–24 on the MMSE. In this small research study, cognition was statistically significant only when participants met the criteria of mild to moderate dementia according to the MMSE. The broader inclusion criteria should not be ignored as this reflects groups in practice, but it is useful to further determine the benefits for the person with dementia. Currently, there is mixed evidence to support variation in the frequency of delivery specified in the original programmes, with findings of a recent study suggesting that a once week 'dose' of CST is ineffective (Cove et al., 2014). This is an issue warranting further exploration, as when implemented in practice, organisations may alter the frequency of delivery in response to practical and logistical constraints (e.g. staff time, availability of transport to get participants to the group).

The changing face of CST

This chapter provides an overview of the delivery of the CST and MCST programmes in everyday practice across dementia care settings and professions, with the addition of outreach support also evaluated. Both CST and MCST are standardised programmes, but it has become apparent that when implemented in real life practitioners tend to make changes to the programme. For example, delivery frequency, the order of individual sessions, session themes, length of programme, and variation of inclusion criteria of group members. This variation has not before been reflected in a research setting.

Previous research has evaluated the change in frequency delivery of the CST programme (Cove et al., 2014), and this was also demonstrated in the observational study (Streater et al., 2016b). Studies such as these are useful to determine the benefits of the altered programme and have highlighted the need for staff members to be aware of the potential impact that variations to the programme may have on outcomes for the person with dementia. Changes in delivery frequency tend to be attributed to a lack of service provisions, which may be unavoidable. However, adapting the programme in certain ways (e.g. changing the frequency of delivery) may lead to people receiving an intervention that has little benefit for them, or receiving an intervention that lacks similarity to the originally devised CST programme.

The observational study allowed broader inclusion criteria for people with dementia to receive the programmes then previously recommended in CST guidelines (Spector et al., 2003), as people scoring above 24 on the MMSE entered the study. The results showed that the programme does not necessarily significantly benefit the person in relation to the outcome measures used. It can be hypothesised that these findings may reflect a 'ceiling effect' whereby there is little room for individuals with higher cognitive function to improve. A ceiling effect may account for lack of significant improvement when measures which are less sensitive to change are used (Cove et al., 2014). It is important to note that the inclusion criteria is dependent on the measure used to determine suitability for participation (e.g. the MMSE versus the CDR). Considering the level of cognitive impairment of those people entering the programme is important; for instance those people at a higher level of functioning might require the staff member to amend the activities in order to increase the likeliness of the programme being of benefit to them, and to avoid adverse effects, such as boredom. In addition, it is recommended that people entering into a group are at a similar level of cognitive functioning to help the group leader pitch session activities appropriately. Of those services that use a broad inclusion criteria for individuals entering the programme, or change aspects of the programme such as the delivery frequency, it is important to collect outcome measures to provide practice-based evidence to justify these alterations (Cove et al., 2014).

Qualitative feedback was gathered from staff members who partially or fully delivered the MCST programme (Box 6.1). The focus groups identified a variety of issues in the delivery of the programmes. The length of the programme, increased cognitive impairment of service users over the duration of their participation in CST and MCST programmes, and required level of staff commitment to deliver the programmes were identified as key issues. It may be that the MCST programme is only appropriate in particular settings and contexts (e.g. day centre) where the person entering the programme is more able at the beginning, and so less likely to fall outside the initial inclusion criteria during the delivery of the programme. In addition, in a setting such as a memory service the service user turnover is generally high; therefore it may not be possible for this type of service to commit to the lengthier MCST programme.

More generally, the qualitative data and informal feedback indicated that session activities are being replaced for others, some programmes are being offered on a rolling basis, and the format of the programme would have been altered if the centre were not involved in the research study. This may be because the programme is easy to understand and deliver, and so people are inclined to alter the programme and be flexible in their approach to its delivery. This does raise the question as to when CST can no longer be considered CST.

Future research

It is difficult to keep track of the adaptations that are being made to the CST and MCST programmes in practice. Further research is required to focus more on the impact of delivery frequency of the programme. Data could be collected in a variety of ways (e.g. service evaluation) to determine the usefulness of any adaptations made to the programme. This data could be used to build the evidence base to support or discourage adaption. In addition, more studies focusing on proactive support services to aid delivery of the programme. This is likely to be happening in practice with peer and clinical supervision, but this is an under researched area and therefore the potential impact of this is unknown.

References

Aguirre E, Spector A, Hoe J et al. (2010). Maintenance Cognitive Stimulation Therapy (CST) for dementia: A single-blind, multi-centre, randomized controlled trial of Maintenance CST vs. CST for dementia. *Trials, 11*(46).

Aguirre E, Spector A, Streater A et al. (2011). *Making a Difference 2.* UK: Hawker Publications, UK.

Barkham M, Firth-Cozens J, Hardy G, Reynolds S, Shapiro D and Warr P. (1989). *Measures of Work Experience for Stress Reduction Research.* SAPU Memo 1049, Department of Psychology, University of Sheffield.

Care Quality Commission. (2014). *Cracks in the Pathway. People's Experiences of Dementia Care.* Newcastle, UK.

Corrigan P, Kwartarini W and Pramana W. (1992). Staff perceptions of barriers to behaviour therapy at a psychiatric hospital. *Behaviour Modification, 16*(1): 132–144.

Cove J, Jacobi N, Donovan H, Orrell M, Stott J and Spector A. (2014). Effectiveness of weekly Cognitive Stimulation Therapy (CST) for people with dementia and the additional impact of enhancing CST with a carer training programme. *Clinical Interventions in Ageing, 9*: 2143–2150.

Craig P, Dieppe P, MacIntyre S et al. (2008). Developing and evaluating complex interventions: The new medical research council guidance. *British Medical Journal, 337*: a1655.

Dagnan D, Grant F and McDonnell A. (2004). Understanding challenging behaviour in older people: The development of the Controllability Beliefs Scale. *Behavioural and Cognitive Psychotherapy, 32*(4): 501–506.

Department of Health. (2005). *Mental Capacity Act.* London, UK: HMSO.

Folstein M, Folstein S and McHugh P. (1975). 'Mini Mental State': A practical method for grading the cognitive state of patients for the clinician. *Journal of Psychiatric Research, 12*(3): 189–198.

Grol R and Grimshaw J. (2003). From best evidence to best practice: Effective implementation of change in patients' care. *The Lancet, 362*: 1225–1230.

Hodge S and Hailey E. (2015). *Second English National Memory Clinics Audit Report.* Royal College of Psychiatrists, Department of Health, UK.

Holton III E, Bates R and Ruona W. (2000). Development of a generalized learning transfer system inventory. *Human Resource Development Quarterly, 11*(4): 333–360.

Hughes C, Berg L, Danziger W et al. (1982). A new clinical scale for the staging of dementia. *British Journal of Psychiatry, 140*(6): 566–572.

Lintern T and Woods B. (2001). *Approaches to Dementia Questionnaire.* Bangor: University of Wales.

Logsdon RG, Gibbons LE, McCurry SM et al. (1999). Quality of life in Alzheimer's disease: Patient and caregiver reports. *Journal of Mental Health and Aging, 5*(1): 21–32.

Orrell M, Aguirre E, Spector A et al. (2014). Maintenance Cognitive Stimulation Therapy for dementia: Single-blind, multicentre, pragmatic randomised controlled trial. *The British Journal of Psychiatry, 204*(6): 454–461.

Orrell, M., Spector, A., Thorgrimsen, L. and Woods, B. (2005). *A pilot study examining the effectiveness of maintenance Cognitive Stimulation Therapy (MCST) for people with dementia. International journal of geriatric psychiatry,* 20(5), pp. 446–451.

Schepers A, Orrell M, Shanahan N and Spector A. (2012). Sense of Competence in Dementia Care Staff (SCIDS) scale: Development, reliability and validity. *International Psychogeriatrics, 24*(7): 1153–1162.

Shanahan N, Orrell M, Schepers A et al. (2013). The development and evaluation of the DK-20: A knowledge of dementia measure. *International Psychogeriatrics, 25*(11): 1899–1907.

Spector A, Gardner C and Orrell M. (2011). The impact of Cognitive Stimulation Therapy groups on people with dementia: Views from participants, their carers and group facilitators. *Aging and Mental Health,* 1–5.

Spector A, Orrell M and Aguirre A. (2011). Translating research into practice: A pilot study examining the use of Cognitive Simulation Therapy (CST) after a one-day training course. *Non-Pharmacological Therapies in Dementia, 1*(1): 63–72.

Spector A, Thorgrimsen L, Woods B et al. (2003). Efficacy of an evidence-based Cognitive Stimulation Therapy programme for people with dementia: Randomised controlled trial. *The British Journal of Psychiatry, 183*(3): 248–254.

Spector A, Thorgrimsen L, Woods B et al. (2006). *Making a Difference: An Evidence-based Group Programme to Offer Cognitive Stimulation Therapy (CST) to People With Dementia.* UK: Hawker Publications.

Streater A, Aguirre E, Spector A and Orrell M. (2016b). Cognitive Stimulation Therapy (CST) for people with dementia in practice: An observational study. *British Journal of Occupational Therapy.*

Streater A, Spector A, Aguirre E and Orrell M. (2016a). Cognitive stimulation therapy for people with dementia in practice: A service evaluation. *British Journal of Occupational Therapy, 79*(9): 574–580.

Streater A, Spector A, Hoare Z, Aguirre E, Russell I and Orrell M. (2017). Staff training and outreach support for Cognitive Stimulation Therapy (CST) and its implementation in practice: A cluster randomised trial. *International Journal of Geriatric Psychiatry*.

Weiss D, Dawis R, England G and Lofquist L. (1967). Manual for the Minnesota Satisfaction Questionnaire. *Minnesota Studies in Vocational Rehabilitation, XXII.*

Chapter 7

Involving family carers in cognitive stimulation therapy

Jenny Cove

Rationale for including carers in CST

As a long-term and often unpredictable condition, dementia not only imposes a significant impact on the life of the person with dementia, but also on those involved in their care. Caregiving is described by Schulz and Martire (2004, p. 240) as:

> the provision of extraordinary care, exceeding the bounds of what is normative or usual in family relationships. Caregiving typically involves a significant expenditure of time, energy, and money over potentially long periods of time; it involves tasks that may be unpleasant and uncomfortable and are psychologically stressful and physically exhausting.

Informal carers (most frequently family members), defined by Brodaty et al. (2003, p. 657) as 'persons providing unpaid care, at home or in a non-institutional environment', commit time, energy, money, and effort to caring. However, caregiving is associated with higher levels of depression, anxiety, and psychotropic drug use (Alzheimer's Association, 2006), decreased quality of life (QoL), diminished self-efficacy, lower life satisfaction, and poorer health outcomes, such as obesity (Vitaliano et al., 2005) and compromised immune systems (Kiecolt-Glaser et al., 1991). Kasuya et al. (2000) define these negative consequences of caregiving as caregiver burden. Significantly, high levels of caregiver burden can also result in poorer outcomes for people with dementia, including decreased QoL and early admission to institutional settings (Etters et al., 2008).

Given that the effects of dementia on both people with dementia and their carers can be great, and can interact with each other, providing combined interventions may result in improved outcomes for both. The value of designing combined interventions has been recognised by Brodaty et al. (2003). These authors note that a key feature of successful interventions was the involvement of people with dementia alongside their carers in structured programmes. Dröes et al. (2006) point out that given the complex and diverse range of problems experienced by people with dementia and their carers, single interventions simply do not met their needs. Interventions which include both can have a greater impact than interventions which target each alone.

Combined interventions for people with dementia and their carers

A systematic review by Smits et al. (2007) has examined the effects of combined intervention programmes for people with dementia and their carers. Twenty-two interventions in 25 reports published between January 1992 and February 2005 were identified. Outcomes for people with dementia reported in the review were: mental health, cognitive functioning, behavioural problems, physical functioning, delayed admission to long-stay care, and mortality. Depressive symptoms were found to improve in people with dementia following participation in combined interventions and time to admission to long-stay care units was delayed. Evidence for the remaining outcomes was mixed. The authors classified outcomes for carers into three groups" mental health, burden, and competence. Only carer general mental health was found to be significantly improved following combined intervention programmes. Results for carer burden and other areas of mental health were inconclusive, while competence appeared to improve in some carers, but not others. Only 18 of the 22 studies reported outcomes for both people with dementia and their carers, and of these 10 reported at least some positive results for both, suggesting that some types of combined interventions are effective for both people with dementia and their carers. However, no discussion of the types of interventions which may be most effective was included. The authors also pointed out that the review was limited by the lack of sufficient power of many of the included studies, the varying degree of quality of the studies, and the limited number of studies available, although it should be noted that only three databases were searched. Although combined interventions appear to delay time until admission to institutional care and improve aspects of both people with dementia and carer mental health, Smits et al. (2007) were unable to make specific recommendations for the development and implementation of intervention programmes because of the inconclusive nature of the results for the remaining outcomes reported.

An unpublished systematic literature review by Cove and Spector (2013) sought to update the systematic review of Smits et al. (2007). Eighteen studies published between February 2005 and March 2013 which included combined intervention programmes for people with dementia and their carers were identified. The 18 papers were categorised according to the type of intervention offered. These were: psychotherapeutic, psychosocial, support group, rehabilitation, or case management interventions. Functional rehabilitation and case management interventions were found to be most effective, while less conclusive evidence for other categories of interventions was found. In line with the findings of Smits et al.'s review (2007), the authors concluded that there is evidence that combined interventions for people with dementia and their carers can be effective; the mixed outcomes reported and variability in the quality of the studies means that definitive conclusions as to the best types of interventions are limited.

Involving carers in cognitive stimulation interventions

Research has shown that involving carers in cognitive stimulation interventions for the person they care for can have positive benefits for both (Onder et al., 2005; Quayhagen and Quayhagen, 2001). Although not designed to offer direct intervention to carers, these studies aimed to involve carers in the delivery of cognitive stimulation. Benefits for people with dementia included improved memory, problem solving, and verbal fluency, while carers experienced enhanced communication and interaction with the person they care for as well as maintenance of their QoL and psychological well-being.

Standard CST does not include any formal carer involvement. However, qualitative data reveals that carers often feel frustrated at not knowing what happens in CST groups, often because the person they care for cannot recall much from the group (Spector et al., 2011). Involving carers more formally would allow them to develop a greater understanding of CST and may potentially encourage them to apply some of the principles and activities of CST in their day-to-day interactions. This in turn may allow people with dementia to receive a higher 'dose' of CST if carers do use its principles and use CST activities between sessions, which might produce additional benefits for people with dementia in line with previous research.

CST training for carers

As CST does not formally include any carer involvement, and no previous study exploring the impact of including carer involvement in the programme was found, Cove et al. (2014) designed a single-blind randomised controlled trial to evaluate whether including carer training in CST led to benefits above and beyond CST alone. This study specifically reported on the outcomes for people with dementia. It is important to note that this study also sought to evaluate the effectiveness of delivering CST once a week for 14 weeks. Although CST was designed to be delivered twice a week for seven weeks, in practice many National Health Service (NHS) departments in the UK run the programme on a once weekly basis due to time and resource constraints. The authors also sought to evaluate this format of delivery as no previous research had done so. However, the content of the CST programme remained unchanged.

Development of the training programme for carers

The training programme was adapted from the CST training programme and training manual Making a Difference 2, (Aguirre et al., 2011). Adaptations were made based on the specific needs of the study, drawing on the knowledge of the research team. An initial version of session 1 of the training programme was piloted prior to the start of the research with a group of nine carers who had a family member with dementia who had recently attend a CST group. Feedback indicated that carers found the content of the training relevant. However, they thought the background information on dementia and the development of CST was too long and reduced the time they could spend learning about the content of CST sessions and how to apply its principles at home with the person for whom they care. Modifications were made based on the feedback from this pilot. The initial background information was condensed and links to websites providing more detailed information were provided in order to allow greater focus on the latter parts of the presentation. Further adaptations to the timing of the session were made following the delivery of the training at the first research site.

Aims of the carer training programme

The aim of the CST carer training programme was not to train carers to deliver CST, but to provide them with training about the nature and rationale of CST, introduce essential skills around interacting with the person they care for and on implementing activities at home using the guiding principles of CST. The objective was to enhance the interactions between the carer and the person they care for in their home environment in such a way that carers felt empowered and could support the experience of the CST group for the person cared for, which was therefore expected to increase the 'dose' of CST that the person with dementia received.

Effectiveness of a CST programme with carer involvement: main trial

Design

A single-blind, randomised control design was used, with three independent conditions: two treatment conditions and a control condition. In treatment condition one, people with dementia received 14 sessions of weekly CST and their carers received CST training (CST plus carer training). In treatment condition two, people with dementia received 14 sessions of weekly CST and carers received no training (CST only). The control condition was a waiting list group: people with dementia did not receive CST, and their carers did not receive training. Those on the waiting list continued with their usual activities. Although participants in the control group were not asked to withhold from participating in any other interventions while on the waiting list, the research team were not aware of any participant who did participate in another psychological intervention during this time. At the end of the study people with dementia in the control group were offered CST and carers of people with dementia in the CST and control group were offered session 1 of the carer training programme. The trial was single-blind: assessors were blinded to treatment allocation. In an attempt to maximise blindness, participants were reminded not to reveal the group they were in before each assessment. It was not possible to conduct a double-blind trial because, as in any psychosocial trial, participants could not be blind to the condition they were in.

Setting

Data collection took place across three sites within South Essex Partnership Trust (SEPT). At one site CST groups were already routinely offered to people with dementia, and at the other two sites CST groups were set up for the purpose of this study. All CST groups were conducted in community settings with transport available to those who needed it. Carer training sessions were similarly conducted in community settings and care for the person with dementia was provided when necessary to facilitate their attendance. Although the same procedures were followed in each site (see below) the research did not run concurrently across sites, and separate CST groups and carer training sessions were held for participants at each site

Sample

People with dementia were recruited from three Memory Assessment Clinics. All people with dementia who had:; (1) been through one of the Memory Assessment Clinics during the previous two years (or who were on the waiting list for CST), (2) met the inclusion criteria, and (3) had a carer who met the inclusion criteria, were invited to take part in the study along with their carer.

Randomisation

Participants were randomised using the block method (Schulz and Grimes, 2002) to achieve equal group sizes and using Random Allocation Software version 1 (Saghaei, 2004). Randomisation was performed separately for each site to ensure participants did not have to travel further than necessary. Randomisation was conducted by the clinician who would be running the CST groups at a particular site. This clinician then informed participating dyads of their group allocation, arranged a date for the initial assessment, and gave them details of CST group dates and carer training session dates where necessary

Inclusion criteria

The Spector et al. (2003) standardised criteria for the psychological treatment of people with dementia (see Chapter 4) were used with the following additional requirements:

1. Lived in the community (i.e. not in a residential setting);
2. Could engage in group activity for at least 45 minutes;
3. Had a carer who was willing to take part in the study (and met inclusion criteria – see below).

The MMSE cut-off score specified in the original Spector et al. (2003) criteria, was altered from 10 or above to 18–30 for this study, as this fitted with the current inclusion criteria for CST used in the services where data collection took place. Point three was added to account for the inclusion of carers in this study. The research team developed a set of inclusion criteria for carers to ensure that they could participate fully in the research. Carers were considered eligible for participation if they:

1 Had a minimum of three contacts per week with the person they cared for and were able to continue this for the period of the research study;
2 Were aged 18 or above;
3 Could speak English;
4 Did not have major physical illness or disability, which could affect participation.

Recruitment

For each of the three research sites, people with dementia and their carers (dyads) who met inclusion criteria were contacted to discuss the study. Information sheets were sent to those who expressed an interest in participating. Dyads were given time to review this information (on average one week) before being contacted to determine if they wished to participate.

Consent

For those who agreed to participate, written informed consent was obtained, in accordance with the provisions of the Mental Capacity Act (2005), from both people with dementia and carers at the first assessment meeting. The person with dementia's General Practitioner (GP) was informed of their participation in the research.

Assessment

Procedure

All participants were assessed at baseline (the two-week period before the intervention) and at follow-up (the two-week period after the intervention ended). Although participants were offered the choice of meeting with researchers at their home, or at their local memory clinic, all participants elected to complete assessments at home. Wherever possible two researchers visited each dyad to conduct assessments so that assessments with the person and their carer could run concurrently, therefore minimising the time commitment for dyads and ensuring the person with dementia was not alone while their carer completed assessments. Carers were asked to provide demographic details for themselves and for the person they cared for at the first assessment.

Outcome measures

The outcome measures for cognition and QoL which showed sensitivity to change in previous CST research were selected (Spector et al., 2003). In addition, the quality of the relationship between the person with dementia and their carer was assessed. This was not previously assessed in CST trials because they did not include carer input.

1 Cognition: Two outcome measures were used to assess cognition – the Mini-Mental State Examination (MMSE; Folstein et al., 1975) and the Alzheimer's Disease Assessment Scale-Cognition (ADAS-Cog; Rosen et al., 1984). The MMSE is a brief, 30-item test with good reliability and validity, assessing a range of cognitive functions including orientation, registration, attention and calculation, recall, language, repetition and complex commands. People with dementia score 1 point for each correct response up to a total of 30, with a score of 0–10 indicating severe dementia, a score of 11–20 indicating moderate dementia and a score of 21 and above indicating mild dementia (Folstein et al., 1975). The ADAS-Cog is a more comprehensive and extensive measure of cognitive function than the MMSE and one of the most commonly used assessments of cognition in clinical trials with people with dementia. Items cover word recall, naming, commands, constructional praxis, ideational praxis, orientation, word recognition, spoken language, comprehension, word-finding and remembering instructions. Scores range from 0–70 with higher scores indicating greater impairment. The ADAS-Cog has high reliability and validity (Rosen et al., 1984).
2 Quality of Life (QoL): QoL for people with dementia was assessed using the Quality of Life-Alzheimer's Disease scale (QoL-AD; Logsdon et al., 1999). The QoL-AD is a brief, 13-item questionnaire delivered in interview format. Response options, and where needed questions, were displayed for people with dementia to follow. People with dementia rate the quality of different aspects of their life. Questions cover the following domains: physical health, energy, mood, living situation, memory, family, marriage, friends, chores, fun, money, self and life as a whole. People with dementia rate each item on a four-point scale whereby a rating of 1 = poor, 2 = fair, 3 = good and 4 = excellent. Scores are in the range of 13–52, with higher scores indicating better quality of life. The QoL-AD has good internal consistency, validity, and reliability (Thorgrimsen et al., 2003).
3 Quality of the caregiving relationship: The quality of the relationship between the person with dementia and their carer was assessed using the Scale for the Quality of the Current Relationship in Caregiving (QCRC; Spruytte et al., 2002). This scale is a 14-item measure assessing relationship quality, including level of criticism and level of warmth. The scale is delivered in interview format with response options and where needed

questions, displayed for people with dementia to follow. Each item is in the form of a statement e.g. 'I blame my relative for the cause of my problems'; 'I feel very good if I am with my relative'. People with dementia rate the degree to which they agree or disagree which each statement on a five-point scale (totally agree, agree, not sure, disagree, totally disagree). The maximum score is 70 with high scores indicating good relationship quality. Good reliability and validity have been demonstrated (Spruytte et al., 2002).

Intervention

CST

The study followed the standardised CST manual (Spector et al., 2005) used by healthcare professionals to deliver CST to people with dementia. Groups were held weekly for 14 weeks, with sessions lasting approximately 45 minutes in accordance with local service provision.

Overview of the CST carer training programme

Carers allocated to the CST plus carer training conditions were asked to attend two training sessions, with an optional workshop offered between these two sessions. The training was delivered in conjunction with the CST programme. Session 1 was a half-day session (three hours) and was delivered to coincide with people with dementia beginning CST. During this session carers were given an overview of dementia and of the development of, and rationale for CST. The programme was outlined and details of individual sessions were described. DVD clips from CST sessions taken from the Making a Difference 2 manual (Aguirre et al., 2011) were also presented. Following this, each of the 18 guiding principles of CST were described and ways of engaging the person at home according to these principles were suggested. Carers were given a workbook which outlined a selection of activities that related to each theme undertaken in the CST programme, which they could select to try with the person between CST sessions. Space was provided for carers to write down their own ideas for relevant activities and they were also encouraged to share their ideas with the group. The workbook also contained a diary and carers were asked to record any activities tried at home with the person for whom they care, along with ratings of the success of these activities. The workbook and diary were developed by the research team based on previous experience of training programmes. Carers were given a copy of the training presentation and a copy of the Making a Difference 2 manual (Aguirre et al., 2011) to take away.

Session 2 was delivered during the final week of the CST programme and lasted approximately one hour. The focus of this session was on maintenance of skills acquired into the future. A brief presentation was given to remind carers of the basic content of CST sessions and the underlying principles of CST. Time was given for answering questions and addressing concerns, and to share ideas of successful activities used at home. An optional workshop was offered at week seven. This was a one-hour question and answer session to give carers the opportunity to discuss any problems they were experiencing and to receive support if they would like, but was not compulsory.

Analyses

The Statistical Package for Social Sciences (SPSS) version 17 was used to analyse data. Intention-to-treat (ITT) analysis was applied using the last observation carried forward (LOCF) method for data missing at follow-up. Scores on the MMSE were found to be normally distributed. However, for the CST group, baseline scores on the QoL-AD and QCRC showed significant skewness and kurtosis. For the control group, scores on the ADAS-Cog showed significant skewness and kurtosis at both time points. Skewness and kurtosis are measures of data distribution and indicate the extent to which data can be considered normally distributed about the mean. In order to accurately apply statistical analysis data sets should be normally distributed. The significant skewness and kurtosis observed meant that the outcome of statistical analyses could not be considered accurate if these were not addressed first to correct them. Therefore, Z-scores were calculated to check for outliers, and subsequently four scores considered as extreme (a z-score of 3 or above) were replaced with the next highest or lowest score. Removal of these extreme scores rendered all outcome measures normally distributed and this was confirmed by calculations of residual scores and Cook's Distance scores for each measure, all of which were within the accepted level needed to assume normality.

One-way Analysis of Variance (ANOVA) and χ^2tests were used to check for differences in demographic characteristics between participants in three conditions at baseline. Outcome measures were analysed using mixed method Analysis of Covariance (ANCOVA) to evaluate the changes in scores over time and across conditions. Use of ANCOVA allows for variability in baseline characteristics (covariates) to be controlled for. The age and gender of the people with dementia were entered as covariates. Effect sizes were calculated using Partial Eta^2 (η_p^2).

Results

Recruitment and attrition

One hundred and sixty-six dyads were identified as suitable for inclusion. Of these, 122 consented to receive information packs, and of these 72 consented to participate and were randomised into one of the three treatment conditions. Four dyads withdrew from the study before the first assessment, therefore no data was available for these participants and they were not included in the final analyses. Nine dyads withdrew from the study between the first assessment and follow-up. There were no significant differences in the proportion of completers and non-completers across the three conditions $\chi^2(2) = 1.042$, $p = 0.594$. Comparison of baseline characteristics of those who withdrew and those who did not, revealed no significant differences. Baseline characteristics explored were age $t(66) = -0.53$, $p = 0.60$, gender $\chi^2(1) = 0.03$, $p = 0.87$, diagnosis $\chi^2(6) = 4.92$, $p = 0.56$, carer age $t(66) = -1.36$, $p = 0.18$, carer gender $\chi^2(1) = 0.52$, $p = 0.47$ and the scores of people with dementia on the four outcome measures: MMSE $t(66) = 0.73$, $p = 0.47$; ADAS-Cog $t(64) = -1.47$, $p = 0.14$; QoL-AD $t(66) = 0.78$, $p = 0.44$; QCRC $t(65) = -0.29$, $p = 0.77$.

Participant characteristics

A description of the characteristics of people with dementia across the three conditions can be found in Table 7.1. Details of education were not consistently collected, and are therefore not included. Across the whole sample, approximately one-quarter of participants had moderate dementia (26.5%) and three-quarters had mild dementia (73.5%). Two-thirds of participants (67.6%) had a diagnosis of Alzheimer's disease (early onset, late onset, or mixed/atypical). The majority of participants were White British (86.8%) and lived in their own home (92.6%). It was most common for participants to be cared for by their spouse (75%) and the majority of participants had not previously taken part in any intervention related to their dementia (89.7%). Of the seven who had done so, three attended a music for memory group, two attended a Parkinson's disease group, one attended an Alzheimer's Society group, and one participant specified only that they attended a non-therapy group. There were no significant differences across the three conditions in any of the participant characteristics. Seventy-eight percent of people with dementia assigned to receive CST attended more than half of the group sessions. There were no differences in the mean number of sessions attended by participants in the CST plus carer training and the CST conditions

Carer attendance at the training programme

Of the 21 carers in the CST plus carer training condition, 14 (66.7%) attended all sessions (sessions 1, 2, and the optional workshop). Two (9.5%) attended sessions 1 and 2, but not the optional workshop, four (19%) attended session 1 only. In total 20 carers attended the first (and main) training session and one (4.8%) did not attend any sessions. Although carers were asked to record all CST activity they used at home, the majority of carers did not, meaning hardly any data about level of use of CST activities or principles were available.

Table 7.1 Baseline characteristics of participants with dementia

	CST plus carer training	*CST*	*Control*	*F/t/χ² value, p-value*
Age, mean (SD)	75.4 (5.56)	76.8 (6.62)	77.8 (7.47)	F = 0.73 ***p = 0.49***
Gender				χ^2 = 1.71
Male (%)	11 (52.4)	15 (62.5)	10 (43.5)	***p = 0.43***
Female (%)	10 (47.6)	9 (37.5)	13 (56.5)	
Ethnicity				χ^2 = 12.78
White British (%)	17 (81.0)	23 (95.8)	19 (82.6)	***p = 0.12***
White Irish (%)	0 (0)	0 (0)	2 (8.7)	
White Other (%)	2 (9.5)	0 (0)	0 (0)	
Black Caribbean (%)	2 (9.5)	0 (0)	2 (8.7)	
Indian (%)	0 (0)	1 (4.2)	0 (0)	
Living Situation				χ^2 = 5.39
Private Accommodation (%)	20 (95.2)	20 (83.3)	23 (100)	***p = 0.25***
Sheltered Housing (%)	0 (0)	1 (4.2)	0 (0)	
Supported Living (%)	1 (4.8)	3 (12.5)	0 (0)	
Dementia Diagnosis Subtype				χ^2 = 17.12
Alzheimer's disease (early onset) (%)	0 (0)	0 (0)	1 (4.3)	***p = 0.15***
Alzheimer's disease (late onset) (%)	15 (71.4)	11 (47.8)	10 (43.5)	
Alzheimer's disease (atypical/mixed) (%)	1 (4.8)	2 (8.7)	6 (26.1)	
Vascular dementia (%)	0 (0)	3 (13.0)	1 (4.3)	
Sub-cortical Vascular dementia (%)	2 (9.5)	1 (4.3)	2 (8.7)	
Dementia in Parkinson's disease (%)	0 (0)	4 (17.4)	1 (4.3)	
Unspecified dementia (%)	3 (14.3)	2 (8.7)	2 (8.7)	
Dementia Severity				χ^2 = 0.08
Mild (%)	15 (71.4)	18 (75.0)	17 (73.9)	***p = 0.96***
Moderate (%)	6 (28.6)	6 (25.0)	6 (26.1)	
Living with Carer				χ^2 = 1.67
Yes (%)	18 (85.7)	19 (79.2)	19 (82.6)	***p = 0.85***
No (%)	3 (14.3)	5 (20.8)	4 (17.4)	
Relationship to Carer				χ^2 = 7.81
Spouse (%)	17 (81.0)	17 (70.8)	17 (73.9)	***p = 0.45***
Partner (%)	0 (0)	0 (0)	1 (4.3)	
Mother/Father (%)	4 (19.0)	5 (20.8)	4 (17.4)	
Mother/Father-in-law (%)	0 (0)	2 (8.3)	0 (0)	
Aunt/Uncle (%)	0 (0)	0 (0)	1 (4.3)	
Age of Carer, mean (SD)	68.81 (10.39)	67.13 (11.26)	70.43 (11.12)	F = 0.54 ***p = 0.59***
No. of medications, mean (SD)	5.19 (4.14)	3.88 (2.62)	5.70 (4.16)	F = 1.53 ***p = 0.22***
Dementia Medication				χ^2 = 1.67
Yes (%)	10 (47.6)	16 (66.7)	13 (56.5)	***p = 0.43***
No (%)	11 (52.4)	8 (33.3)	10 (43.5)	
Attended previous dementia				χ^2 = 1.01
intervention	1 (4.8)	3 (12.5)	3 (13.0)	***p = 0.60***
Yes (%)	20 (95.2)	21 (87.5)	20 (87.0)	
No (%)				
No. of CST sessions attended, mean (SD)	10.95 (3.64)	10.50 (4.53)	N/A	*t* = 0.37 ***p = 0.72***

Outcomes for people with dementia

There were no significant baseline differences across the three conditions on any of the outcome measures: MMSE, $F(2,67) = 0.16, p = 0.85$; ADAS-Cog, $F(2,65) = 0.05, p = 0.96$; QoL-AD, $F(2,67) = 0.69, p = 0.51$; QCRC, $F(2,66) = 0.22, p = 0.81$. Mean scores at baseline and follow-up for each outcome measure for each condition are displayed in Table 7.2, which also displays between-group effects and effect sizes from the ANCOVA analysis.

There were no changes in cognition as assessed by the MMSE over time, $F(1,63) = 0.81, p = 0.37$ ($\eta_p^2 = 0.01$) and no significant differences between the three groups at follow-up, $F(1,63) = 0.84$, $p = 0.92$ ($\eta_p^2 = 0.003$). Although there was a significant decline in cognition between baseline and follow-up across the whole group as assessed by the ADAS-Cog, $F(1,61) = 4.38$, $p = 0.04$, this effect was very small ($\eta_p^2 = 0.07$) and there were no between-group differences on this measure at follow-up, $F(1,61) = 0.02$, $p = 0.98$ ($\eta_p^2 = 0.001$). There were no between-group differences on any of the 12 subscales of the ADAS-Cog. There were no changes in QoL (QoL-AD) over time, $F(1,61) = 0.003, p = 0.96$ ($\eta_p^2 = 0.0001$) and no differences between the three groups at follow-up, $F(1,63) = 0.82, p = 0.44$ ($\eta_p^2 = 0.03$). Similarly, there were no changes in the QCRC over time, $F(1,62) = 1.68, p = 0.20$ ($\eta_p^2 = 0.03$) and no between-group differences at follow-up, $F(1,62) = 0.97, p = 0.39$ ($\eta_p^2 = 0.03$).

Table 7.2 Mean Scores at baseline and follow-up for each outcome measure

	Baseline			*Follow-Up*			*ANCOVA between-group difference*	η_p^2
	CST plus carer training	*CST*	*Control*	*CST plus carer training*	*CST*	*Control*		
Mini-Mental State Examination	22.33 (3.54)	22.71 (3.76)	22.91 (3.01)	22.19 (4.48)	22.38 (4.75)	22.13 (3.40)	F = 0.84 p = 0.92	0.003
Alzheimer's Disease Assessment scale – Cognition	18.35 (7.1)	18.13 (8.24)	17.68 (6.51)	20.10	19.04	20.09	F = 0.02 p = 0.98	0.001
Quality of Life – Alzheimer's Disease scale	36.43 (6.06)	36.42 (5.44)	34.78 (5.43)	36.45	35.65	35.32	F = 0.82 p = 0.44	0.03
Scale for the Quality of the Current Relationship in Caregiving	57.38 (6.49)	57.09 (6.91)	56.13 (6.53)	57.90	55.65	56.41	F = 0.97 p = 0.39	0.03

Discussion and reflections

The study aimed to determine the effects of enhancing CST with a carer training programme. No improvements in cognition, QoL, or the quality of the caregiving relationship were observed for people with dementia who received CST plus carer training, when compared to the CST only and the no treatment control group. The study also examined the effects of delivering CST on a weekly basis and found no evidence to suggest that this format is effective. No differences in outcomes for people with dementia who received CST (and whose carers did not receive any training) and those in the control group were observed.

Reflecting on the results of the trial

The results of the current study indicate that enhancing CST with a carer training programme does not result in improved outcomes for people with dementia. Involving carers in CST in this way did not have positive outcomes for people with dementia, and therefore services should carefully consider whether such adaptations to the original programme are an effective use of time and resources. However, it is important to consider several other possible explanations of the result observed.

Format of CST

In this study CST was delivered once a week for 14 weeks rather than twice a week for seven weeks. This was because the research also sought to determine the effectiveness of a weekly format. There is strong evidence for the efficacy of twice-weekly CST, and this format is recommended in the NICE guidelines (NICE, 2007). Twice-weekly CST provides a more intensive treatment 'dose' and this may be a necessary ingredient to ensure effective outcomes. Although the structure and content of the once-weekly CST programme was the same as that utilised in the twice-weekly paradigm, simply delivering the same programme with the same session content was not sufficient to achieve change without the intensity of the session delivery. New learning or maintenance of existing capacities may require a more frequent level practice or repetition to be successful than once-weekly CST is able to achieve. It may therefore be the case that the carer training programme did not result in any improved outcomes for people with dementia because the CST they received was not effective.

Validity of the carer training programme

One possibility as to why the carer training programme appears to have been ineffective is that it was not substantial enough and failed to achieve its aims of providing people with dementia with a higher 'dose' of CST. The training programme was developed by the research team and modified based on limited feedback from a small pilot study, and as such may not have been a good enough programme to achieve its aims. The maximum number of hours training received by carers was five, and this may simply not have been enough to ensure any differences occurred in their interactions or activities undertaken with the person for whom they care. No data as to whether the training had successfully changed carers' knowledge or behaviour were collected, so it is not possible to determine whether the training programme was valid.

Changes in carers' interactions with the person for whom they care

A second possibility is that, even if the training programme was a valid and useful one, carers may not have implemented any changes in their interactions with the person for whom they care following the training. Almost no data was available as to the extent to which carers used any of the recommended activities or adapted their interactions according to the CST principles because the majority of carers did not fill in the weekly diary given to them to record such activity. One possibility then is that carers were not using the CST at home and therefore people with dementia in this group did not receive a higher 'dose' of the intervention than those in the CST group as planned. This may explain why involving carers in the intervention appears to have had no more impact for people with dementia than receiving CST alone. Even if carers did interact differently with the person for whom they care having learned about dementia and the key principles of CST, it is possible that the outcome measures chosen were not appropriate to detect the impact of such changes for the person with dementia as the constructs assessed may not have been influenced by changes in carer behaviour.

Participants' level of cognitive functioning

One further explanation for the lack of positive outcomes observed is that people with dementia in the current study were already functioning at their optimum level, particularly in terms of their cognitive abilities. Cognitive functioning, as assessed by the MMSE and the ADAS-Cog, was higher in the present study than in previous trials. Mean MMSE scores in both the study by Spector et al. (2003) and that by Aguirre et al. (2013) were lower (14.4 and 16.7 respectively) than that observed in the current study (22.66). Similarly, on the ADAS-Cog people with dementia in the current study scored, on average, 18.05, compared with 27 and 34.4 in Spector et al. (2003) and Aguirre et al. (2013) respectively. According to the criteria set out by Folstein et al. (1975), using MMSE scores reveals that participants in the two previous studies were on average in the moderate range of dementia, while people with dementia in the current study were, on average, in the mild range. Previous studies may have observed improvements in cognition because people with dementia had already deteriorated to a level at which there was potential for improvement. This conclusion is similar to that of Hall et al. (2013) who observed no change from baseline in cognition as assessed by the MMSE. The average baseline MMSE score in their study was closer to that of the current study, and supports the possibility that initial higher levels of cognitive functioning may not leave scope for any improvements to be achieved. However, it is possible that the impact of CST continues to take effect, particularly for those people with dementia whose carers received CST training, and who could effectively be receiving a longer-term 'dose' of CST. As the current study did not include a long-term follow-up assessment, it is not possible to determine if this may be the case.

Sensitivity of outcome measures

A further possibility is that there were differences between the groups in the current study, which were not adequately assessed. Although Hall et al. (2013) did not observe any improvement in cognition as assessed by the MMSE, they did observe some improvements in cognition on other measures. However, these were more comprehensive, domain-specific measures than either the MMSE or the ADAS-Cog. It could therefore be that ceiling effects on the MMSE and ADAS-Cog were observed in the current study, while more sensitive measures would have allowed differences to be detected. Furthermore, of the two previous studies which have measured QoL only one (Spector et al., 2003) found improvements following CST on the QoL-AD (the measure of QoL used in the current study). Aguirre et al. (2013) found improvements in QoL on the Dementia Quality of Life measure (DEMQOL; Smith et al., 2005), but not on the QoL-AD. The two measures may, the authors argue, be measuring two different aspects of QoL. The current study therefore may not have assessed all aspects of QoL and could have missed improvements due to a limited assessment of this outcome.

Range of outcomes assessed

It is also possible that people with dementia experienced benefits following CST that were not measured in this study. The outcome measures were selected based on those for which Spector et al. (2003) found improvements in their study, meaning that no measures of communication, behaviour, global functioning, mood, or anxiety were included. However, as stated there were differences in participants' cognitive functioning between the current study and that of Spector et al. (2003), and the majority of participants in their study lived in residential settings while all participants in the current study were community-based. It is possible that people with dementia in the current study may have experienced positive outcomes in these domains, or other domains not assessed. For example, the qualitative study by Spector et al. (2011) revealed that people with dementia experienced a range of benefits following CST not assessed in the quantitative studies of Spector et al. (2003), Aguirre et al. (2013) and Hall et al. (2013), including increased confidence and sense of achievement.

Consideration of the quality of the trial

There were several limitations to the current study. Although attempts to ensure that all assessors were blind to participants' group allocation were made, no formal measure of the integrity of the blinding process was included. One way to measure the integrity of blinding is to ask assessors to indicate which group they think a participant is in and how confident they are in this perception. As this was not done, it was not possible to determine the extent to which observer biases were introduced to assessments in the current study.

Secondly, no monitoring of treatment fidelity was undertaken, hence the extent to which CST sessions were implemented as planned and the consistency with which they were implemented is unknown. Adherence checks, for example the completion by facilitators of a checklist to measure adherence to the intervention at the end of each session, would have allowed for an estimation of the level of adherence to the CST programme to be made and thus increase confidence that the intervention received by people with dementia was the intended intervention.

Thirdly, although it was originally planned that the same assessor would complete baseline and follow up assessments for the same participants, in practice this was not possible. This was due to the availability of assessors and the loss of blinding of one assessor in particular, meaning she was unable to complete the majority of follow up assessments. This introduces the possibility that systematic differences in the way assessors delivered assessments may have resulted in biases across participants' pre- and post-assessments. However, given the proven inter-rater reliability of both the MMSE and ADAS-Cog, the difference in assessors is unlikely to have resulted in significant bias in assessment outcomes.

Finally, although the study was powered to detect large effect sizes, the relatively small sample size may have meant it was under-powered to detect smaller effects that exist.

Clinical implications

At present this study does not provide evidence to suggest that enhancing CST with a carer training programme should be recommended in practice. However, given the limitations discussed above and possible explanations for the results achieved, it is suggested that services considering including a carer-training programme as part of their CST service should undertake service-level monitoring of outcomes to: (1) ensure that those who participate are benefiting, (2) provide justification for including a carer training programme, and (3) provide service-level data that can be used to further explore the effectiveness of such a programme.

Future research

The findings of the current study provided no evidence for the effectiveness of enhancing CST with a carer-training programme and were in contrast to those of previous research indicating the effectiveness of CST. However, as the format of the CST in this study was different from that used in previous research, it is recommended that the study be replicated using the traditional twice-weekly CST format in order to determine whether carers can maintain the observed benefits of twice-weekly CST in the longer term. It is also recommended that the current study be replicated using a wider range of outcome measures to capture possible benefits missed by the study, for example mood, communication, and behaviour. At the same time, qualitative studies with people with dementia to explore the impact involving their carers in a carer-training programme, for example the impact on participants' confidence, self-efficacy, sense of achievement, and relationship with their carer, could be considered. This would allow a more subjective exploration of the benefits CST enhanced with carer training.

Further development of the carer-training programme will also be of benefit. The carer-training programme was developed to be a brief, low intensity intervention to see if this would provide an increased 'dose' of CST for people with dementia. As this appears not to have been the case, a more intensive programme may be necessary to achieve the desired effects. The development and evaluation of such a programme should form a focus of future research efforts. The validity of any developed programme should also be explored, for example through the use of measures of carers' knowledge of dementia.

Conclusions

While there is currently no evidence from this study to suggest that enhancing CST with carer training offers additional benefits to people with dementia, this is the first study of its kind, and therefore caution should be exercised when interpreting the results. While services should consider these outcomes carefully alongside consideration of the time and resources taken to run CST carer-training programmes when deciding whether to include such programmes, continued collection of outcome data will allow for ongoing monitoring of the progress of participants to ensure benefits are being achieved, and would also contribute to the further evaluation CST carer training programmes. Further research should evaluate the impact of enhancing the traditional format of twice-weekly CST with a carer-training programme and seek to explore a wider range of outcomes, as well as including a qualitative exploration of the benefits for people with dementia of CST enhanced with a carer-training programme.

References

Aguirre, E., Woods, R.T., Spector, A. and Orrell, M. (2013). *Cognitive stimulation for dementia: a systematic review of the evidence of effectiveness from randomised controlled trials. Ageing research reviews,* 12(1), pp. 253–262.

Aguirre, E., Spector, A., Streater, A., Hoe, J., Woods, B., and Orrell, M. (2011). *Making a Difference 2.* UK: Hawker Publications.

Alzheimer's Association (2006). *National Site.* Retrieved March 20, 2013, from www.alz.org/

Brodaty, H., Green, A., and Koschera, A. (2003). Meta-analysis of psychosocial interventions for caregivers of people with dementia. *American Geriatric Society, 51,* pp. 657–664.

Cove, J., Jacobi, N., Donovan, H., Orrell, M., Stott, J., and Spector, A. (2014). Effectiveness of weekly Cognitive Stimulation Therapy for people with dementia and the additional impact of enhancing Cognitive Stimulation Therapy with a carer training program. *Clinical Interventions in Ageing, 9,* pp. 2143–2150.

Cove, J., and Spector, A. (2013). *The Effectiveness of Combined Interventions for People With Dementia and Their Carers.* Unpublished Clinical Psychology Doctoral Thesis. Clinical, Education and Health Psychology Department, University College London.

Dröes, R., Meiland, F., Schmitz, M., and van Tilburg, W. (2006). Effects of the meeting centre support program on informal carers of people with dementia: Results from a multi-centre study. *Aging and Mental Health, 10,* pp. 112–124.

Etters, L., Goodall, D., and Harrison, B.E. (2008). Caregiver burden among dementia patient caregivers: A review of the literature. *Journal of the American Academy of Nurse Practitioners, 20,* pp. 423–428.

Folstein, M.F., Folstein, S.E., and McHugh, P.R. (1975). Mini-mental state: A practical method for grading the cognitive state of patients for the clinician. *Journal of Psychiatric Research, 12,* pp. 189–198.

Hall, L., Orrell, M., Stott, J., and Spector, A. (2013). Cognitive Stimulation Therapy (CST): Neuropsychological mechanisms of change. *International Psychogeriatrics, 25,* pp. 479–489.

Kasuya, R.T., Polgar-Bailey, P., and Takeuchi, R. (2000). Caregiver burden and burnout: A guide for primary care physicians. *Postgraduate Medicine, 108,* pp. 119–123.

Kiecolt-Glaser, J.K., Dura, J.A., Speicher, C.E., Trask, J., and Glaser, R. (1991). Spousal caregivers of dementia victims: Longitudinal changes in immunity and health. *Psychosomatic Medicine, 53,* pp. 345–362.

Logsdon, R., Gibbons, L.E., McCurry, S.M., and Teri, L. (1999). Quality of life in Alzheimer's disease: Patient and carer reports. *Journal of Mental Health and Aging, 5,* pp. 21–32.

Mental Capacity Act, 2005. London: Stationery Office.

NICE-SCIE. (2007). *Dementia: Supporting People With Dementia and Their Carers in Health and Social Care.* NICE Clinical Guideline 42. London: National Institute for Health and Clinical Excellence.

Onder, G., Zanetti, O., Giacobini, E., Frisoni, G., Bartorelli, L., Carbone, G., Lambertucci, P., Silveri, M., and Bernabei, R. (2005). Reality orientation therapy combined with cholinesterase inhibitors in Alzheimer's disease: Randomised control trial. *British Journal of Psychiatry, 187,* pp. 450–455.

Quayhagen, M., and Quayhagen, M. (2001). Testing of a cognitive stimulation intervention for dementia caregiving dyads. *Neuropsychological Rehabilitation, 11,* pp. 319–332.

Rosen, W.G., Mohs, R.C., and Davis, K.L. (1984). A new rating scale for Alzheimer's disease. *American Journal of Psychiatry, 141,* pp. 1356–1364.

Saghaei, M. (2004). Random allocation software for parallel group randomized trials. *BMC Medical Research Methodology, 4,* p. 26.

Schulz, K., and Grimes, D. (2002). Blinding in randomised trials: Hiding who got what. *Lancet, 359,* pp. 696–700.

Schulz, R., and Martire, L.M. (2004). Family caregiving of persons with dementia: Prevalence, health effects and support strategies. *The American Journal of Geriatric Psychiatry, 12,* pp. 240–249.

Smith, S.C., Lamping, D.L., Banerjee, S., Harwood, R., Foley, B., Smith, P., Cook, J.C., Murray, J., Prince, M., Levin, E., Mann, A., and Knapp, M. (2005). Measurement of health-related quality of life for people with dementia: Development of a new instrument (DEMQOL) and an evaluation of current methodology. *Health Technology Assessment, 9,* pp. 1–112.

Smits, C., de Lange, J., Droes, R.-M., Meiland, F., Vernooij-Dassen, M., and Pot, A.M. (2007). Effects of combined intervention programmes for people with dementia living at home and their caregivers: A systematic review. *International Journal of Geriatric Psychiatry, 22,* pp. 1181–1193.

Spector, A., Gardner, C., and Orrell, M. (2011). The impact of Cognitive Stimulation Therapy groups on people with dementia: Views from participants, their carers and group facilitators. *Ageing and Mental Health, 15,* pp. 945–949.

Spector, A., Thorgrimsen, L., Woods, B., and Orrell, M. (2005). *Our Time: An Evidence-based Programme to Offer Cognitive Stimulation to People With Dementia.* Cedar Falls, IA: Freiberg Press.

Spector, A., Thorgrimsen, L., Woods, B., Royan, L., Davies, S., Butterworth, M., and Orrell, M. (2003). Efficacy of an evidence-based Cognitive Stimulation Therapy programme for people with dementia: Randomised controlled trial. *British Journal of Psychiatry, 183,* pp. 248–254.

Spruytte, N., Van-Audenhove, C., Lammertyn, F., and Storms, G. (2002). The quality of the caregiving relationship in informal care for older adults with dementia and chronic psychiatric patients. *Psychology & Psychotherapy: Theory, Research & Practice, 75,* pp. 295–311.

Thorgrimsen, L., Selwood, A., Spector, A., Royan, L., Lopez, M.M., Woods, B., and Orrell, M. (2003). Whose quality of life is it anyway? The validity and reliability of the Quality of Life – Alzheimer's Disease (QOL-AD) scale. *Alzheimer's Disease and Associated Disorders, 17,* pp. 201–208.

Vitaliano, P.P., Echeverria, D., Yi, J., Phillips, P.E.M., Young, H., and Siegler, I.C. (2005). Psychophysiological mediators of caregiver stress and differential cognitive decline. *Psychology and Aging, 20,* pp. 402–411.

Part III

The CST process

How does it work?

Chapter 8

People's experiences of cognitive stimulation therapy

A qualitative understanding

Phuong Leung

Introduction

A recent review found that carer involvement in psychosocial interventions may enhance mutual understanding, communication, relationship quality, and well-being for both people with dementia and their carers (Moon and Adams, 2013). However, evidence suggests that the inclusion of carers in cognitive training interventions (Zarit, Zarit, and Reever, 1982) and Cognitive Stimulation (CS) (Milders et al., 2013) could be very challenging as some carers experienced increasing depressive symptoms when they participated in the cognitive stimulation intervention alongside their relatives.

A recent systematic review by Leung, Orgeta, and Orrell (2017a) evaluating the effects of carer involvement in cognition-based interventions (CBIs) for people with dementia on carer well-being, used a conceptual framework to explore the effects of carer involvement in the individual CST (iCST) intervention. This conceptual framework consists of the binding ties theory (Townsend and Franks, 1995), the enrichment process theory (Cartwright et al., 1994), and the scaffolding process theory (Cavanaugh et al., 1989). These theories are proposed as mediators of the relationship between carer involvement in CBIs and carer well-being. In dementia care, interpersonal interactions and mutual understanding help carers to adapt to the changing needs of caring for someone with dementia. As a result, this enhances the caregiving relationship (Townsend and Franks, 1995). Studies show that carers who have difficulty adapting to the changes of care demands experience a decline in the caregiving relationship (Yang et al., 2014). Cartwright and colleagues (1994) suggest that the enrichment process provides carers with opportunities to share meaningful and pleasurable activities with people with dementia. However, the enrichment process only occurs within the context of an existing positive relationship, or when carers are motivated to improve the relationship quality. During the trajectory of dementia, cognitive support by the carer can play a vital role in terms of improving cognitive performance and enhancing the competence of people with dementia to accomplish their goals. Thus, it enhances the quality of the caregiving relationship (Cavanaugh et al., 1989). These mediators

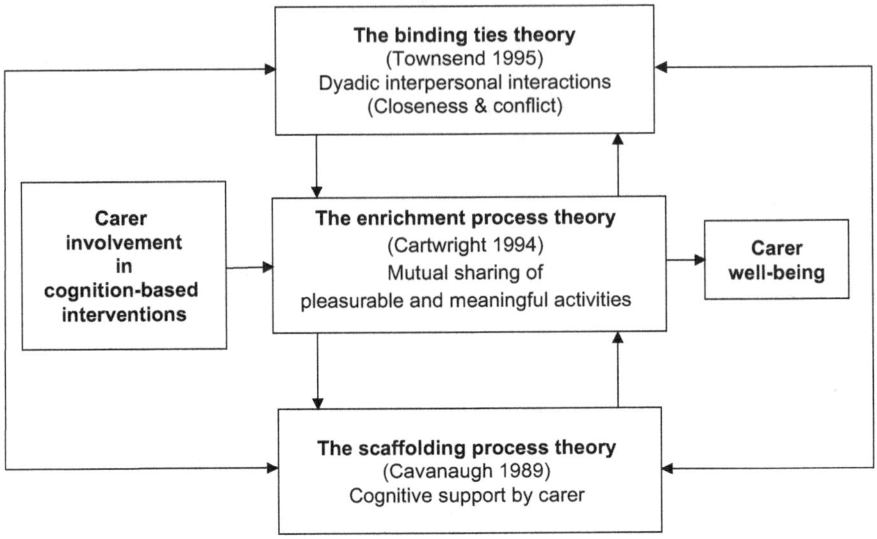

Figure 8.1 A conceptual framework of carer involvement in cognition-based interventions for people with dementia

are interrelated and focus on positive aspects of carer involvement in CBIs (Figure 8.1).

Many RCTs have evaluated the effects of CBIs for people with dementia (Bahar-Fuchs et al., 2013; Woods et al., 2012). However, little is known about the experiences and perspectives of people with dementia and their carers participating in group CST and iCST. The use of qualitative methods in the feasibility of studies prior to RCTs or nested to RCTs is recommended by the Medical Research Council (Craig et al., 2008; O'Cathain et al., 2014)

Furthermore, nesting qualitative methods in the RCTs of complex interventions is increasingly recognised as adding value to research studies, providing opportunities to have a better understanding of the effects of interventions and fully utilising participants' experiences (Lewin et al., 2009). These methods help in understanding the experiences, benefits, and limitations of interventions (das Nair and Lincoln, 2013; Lewin et al., 2009).

Aim

This chapter aims to evaluate the qualitative studies exploring the experiences and perspectives of people with dementia and family carers participating in CST groups and the carer-delivered iCST development phase and iCST trial.

Method

We reviewed three qualitative studies which included CST groups (Spector et al., 2011), the iCST development phase (Yates et al., 2015), and the carer-delivered iCST post-trial (Leung et al., 2017b)

Analysis

A method of thematic analysis was used to code data from each study whereby emerging themes were identified and interpreted within the context of existing literature. The relationship of the data and construct synthesis were explored by using open codes to text, identified themes, and documented supporting evidence in the form of quotes.

Results

Study population

CST groups

A total of 38 participants living in the community were recruited from three existing CST groups running in greater London, of which 17 were people with dementia, and 14 carers (Spector et al., 2011). Seventeen participants with dementia and 14 carers were recruited from three CST groups run by National Health Service (NHS) staff, and one by a charitable organisation. All participants with dementia had Alzheimer's disease (AD), except for one who had Lewy Body dementia. Their mean age was 82 years and a mean MMSE score at baseline assessment was 21, indicating mild dementia. Five were male and 12 were female. In the carer group, 11 were relatives, one was a friend, one a neighbour, and one a paid carer.

iCST development phase and iCST post-trial

Qualitative data was gathered during the iCST development phase and post-trial. In the development phase, 18 people with dementia and 14 carers were consulted in a series of six focus groups. An additional 10 dyads (people with dementia and their carers) took part in interviews (Yates et al., 2015). Post-trial, a subsample of 23 dyads of people with dementia and their carers was selected from 178 dyads randomised to the intervention group (Orgeta et al., 2015). Fourteen carers and 18 people with mild dementia took part in the development phase focus groups, and 10 dyads (carers and people with dementia) took part in interviews. The mean age of participating people with dementia at the development phase was 84.4 years, and 67.8 years for carers. The post-trial qualitative interviews involved 10 dyads recruited from London, four from Manchester, five from Norfolk and Suffolk, and four from Dorset. The mean age of participating people

Table 8.1 Demographic characteristics of people with dementia and family carers

	People with dementian = 22	*Carersn = 23*
	Mean (SD) Mean [%]	*Mean (SD) Mean [%]*
Age	74.7 (6.00)	65.9 (13.68)
Age range	65 to 84	32 to 86
Gender		
Male	16 [73]	4 [17]
Female	6 [27]	19 [83]
Ethnicity		
White British	15 [68]	20 [87]
Other White European	4 [18]	2 [9]
Caribbean	3 [14]	1 [4]
Education		
School leaver (14–17)	12 [55]	10 [43]
School leaver (18 years of age)	4 [18]	2 [9]
Higher education	4 [18]	6 [26]
Further education	2 [9]	5 [22]
Mean MMSE at baseline	22.5 (3.38)	
Mean number of iCST sessions completed	49 (18.38)	
iCST session range	18 to 75	

with dementia was 74.7 years, and the average age of carers was 65.9 years. People with dementia taking part in the qualitative study had a mean MMSE score of 22.5 at baseline assessment, which is indicative of mild dementia (Table 8.1). There were 17 spousal carers, five adult-child carers, and one sibling carer.

Inclusion criteria

CST groups

People with dementia were recruited if they met the Spector et al. (2003) inclusion criteria (see Chapter 4). Carers were considered eligible for inclusion in the study if they had at least once weekly face-to-face contact with the person with dementia for whom they were named as carer.

iCST development phase and iCST post-trial

People with dementia were eligible to participate in the iCST development phase and post-trial interviews if they met the inclusion criteria for iCST specified in Chapter 5. Carers were eligible to participate in the iCST development interviews

(Yates et al., 2015), and post-trial interviews (Orgeta et al., 2015) if they were currently caring for a person with dementia at least three hours per week.

The interventions

People with dementia interviewed about their experience of CST had participated in the group programme (described in Chapters 1 and 4). People with dementia and their carers were consulted during the development phase of iCST study to test if the intervention was feasible and met the needs of people with dementia and their carers (described in Chapter 5).

A subgroup of people with dementia and their carers who participated in the iCST trial were interviewed about their experiences and perspectives of iCST. The iCST intervention consisted of one-to-one structured cognitive stimulation sessions delivered by carers at home (see Chapter 5 for a detailed description of iCST).

Ethical consideration

The CST groups study received the Ethical and Research Governance approval from the Leicestershire, Northamptonshire, and Rutland Research Ethics Committee. The iCST study was approved by the East London 3 Research Ethics Committee. People with dementia and family carers gave written informed consent to participate in both studies.

Data collection

CST group

People with dementia and their carers were consulted in focus groups and individual interviews. The interview schedule included some open questions about the general impact of the group, as well as questions focusing on specific areas (memory, language, mood, communication, functional abilities, and sociability). The same question sets were used for people with dementia and carers except for small adjustments where appropriate. All participants took part in the focus groups as well as the individual interviews. All materials were either video recorded (focus groups) or audio recorded (individual interviews), and were transcribed verbatim. All data were collected within two weeks of the final CST session.

iCST development phase and iCST post-trial interviews

Data collection methods for the development phase focus groups and interviews are described in Chapter 5. The post-trial semi-structured in-depth interviews were fully audio recorded. The iCST manual and activity workbook were used as a visual aid to help the person with dementia and their carer to recall their experiences of doing the activities. Interview topics were derived from the literature of CST (Woods et al., 2012) and interpersonal interactions (Townsend

Table 8.2 Key topic questions

1. Introduction to the topic of mental stimulation
• What is mental stimulation?
• Why mental stimulation is important?
• What types of activities are mentally stimulating?
2. Experiences of taking part in iCST
• How would you describe your experiences of taking part in iCST?
• What did you find helpful in taking part in iCST? What about your relative?
• Have you experienced any changes in everyday life as a result of taking part in iCST? If yes, what has changed for you and your relative?
• Have you experienced any changes in your relationship with your relative? If yes, what has changed for you?
3. Barriers to offering iCST
• What is likely to hinder you in offering iCST to your relative? Any specific factors?
• What is likely to help you succeed in offering iCST to your relative in the future? Any specific factors?

(Both the person with dementia and their carer were asked to respond to key topics 1 and 2. Only the carer was asked to respond to key topic 3)

and Franks, 1995), mutual sharing of pleasurable and meaningful activities (Cartwright et al., 1994), and cognitive support (Cavanaugh et al., 1989). People with dementia and their carers were asked separately to describe their experiences of participating in the iCST intervention. Initially open-ended questions were used followed by questions focusing on specific areas such as mentally stimulating activities, memory, everyday life activities, and relationship quality (Table 8.2).

Data analyses

CST groups, iCST development phase, and iCST post-trial were analysed using framework analysis, which was developed to meet specific information needs and outcomes within a short timescale (Ritchie and Spencer, 1993). It includes five key stages: (1) familiarisation, identifying a thematic framework, (2) indexing, (3) charting, (4) mapping, and (5) interpretation (Ritchie and Spencer, 1993). The interviews were transcribed professionally. Two researchers independently read interview transcripts thoroughly to become familiar with the broad themes. Researchers discussed, compared, and contrasted styles of summarising in the early stages of the analysis process to ensure consistency (Ritchie et al., 1993).

Findings from the thematic analysis

Across the three studies, three main themes were identified: 'concepts of mental stimulation', 'experiencing changes in everyday life', and 'carer adherence to the intervention' alongside 12 sub-themes (Table 8.3).

Table 8.3 Main themes and sub-themes emerged from the interviews

Main themes	*Sub-themes*
Concept of mental stimulation	• Effects of mentally stimulating activities • Types of mentally stimulating activities
Experiencing changes in everyday life	• Opportunities for mental stimulation • Improvement in concentration and alertness • Opportunities to communicate • Enjoyment and pleasant activities • Being active in everyday life • Provided supportive/non-threatening group environment • Brought the carer and person with dementia closer 'together' • Carers' awareness of the 'needs' of the person with dementia
Carer adherence to the intervention	• Barriers to implementing the intervention • Factors to increase the intervention adherence

Theme 1: concepts of mental stimulation

Effects of mentally stimulating activities

Most people with dementia perceived mental stimulation as an activity that provided opportunities to keep 'the brain going', think, and reflect. They also emphasised the importance of being mentally active, using the term 'use it or lose it.'

> It gives an opportunity to think, reflect, review words, and understand them, to reflect on what you want to say and what you're hearing somebody else saying and about the whole situation.
>
> (Person with dementia – iCST post-trial)

People with dementia emphasised the importance of mental stimulation, citing benefits such as keeping up to date with everyday events, increasing sense of well-being, learning, improving the mind, and preventing cognitive deterioration.

> save us going backwards this is an advance on anything that will help us talk and improve our thoughts.
>
> (Person with dementia – iCST development phase focus group)

People with dementia spoke about mentally stimulating activities as a way of occupying their time in a meaningful way, linking being active to the ability to retain a sense of self.

> Can't give you a proper reason but it gives you an activity, doesn't it? There's activity there, and without it you're nothing.
>
> (Person with dementia – iCST development phase)

In the development phase, some carers suggested that mental stimulation provided opportunities to be in the present, link with the past, and take in new information. They also noted several benefits of mentally stimulating activities such as improvements in mood and increasing alertness.

> I mean, we go to the theatre, we come home, not even two minutes after we've left there, she doesn't remember we've ever been, but that buoyant feeling is good.
>
> (Carer – iCST development phase focus group)

Types of mentally stimulating activities

People with dementia and their carers identified a broad range of mentally stimulating activities (Table 8.4). Engaging in conversation and games/puzzles were amongst the most popular suggested activities. Both people with dementia

Table 8.4 Types of mentally stimulating activities

• Art & Craft	Painting, drawing, making masks, or making cards
• Conversation & communication	Talking to others, discussing politics or current affairs
• Cultural interests	Going to the theatre or a concert
• Music	Playing piano, accordion, singing, or listening to music
• Outdoor activities	Social outings, walking, walking a dog, driving, or cycling
• Physical activities	Exercise, bowling, leisure games
• Practical tasks	Shopping, cooking, gardening
• Problem solving	Managing and organising
• Quizzes/games	Word games, board games, crossword, word search, or dominoes
• Reading	Reading books, poems, or newspaper
• Religion	Going to church or praying
• Reminiscing	Sharing meaningful past events
• Social contact	Family, friends, and community (i.e. attending meetings or being involved in voluntary work)

and carers suggested practical tasks and outdoor activities helped them to stay mentally active and enhance their well-being.

> I like making things with my hands, just to keep my mind stimulated.
>
> (Person with dementia – iCST post-trial)

They also described the importance of maintaining a sense of connection to family, friends, and community such as having grandchildren around, or being involved in voluntary work.

Theme 2: experiencing changes in everyday life

Opportunities for mental stimulation

Participants in CST groups reported memory improvements, and half reported either a specific improvement in retaining new information or a non-specific memory improvement.

> Yes remembering the recent events have been a lot more simple and a lot more logical than it was certainly.
>
> (Person with dementia – CST)

One in three carers of participants attending group CST noticed a more general memory improvement.

> she seems to be retaining more information. And she's able, although its sometimes difficult for her to trawl and drag up the information, she seems to want to do it a bit more and she'll store some information.
>
> (Carers – CST)

Seventy percent of people with dementia (n = 16) and 65% of carers (n = 16) reported that iCST provided opportunities for general mental stimulation and described their experience as helping them to 'think better.' Taking part in the iCST intervention also appeared to motivate people with dementia to keep their mind active and look for more information about mental stimulation outside the sessions. Importantly, the sessions helped them to realise that their memory was not completely lost and motivated them to stay mentally active.

> The course has re-stimulated me to think [and] It does sharpen up what you are doing.
>
> (Person with dementia – iCST post-trial)

However, nearly twenty percent of the people with dementia (n = 4) did not find iCST stimulating enough and said the activities were too easy.

> Silly things (the activities) they're asking you, they didn't help me think better.
>
> (Person with dementia – iCST post-trial)

> I didn't gain much from it, because a lot of it wasn't appropriate for my particular stage of difficulty . . . you must have so many people at different stages, with different needs.
>
> (Person with dementia – iCST post-trial)

Improvement in concentration and alertness

Most carers participating in CST groups reported improvement in terms of the person with dementia's concentration and daily life skills, as well as a change in their alertness and brightness. There was also a consensus that participants were engaging in more activities such as personal care, conversations, and watching television.

> Mum had been more engaged with the activities they offer there. . . . She doesn't particularly seem to seek other peoples' company I mean she tolerates people but I know for a fact that she's been enjoying bingo and they had a singer going round singing songs from the old days and apparently mum had a whale of a time.
>
> (Carers – CST)

Carers participating in the iCST study also noticed that participating in mentally stimulation activities might lead to non-specific memory improvements such as feeling alert, and raising 'general awareness of what is happening'. It also motivated people with dementia to maintain or learn new skills in daily life and increased their confidence.

> One time we made the bread, I turned around and he was washing up . . . I noticed that if something has come off, it gives him more confidence, he has a little bit more about him, you know, he is not just shrivelling away, he comes out of himself.
>
> (Carer – iCST post-trial)

A carer showed a photo of the cake which was made by her husband during the iCST cooking session.

> I'm going to show you that (a photo of the cake), he made that, he's never made a cake in his life (iCST cooking session).
>
> (Carer – iCST post-trial)

Most CST participants reported that they were concentrating more and noticed a subsequent improvement in memory. They also felt that the action of talking in the group facilitated remembering.

> Well it always makes a change when you have to concentrate on something it's more helpful for your memory . . . I think it makes you concentrate more in everything you're doing really.
>
> (Person with dementia – CST)

Opportunities to communicate

Most participants said that CST groups provided the opportunity to hear each other's views, which was interesting and helped to broaden their outlook on life. This gave them a sense of achievement.

> I've had feedback about how much she's been involved, what she's given to the group and how much she's talked and participated and chatted with other people and I just think that's brilliant. It is short lived but just for that moment that hour and half or whatever it's been superb you know, knowing that mum's been interested enough to give her views and share her views and listen to other people.
>
> (Carer – CST)

> it was just good to be able to go and discuss the things so you felt that at least you'd done something you know I wasn't wasting my time.
>
> (Person with dementia – CST)

Some participants reflected on the contrast between CST groups and feelings of loneliness and a passive state of mind when at home.

> Well yes you get other people's point of view. If you are by yourself at home all the time you haven't got anyone to discuss anything with. Well its better than stagnating at home saying nothing to anyone all day isn't it.
>
> (Person with dementia – CST)

Participants reported that they enjoyed the conversational aspect of CST groups and felt that they were able to talk more easily in the group environment. Furthermore, a third of carers said their relatives showed improvements in their verbal skills outside the CST groups, more willingness to engage in conversation, and more fluency in conversations.

> She's clearer on the telephone. Clearer I suppose in the way she holds the conversation it's not that she speaks differently it's just that the flow of the conversation is a little easier.
>
> (Carer – CST)

Some carers stated that the person did not talk much about what happened within the sessions, which they described as frustrating.

> He wasn't always able to tell me, he perhaps couldn't usually say exactly what they were doing but you know, just get an idea if someone's been enjoying themselves and had a good time.
>
> (Carer – CST)

Although iCST was delivered in a one-to-one setting, most people with dementia said iCST provided them with opportunities to engage in conversations and discussions, which they would not normally do. Carers also stated that the design and structure of iCST helped them to frame conversations.

> Just opening topics of conversation, maybe listening to her, encouraging her to express herself and talk about things.
>
> (Carer – iCST post-trial)

Enjoyment and pleasant activities

Most carers felt that attending the CST groups made people with dementia feel more positive, relaxed, confident, and that they looked forward to attending sessions every week.

> Well first thing it was fun, because nobody, well it was serious but it was enjoyable, yes it was enjoyable. . . . There was an awful lot of laughing.
>
> (Person with dementia – CST)

> It made me a bit more confident, you know at the beginning I was a bit hesitant to say much, well you just think well if I've got something to say then I'll say.
>
> (Person with dementia – CST)

Eighty-two percent of people with dementia (n = 19) participating in iCST found the sessions were enjoyable. They described the activities as pleasurable, entertaining, and interesting. For some people with dementia, the feelings of enjoyment and achievement were more salient than their memory of specific activities.

> I have felt I have done something when it is time to pack up and put the things away . . I enjoy doing them . . . feel you've accomplished something.
>
> (Person with dementia – iCST post-trial)

> Yeah even though like things might not stay with me, but it's brilliant.
>
> (Person with dementia – iCST post-trial)

iCST provided carers with opportunities to interact with the person with dementia who felt their involvement was not a burden.

> It did give him (the person with dementia) an interest for that little while when we did it . . . It was more fun than a burden.
>
> (Carers – iCST post-trial)

> No not at all a burden. He (the person with dementia) kept saying, will we be doing a session this afternoon because afternoon can be that gap when you can think how am I going to fill in this afternoon. I can read, I love reading.
>
> (Carers – iCST post-trial)

Being active in everyday life

Most people with dementia who took part in CST groups or iCST reported that being involved in the sessions added value to their daily life. For instance they felt encouraged to take up new activities, felt motivated, and that their awareness of 'things around' them increased. For some people with dementia taking part in iCST was an 'obligation', which encouraged them to seek out and engage in other activities such as hobbies they enjoyed in the past, or new events and interests.

> It's made me start thinking about doing what I used to do which was painting . . . I think I could do more painting, and that might make me better, you know, and I can get up and do things more easily.
>
> (Person with dementia – iCST post-trial)

Carers who delivered iCST experienced changes in their everyday life such as having 'more of a focus' or looking for further information related to mentally stimulating activities to do with their relative. Their involvement in the intervention gave them a break from routine care tasks and focused them on mutual sharing of pleasurable and mentally stimulating activities with their relative.

Supportive/non-threatening environment of CST groups

Most participants found group CST was a non-threatening and supportive environment which fostered a sense of togetherness and friendship. Participants were able to support each other and also felt supported by the group facilitators.

> It was like that you could feel yourself becoming close to people, it's a nice feeling. That's what I feel anyway and you never felt threatened.
>
> (Person with dementia – CST)

> Well the first enter everybody is smiling that is main thing. Cause if you see one face, is smiling everybody, no one short.
>
> (Person with dementia – CST)

Attending CST groups also provided people with dementia opportunities to share their experiences.

> Yes the trouble shared is a trouble halved as they say, yes, you think there's other people out there and geographically not far away could be next door, so yeah I think it helped all of us to know that we're on the same boat on the same road, yes that was a very good part of it.
>
> (Person with dementia – CST)

Bringing the carer and person with dementia 'together'

Many people with dementia felt that iCST activities brought them closer with their carers. Taking part in iCST activities enabled them to 'do things together' and to see 'another side of [the] carer' such as 'being very patient.' Carers also found doing iCST together with their relative provided them with opportunities to engage in enjoyable mentally stimulating activities and enhanced the quality of their relationship.

> It's keeping the relationship going and although I can see that there can be changes in the relationship, doing this kind of activities together cements it and makes you stay involved in each other's lives.
>
> (Carer – iCST post-trial)

Carers awareness of the needs of the person with dementia

Engaging in iCST provided carers with opportunities to interact with the person and gain a better understanding of their cognitive needs. Interactive cognitive support enabled carers to be aware of situations people with dementia might encounter in everyday life.

> but the main changes were in how I was probably relating to her and thinking about how she would understand things, and how that could be in everyday situations . . . The change is probably more about me that I noticed about her.
>
> (Carer – iCST post-trial)

Theme 3: carer adherence to the intervention

Barriers to implementing the intervention

During the development phase of iCST, most carers agreed that completing three sessions a week would be feasible, but perhaps not always possible depending on factors such as motivation (both the carer and person with dementia), mood, or needing to prioritise other tasks.

> I can imagine saying to him 'come on we'll have a game of skittles' and he'd say 'oh I don't feel up to it at the moment'. There's all those factors to consider really so then, by the time you come to do it on that day, something else has gone on and it hasn't happened. So I think the flexibility here is important.
>
> (Carer – iCST development phase focus group)

Carers delivering iCST in the main trial reported that it was difficult to fit in the activities because of time constraints such as having in a full-time/part-time paid job, role strain, or other family commitments.

> We might have had a problem with identifying the time to sit down and organise ourselves.
>
> (Carer – iCST post-trial)

Some carers found it difficult to be positive as they perceived dementia as a progressive condition.

> It is so easy to be negative and very difficult to be positive because you know when you are working with somebody, he isn't going to get better.
>
> (Carer – iCST post-trial)

Physical health problems or decreased emotional well-being also affected engagement for people with dementia.

> Only the period when he was reluctant and I suppose that was also tied to him having an emotional response to his condition.
>
> (Carer – iCST post-trial)

A few carers found their approach and communication skills in delivering the sessions could hinder engagement with the person with dementia.

> That is a bit of a disadvantage in a way because I have started off this and for goodness sake take your teachers voice I was thinking off because I was teaching him like a little boy in school.
>
> (Carer – iCST post-trial)

In terms of support carers received to deliver iCST and its impact on adherence, carers found the purpose of the intervention was insufficiently explained.

> Maybe there could have been a little bit more explanation behind how to and what the purpose of this.
>
> (Carer – iCST post-trial)

Factors to increase the intervention adherence

Carers suggested having more help to deliver the intervention from other people would improve adherence.

> Involvement with other people it would be a great aid.
>
> (Carer – iCST post-trial)

Peer support was also seen as an extra source of support.

> Another way of looking at it I suppose is there anyone else in the district who is doing the same thing.
>
> (Carer – iCST post-trial)

Some carers emphasised that it was essential to prioritise their daily tasks to fit in the iCST intervention.

> Having to fit it in and knowing that we were going to do it that day . . . that is a key thing that the carer needs to be aware of their input to stimulate the person is really crucial.
>
> (Carer – iCST post-trial)

Discussion

This chapter aimed to evaluate three qualitative studies exploring the experiences and perspectives of people with dementia and their family carers participating in CST groups, the iCST development phase, and iCST post-trial. The findings suggest that CST groups and the carer-delivered iCST intervention may benefit people with dementia and their carers' lives in a variety of ways. Participants could relate to the concept of mental stimulation and identified a range of mentally stimulating activities. Their appraisal that mental stimulation was meaningful appeared to help them to be motivated and stay mentally active. Although CST and iCST aim to improve cognition and QoL in people with dementia, the interventions are delivered in different settings. In the study by Spector et al. (2011), CST was delivered in a group setting and facilitated by trained staff, while in the studies by Yates et al. (2015) and Leung et al. (2017b), iCST was delivered on a one-to-one basis at home by family carers. Nevertheless, the findings show that both attending CST groups and participating in iCST sessions provided people with opportunities to engage in general and intellectual stimulating activities which they felt helped them to 'think better'. These results are supported by previous studies (Onder et al., 2005; Spector et al., 2003).

Dementia is a chronic neurodegenerative brain disease that causes a decline in memory, communication, loss of independence, and withdrawal from social activities (Alzheimer's Association, 2015). CST groups provided a social environment which may help people with dementia to enhance their abilities to communicate and improve their sense of competence. The most commonly reported cognitive changes were an improvement in concentration and alertness. Participating in CST groups and iCST enabled people with dementia to be more alert and focus in their everyday conversations. This finding is consistent with a previous studies by Brataas et al. (2010). People with dementia taking part in CST groups reported that they were more attentive to the surrounding environment which helped them to engage in activities. People with dementia and their carers felt that iCST provided a direction that motivated them to seek for new information and mentally stimulating activities such as looking for resources to enhance their current activities. Some people with dementia revisited past hobbies such as painting, or participated in daily activities (e.g. preparing or cooking meals). Staying 'alert' and having 'a focus' may have been seen by people with dementia as an opportunity to maintain daily skills and generally remain 'engaged' in everyday activities.

People with dementia and family carers valued CST and iCST sessions as a tool which enabled them to initiate conversations and provided a framework for communication. Taking part in group CST and iCST appeared to strengthen interpersonal communication skills, which may be owing to the key principles of CST (Spector et al., 2003). People participating in group CST reported a feeling of not being alone through sharing common difficulties and finding it easier to hold conversations both within and outside of the group. This finding suggests that having the opportunity to take part in pleasurable and mentally stimulating activities in a supportive, non-threatening environment as part of CST may have a positive impact on confidence.

Most people with dementia and family carers found that CST groups and iCST offered opportunities to be involved in enjoyable and pleasant activities, revisiting, or focusing on new interests and hobbies. This finding provides further evidence of the importance of taking part in enjoyable activities so that people with dementia remain engaged (Cartwright et al., 1994; Hellström et al., 2007). The results are consistent with the enrichment process theory that even though people with dementia might not remember details of the activities, they were able to reflect on 'feelings of enjoyment' and 'feeling good' (Cartwright et al., 1994; Nygard, 2006). People with dementia felt motivated by taking part in group CST and iCST interventions as they realised that their memory was not completely lost (Moebs et al., 2015; Thomas and Velthouse, 1990). Indeed, participants wanted to 'fight back' as much as they could by remaining mentally active (Clare, 2002; Genoe and Dupuis, 2014). Furthermore, most participants felt that taking part in CST groups made them feel more positive, relaxed and confident; they looked forward to attending the group every week.

Engaging in the iCST intervention helped carers to have a break from routine care tasks and build a rapport with their relative (Roland and Chappell, 2015). iCST provided opportunities for people with dementia and their carers to 'become closer' and further strengthen their caregiving relationship. This finding is consistent with the quantitative result of the RCT that participating in iCST enhances the quality of the caregiving relationship from the person with dementia's perspective (Orgeta et al., 2015).

Participating in iCST sessions provided people with dementia with opportunities to share pleasurable and mentally stimulating activities with their carers and experience a sense of self-worth. The post-trial qualitative interviews showed that iCST gave carers a chance to interact with their relative which raised their awareness of dementia as a disease. Some carers found that iCST enabled them to gain a better understanding of the cognitive needs of their relative in everyday life, which is consistent with scaffolding theory that cognitive support helps carers to be sensitive to the cognitive needs of the person with dementia (Cavanaugh et al., 1989). Furthermore, cognitive support by carers can help people with dementia to stay mentally active, improve the relationship quality (Fauth et al., 2012; Genoe and Dupuis, 2014; Phinney, 2006; Townsend and Franks, 1995), and enhance carer well-being (Moon and Adams, 2013).

Carers delivering iCST identified several barriers to implementing the intervention. They found it hard to fit iCST into a busy schedule (Yates et al., 2015). This might relate to them having little time or energy for pleasurable activities (Adams, 2008; Campbell et al., 2008). Carers found engaging people with dementia in iCST could be particularly challenging because of the progressive nature of the illness. Poor physical health or decreased emotional well-being was considered as a barrier to people with dementia participating in mentally stimulating activities (Choi and Twamley, 2013). Some carers did not feel skilled enough to deliver the intervention which could impact on the intervention adherence (Chee et al., 2007). Carers suggested that having extra support by involving other people in delivering the intervention and prioritising their daily tasks would help to reduce role strain (Lopez-Hartmann et al., 2012) which might improve adherence to the intervention.

Limitations

The qualitative study of CST identified several limitations. Firstly, participants typically reported the general benefits of attending rather than specific benefits of CST activities. Therefore, the findings did not provide any insight into whether people thought that some activities were more beneficial than others. There can be inherent difficulties with asking people with memory problems to remember their experiences in detail. There was also considerable variation in the amount of contact between carers and group participants, which may have impacted on the knowledge about the extent to which any improvements generalised to everyday life.

The iCST qualitative post-trial interviews may have been susceptible to bias as most participants who were interviewed had done well with the intervention.

By not approaching dyads who did not complete any sessions or reported poor compliance (i.e. 10 sessions or less) (Prick et al., 2014), the external validity of the study could have been affected. Furthermore, the data may have been affected by social desirability bias as participants tended to have positive perceptions of the intervention.

The qualitative findings indicated that although most people with dementia and carers enjoyed the sessions, others were less satisfied as they found the iCST sessions were not challenging enough. This was particularly the case for those with mild dementia. Future research should investigate issues of suitability of cognitive stimulation interventions and the importance of matching activities to personal preferences and level of stimulation.

Conclusion

Despite the cognitive difficulties people with dementia typically experience, these studies have shown that their experiences and perspectives can contribute towards establishing a credible framework for understanding group and individual processes in CST to support quantitative findings (Spector et al., 2003, 2010; Orgeta et al., 2015).

Qualitative data helps to explain exactly how CST delivered in a group setting, and individually at home, can be effective in improving cognition and communication. From a clinical perspective, group CST and iCST may be a useful tool to help people with dementia and their carers to communicate. The findings also support a conceptual framework of carer involvement in CBIs for people with dementia where interpersonal interactions, mutual sharing of pleasurable and mentally stimulating activities, and carer's cognitive support mechanisms are conceptualised as mediators of carer well-being.

References

Adams, K. B. (2008). Specific effects of caring for a spouse with dementia: differences in depressive symptoms between caregiver and non-caregiver spouses. *International Psychogeriatrics*, *20*(3), 508–520.

Alzheimer's Association. (2015). 2015 Alzheimer's disease facts and figures. *Alzheimers Dement*, *11*(3), 332–384.

Bahar-Fuchs, A., Clare, L., and Woods, B. (2013). Cognitive training and cognitive rehabilitation for mild to moderate Alzheimer's disease and vascular dementia. *Cochrane Database of Systematic Reviews*, *6*, CD003260.

Brataas, H. V., Bjugan, H., Wille, T., and Hellzen, O. (2010). Experiences of day care and collaboration among people with mild dementia. *Journal of Clinical Nursing*, *19*(19–20), 2839–2848.

Campbell, P., Wright, J., Oyebode, J., Job, D., Crome, P., Bentham, P., and Lendon, C. (2008). Determinants of burden in those who care for someone with dementia. *International Journal of Geriatric Psychiatry*, *23*(10), 1078–1085.

Cartwright, J. C., Archbold, P. G., Stewart, B. J., and Limandri, B. (1994). Enrichment processes in family caregiving to frail elders. *ANS Advances in Nursing Science, 17*(1), 31–43.

Cavanaugh, J. C., Dunn, N. J., Mowery, D., Feller, C., Niederehe, G., Fruge, E., and Volpendesta, D. (1989). Problem-solving strategies in dementia patient-caregiver dyads. *Gerontologist, 29*(2), 156–158.

Chee, Y. K., Gitlin, L. N., Dennis, M. P., and Hauck, W. W. (2007). Predictors of adherence to a skill-building intervention in dementia caregivers. *Journals of Gerontology Series A – Biological Sciences and Medical Sciences, 62*(6), 673–678.

Choi, J., and Twamley, E. W. (2013). Cognitive rehabilitation therapies for Alzheimer's disease: a review of methods to improve treatment engagement and self-efficacy. *Neuropsychology Review, 23*(1), 48–62.

Clare, L. (2002). We'll fight it as long as we can: coping with the onset of Alzheimer's disease. *Aging and Mental Health, 6*(2), 139–148.

Craig, P., Dieppe, P., Macintyre, S., Michie, S., Nazareth, I., and Petticrew, M. (2008). Developing and evaluating complex interventions: the new Medical Research Council guidance. *BMJ, 337*, a1655. doi:10.1136/bmj.a1655

das Nair, R., and Lincoln, N. B. (2013). The effectiveness of memory rehabilitation following neurological disabilities: a qualitative inquiry of patient perspectives. *Neuropsychological Rehabilitation, 23*(4), 528–545.

Fauth, E., Hess, K., Piercy, K., Norton, M., Corcoran, C., Rabins, P., and Tschanz, J. (2012). Caregivers' relationship closeness with the person with dementia predicts both positive and negative outcomes for caregivers' physical health and psychological well-being. *Aging & Mental Health, 16*(6), 699–711.

Genoe, M. R., and Dupuis, S. L. (2014). The role of leisure within the dementia context. *Dementia* (London), *13*(1), 33–58.

Hellström, I., Nolan, M., and Lundh, U. (2007). Sustaining couplehood 'Spouses' strategies for living positively with dementia. *Dementia, 6*(3), 383–409.

Leung, P., Orgeta, V., and Orrell, M. (2017a). The effects on carer well-being of carer involvement in cognition-based interventions for people with dementia: a systematic review and meta-analysis. *International Journal of Geriatric Psychiatry*. doi:10.1002/gps.4654

Leung, P., Yates, L., Orgeta, V., Hamidi, F., and Orrell, M. (2017b). The experiences of people with dementia and their carers participating in individual Cognitive Stimulation Therapy. *International Journal of Geriatric Psychiatry*.

Lewin, S., Glenton, C., and Oxman, A. D. (2009). Use of qualitative methods alongside randomised controlled trials of complex healthcare interventions: methodological study. *BMJ, 339*, b3496.

Lopez-Hartmann, M., Wens, J., Verhoeven, V., and Remmen, R. (2012). The effect of caregiver support interventions for informal caregivers of community-dwelling frail elderly: a systematic review. *International Journal of Integrated Care, 12*, e133.

Marshall, M. N. (1996). Sampling for qualitative research. *Family Practice, 13*(6), 522–526.

Milders, M., Bell, S., Lorimer, A., MacEwan, T., and McBain, A. (2013). Cognitive stimulation by caregivers for people with dementia. *Geriatric Nursing, 34*(4), 267–273.

Moebs, I., Gee, S., Miyahara, M., Paton, H., and Croucher, M. (2015). Perceptions of a cognitive rehabilitation group by older people living with cognitive impairment and their caregivers: a qualitative interview study. *Dementia (London)*. doi:10.1177/1471301215609738

Moon, H., and Adams, K. B. (2013). The effectiveness of dyadic interventions for people with dementia and their caregivers. *Dementia* (London), *12*(6), 821–839.

Nygard, L. (2006). How can we get access to the experiences of people with dementia? Suggestions and reflections. *Scandinavian Journal of Occupational Therapy, 13*(2), 101–112.

O'Cathain, A., Goode, J., Drabble, S. J., Thomas, K. J., Rudolph, A., and Hewison, J. (2014). Getting added value from using qualitative research with randomized controlled trials: a qualitative interview study. *Trials, 15*, 215. doi:10.1186/1745-6215-15-215

Onder, G., Zanetti, O., Giacobini, E., Frisoni, G. B., Bartorelli, L., Carbone, G., Bernabei, R. (2005). Reality orientation therapy combined with cholinesterase inhibitors in Alzheimer's disease: randomised controlled trial. *British Journal of Psychiatry, 187*, 450–455.

Orgeta, V., Leung, P., Yates, L., Kang, S., Hoare, Z., Henderson, C., and Orrell, M. (2015). Individual Cognitive Stimulation Therapy for dementia: a clinical effectiveness and cost-effectiveness pragmatic, multicentre, randomised controlled trial. *Health Technology Assessment, 19*(64), 1–108.

Phinney, A. (2006). Family strategies for supporting involvement in meaningful activity by persons with dementia. *Journal of Family Nursing, 12*(1), 80–101.

Prick, A.-E., de lange, J., Van't Leven, N., and Pot, A. M. (2014). Process evaluation of a multicomponent dyadic intervention study with exercise and support for people with dementia and their family caregivers. *Trials, 15*. doi:10.1186/1745-6215-15-401

Ritchie, J., and Spencer, L. (1993). Qualitative data analysis for applied policy research. In *Analysing Qualitative Data*, edited by A. Bryman and R. Burgess. London: Routledge, 173–194.

Roland, K. P., and Chappell, N. L. (2015). Meaningful activity for persons with dementia: family caregiver perspectives. *American Journal of Alzheimer's Disease and other Dementias, 30*(6), 559–568.

Spector, A., Gardner, C., and Orrell, M. (2011). The impact of Cognitive Stimulation Therapy groups on people with dementia: views from participants, their carers and group facilitators. *Aging & Mental Health, 15*(8), 945–949.

Spector, A., and Orrell, M. (2010). Using a biopsychosocial model of dementia as a tool to guide clinical practice. *International Psychogeriatrics, 22*(6), 957–965. doi:10.1017/s1041610210000840

Spector, A., Thorgrimsen, L., Woods, B., Royan, L., Davies, S., Butterworth, M., and Orrell, M. (2003). Efficacy of an evidence-based Cognitive Stimulation Therapy programme for people with dementia – Randomised controlled trial. *British Journal of Psychiatry, 183*, 248–254.

Thomas, K. W., and Velthouse, B. A. (1990). Cognitive elements of empowerment: an 'interpretive' model of intrinsic task motivation. *Academy of Management Review, 15*(4), 666–681.

Townsend, A. L., and Franks, M. M. (1995). Binding ties: closeness and conflict in adult children's caregiving relationships. *Psychology and Aging, 10*(3), 343–351.

Woods, B., Aguirre, E., Spector, A. E., and Orrell, M. (2012). Cognitive stimulation to improve cognitive functioning in people with dementia. *Cochrane Database of Systematic Reviews, 2*, CD005562.

Yang, C. T., Liu, H. Y., and Shyu, Y. I. L. (2014). Dyadic relational resources and role strain in family caregivers of persons living with dementia at home: a cross-sectional survey. *International Journal of Nursing Studies, 51*(4), 593–602.

Yates, L. A., Leung, P., Orgeta, V., Spector, A., and Orrell, M. (2015). The development of Individual Cognitive Stimulation Therapy (iCST) for dementia. *Clinical Interventions in Aging, 10*, 95–104.

Zarit, S. H., Zarit, J. M., and Reever, K. E. (1982). Memory training for severe memory loss: effects on senile dementia patients and their families. *Gerontologist, 22*(4), 37.

Chapter 9

Neuropsychological aspects of cognitive stimulation therapy

Bridget T.Y. Liu, Antony C.L. Au, and Gloria H.Y. Wong

Introduction

The efficacy of CST in enhancing cognition in people with mild-to-moderate Alzheimer's disease (AD) is established (Woods et al., 2012). Its exact mechanisms of action at cognitive and neurobiological levels are to be determined. To date, only a handful of studies have tried to explore the mechanisms of change at the neuropsychological level. Knowledge of how non-pharmacological interventions lead to changes will facilitate further improvement in design (Craig et al., 2008), with potential implications on participant selection, such as the best time window or disease stages to intervene.

CST involves engaging the person in enjoyable cognitive activities that do not primarily consist of practice of specific cognitive domains. It was developed based on the observed cognitive benefits in reality orientation, with an additional social element (Spector et al., 2010) (see Chapter 4). These characteristics of CST converge with the theoretical framework of a general cognitive reserve, neuroplasticity, and recent development in understanding brain functioning from a large-scale brain network perspective. This chapter outlines briefly the current theories and evidence that contribute to a neuropsychological understanding of CST, with exploratory results from an MRI study testing this neuropsychological framework in a group of Hong Kong Chinese people with mild dementia.

Theoretical background

Concepts of reserve and neuroplasticity

The pathogenesis of AD is recognised as a process involving an amyloid cascade that leads ultimately to neuronal death (for a concise review, see Ballard et al., 2011). Structural brain pathology, however, does not fully account for the variability in clinical manifestation and cognitive performance (Stern, 2002). The discrepancy invokes the concept of reserve, which involves both passive and active models, and provides a perspective for understanding the possible mechanisms of non-pharmacological interventions that target cognitive functioning.

Reserve can be classified into cognitive reserve and brain reserve, which are viewed as parallel mechanisms for coping with brain damage (Stern, 2002). It can also be considered as a passive or active coping process. The passive process of brain reserve mainly involves a larger reserve to start with, so that the person can sustain greater damage before cognitive impairment manifest, such as having a larger number of neurons, synapses, or redundant neural networks. In the active process of cognitive reserve, people who process tasks more efficiently can cope better with brain damage, by having a more efficient cognitive paradigm, or by recruiting compensatory strategies (Stern, 2012). By using proxy measurements of cognitive reserve (intelligence, occupation, and education), a systematic review of 22 studies that followed 29,000 people over 7.1 years found a lower risk of dementia (odds ratio [OR] = 0.54). The study also noted complex mental activity in late life as an independent predictor of a lower dementia risk (Valenzuela and Sachdev, 2006).

At the physiological level, cognitive reserve is presumed to manifest in synaptic organisation or the use of brain networks, the latter may include more efficient recruitment of the same network, or ability to recruit alternate networks (Stern, 2002). A related concept here is neuroplasticity, which refers to the ability of our nervous system to modify its organisation in response to environmental pressure, physiological changes, and experience (Pascual-Leone et al., 2005). It can be observed functionally in the changes of activation pattern of different brain regions, and structurally in neuronal and synaptic changes (Ganguly and Poo, 2013).

Neuroplasticity is the mechanism for development and learning (Pascual-Leone et al., 2005). Connectivity of brain networks, in particular topologically complex or globally distributed brain networks, undergo reconfiguration during learning (Bassett et al., 2011). As behaviourally relevant experience may reshape connectivity (activity-dependent plasticity) (Ganguly and Poo, 2013), we can postulate how non-pharmacological interventions that focus on strengthening established connections (e.g. recall of episodic memory in reminiscence therapy) have different effects on neuroplasticity or cognitive reserve compared with strategies that emphasise learning and novel experience (e.g. cognitive training, cognitive stimulation, and cognitive rehabilitation).

Brain network connectivity in Alzheimer's disease

Among the many large-scale brain networks that have been identified, the default mode network (DMN) and central executive network (CEN) are particularly implicated in mild cognitive impairment and AD (Bullmore and Sporns, 2012), which also represent brain regions first affected by amyloid deposition and grey-matter atrophy in AD (Buckner et al., 2005; Buckner et al., 2008). Anomalies in these networks are thought to be responsible for the disruption of general cognition and memory (Bullmore and Sporns, 2012).

The DMN is a long-distance, inter-modular network anchored in the (1) anterior cingulate cortex (ACC) and medial prefrontal cortex (MPFC); (2) posterior cingulate cortex (PCC), the precuneus, and retrosplenial cortex; and (3) bilateral parietal lobule (Raichle et al., 2001). Several other areas have also been suggested, such as the hippocampal formation and medial temporal cortex (Buckner et al., 2008). The DMN is most active during restful waking and supressed during attention-demanding cognitive tasks (Raichle et al., 2001; Greicius et al., 2003). Two main hypotheses of the function of this network are: the (1) internal mentation hypothesis, which postulates the DMN as supporting internal mentation (e.g. manipulation of episodic, autobiographical, semantic memory to develop future plans, self-referential thinking, and social function), and (2) the sentinel hypothesis, which suggests that it supports exploratory monitoring of the environment when focused attention is relaxed (Buckner et al., 2008; Greicius et al., 2003; Greicius et al., 2009). Age-associated changes of the DMN have been observed in cognitively healthy older persons, and these changes are accelerated in people with AD, even after controlling for atrophy, and are correlated with cognitive performance (Jones et al., 2011), suggesting it to be a relevant marker for cognitive reserve.

The CEN is anchored in the dorsolateral prefrontal cortex (dlPFC) and posterior parietal cortex (PCC) (Seeley et al., 2007). The CEN is responsible for high-level cognitive functions, including attention control and working memory (see Bressler and Menon, 2010). The CEN also appears to regulate the DMN (Bressler and Menon, 2010). In people with AD, there is evidence that the CEN is involved in semantic and episodic memory tasks, as opposed to the temporal cortices involvement observed in cognitively healthy controls, suggesting a compensatory role of executive function (Grady et al., 2003). This is in line with the cognitive reserve theory of recruiting alternate networks to cope with brain damage (Stern, 2002).

By studying the functional connectivity of these networks, that is the synchronised blood-oxygen-level-dependent (BOLD) activity across the brain areas implicated, we can observe a record of previous coactivation of these areas, with regions that have been modulated together during task showing spontaneous correlations in resting state (Fox and Raichle, 2007). Resting-state functional MRI (RS-fMRI) can therefore be a tool for studying DMN and CEN connectivity as an index of cognitive reserve, and potentially for observing changes in cognitive reserve after non-pharmacological interventions such as CST.

Cognitive interventions for AD

Domain-specific versus cross-modality design

Non-pharmacological interventions targeting cognition include cognitive training, cognitive rehabilitation, and CST (NICE, 2011). Both cognitive training and cognitive rehabilitation are domain-specific: cognitive training commonly involves guided practice using a set of standard tasks designed for a particular cognitive function, such as working memory; cognitive rehabilitation involves strategies to enhancing residual cognitive skills and cope with deficits in specific cognitive domains (Prince et al., 2015).

Unlike these approaches, CST is essentially a cross-modality intervention. The main principle in CST is to provide opportunities for enjoyable mental exercises at an optimal level. The design of CST is ecological in the sense that it involves real-world social interactions and cognitive processing in a group game/discussion format. The key principles and format of CST ensure integration of (1) complexity, (2) novelty, and (3) diversity, which have been proposed as the required components in cognitive programmes to allow transferrable, generalised cognitive gains (Moreau and Conway, 2014). The relevant key principles in CST include: new ideas, thoughts and associations; providing triggers to aid recall; implicit learning; stimulating language; and stimulating executive function (Spector et al., 2006). Each session has a different theme to ensure diversity, and the group setting also provides a rich environment for social cognition and language use, which involve complex cognitive processes. Current evidence, albeit limited, does support generalised, non-domain-specific cognitive gains from CST.

Current evidence of CST mechanisms

Only a handful of studies have investigated the neuropsychological mechanisms of CST. In an earlier randomised controlled trial (n = 56) of a general cognitive stimulation approach, Breuil et al. (1994) found improvements in memory and learning after 10 sessions over five weeks, as assessed using the Word List Memory Test (WLMT) in the Consortium to Establish a Registry for Alzheimer's Disease (CERAD) (Morris et al., 1989). Cognitive benefits were correlated with a higher baseline general cognitive score and lower education.

Two more recent studies have investigated mechanisms of action adopting a standard CST protocol as outlined by Spector et al. (2003). Using the data from a randomised controlled trial (RCT) of 201 people with dementia (Spector et al., 2010), a generalised improvement in cognition was detected, using the cognition subscale of the Alzheimer's Disease Assessment Scale (ADAS-Cog) (Rosen et al., 1984). The study also noted changes in the language subscale, but not on other subscales. The authors concluded that CST may impact on general cognition by enhancing language, which is achieved through new semantic links created in the process (Spector et al., 2010). Using a different set of neuropsychological assessments, Hall et al. (2013) arrived at similar conclusions. In a smaller sample of 34 people with dementia, changes were observed post-intervention in memory, comprehension of syntax, and orientation post-intervention. The authors speculated that the language-based nature of CST may enhance pathways responsible for processing of syntax, and facilitate verbal recall by creating new semantic links to confer generalised cognitive benefits (Hall et al., 2013).

Putative brain mechanisms of CST

Based on the above initial evidence and theoretical framework, we predicted that CST enhances cognition in people with dementia through a generalised effect on cognition, and that the improvements may be related to brain reserve and cognitive reserve. Specifically, we explored the following research questions:

1 Does baseline brain and cognitive reserve predict cognitive gains from CST?
2 Does CST enhance cognition by changes in cognitive reserve?

We postulated that, as noted in earlier studies, the cognitive benefits with CST are mediated by improvements in general memory, learning, and language functions. People who have a larger reserve, as reflected in their baseline brain/cognitive reserve proxies (grey matter volume, higher education, better work attainment, and more intact large-scale brain networks), may benefit more from CST. We also explored whether cognitive improvements after CST are related to an increase in network connectivity in brain networks that support memory and general cognition.

Exploring neuropsychological mechanisms of CST: an MRI study

Design

We conducted a pilot prospective follow-up study in a small sample of Hong Kong Chinese people with mild dementia, measuring outcomes before and after receiving an evidence-based protocol of group CST (Spector et al., 2003) with cultural adaptation for Hong Kong (Wong, 2015). The whole sample underwent neuropsychological assessments, while brain MRI was conducted in a subsample of participants.

Participants

Participants were 30 people with dementia receiving CST for the first time, recruited from five elderly community care and residential care facilities operated by nongovernmental organisations (NGOs). Among them, 20 eligible participants were recruited to the MRI part of the study. We adopted the inclusion criteria used in the initial CST study (Spector et al., 2003), with additional criteria on cognitive performance level to minimise sample heterogeneity in this small sample pilot study and for eligibility to the MRI study.

Inclusion criteria for neuropsychological assessment:

- A clinical diagnosis of dementia made by a medical doctor;
- An early stage of dementia as indicated by a Cantonese Mini-Mental State Examination (MMSE) score of over 18 (Chiu et al., 1994);

- Absence of other psychiatric disorders, including major depression, schizophrenia, bipolar disorder, anxiety disorders, and intellectual disability;
- Able to communicate and understand communication;
- Able to see and hear well enough to participate in a meaningful assessment; and
- Both the persons with dementia and their caregivers able to give informed consent.

Inclusion criteria for MRI:

- Right-handedness assessed using the Edinburgh Handedness Inventory (Oldfield, 1971);
- No contraindications to MRI, including presence of cardiac pacemakers, incompatible metal implants, history of stroke or heart attack, head trauma leading to loss of consciousness, and claustrophobia.

Potentially eligible participants were referred by their NGO staff and invited for a screening assessment to determine eligibility. The research procedure was explained to their caregiver, and informed consent was provided by both the participant and their caregiver. The study has obtained ethics approval from the Ethics Committee of The University of Hong Kong.

Assessments and procedures

Participants were assessed at baseline before receiving 14, 45 minute sessions of twice-weekly CST (Spector et al., 2003). The protocol was culturally adapted for Hong Kong Chinese (Wong, 2015), including modifications on activities not applicable to Chinese culture (e.g. word games involving alphabets). The group CST facilitators in this study received CST training provided by one of the authors (GHYW) who has a formal training background in psychology and psychiatry. Upon completion of the 14 CST sessions, participants underwent the same set of behavioural assessment and brain MRI scan. All behavioural measures were conducted by researchers with a formal training background in psychology.

Behavioural measurements

Participants and their caregivers were interviewed to collect information on their demographics (age and gender) and proxies for cognitive reserve (years of education and work) at baseline. Assessments of cognitive performance, mood, and communication were performed at baseline and completion of the 14 CST sessions.

Cognitive performance was measured using the ADAS-Cog (Rosen et al., 1984). The ADAS-Cog contains 11 questions measuring a range of cognitive domains, which can be divided into three subscales of (1) memory and learning;

(2) language; and (3) praxis. The entire scale has a range of score from 0 to 70, where a higher score denotes worse performance. With repeated measures, cognitive improvement can be defined as a change in score of ≥ 0 point (no deterioration) or ≥ 4 points (clinical improvement) comparing post-intervention with baseline score (Spector et al., 2003).

Mood was assessed using the Cornell Scale of Depression in Dementia (CSDD) (Alexopoulos et al., 1988). The CSDD is a comprehensive interview tool that captures the clinical impression based on informant and patient interviews. Scores ranging from 0 to 2 were given to each of the 19 items in the scale. Communication was assessed using the Holden Communication Scale (HCS) (Holden and Woods, 1995). The HCS measures social behaviour and communication; it was completed by staff facilitators of the CST groups in this study via interview conducted by study researchers.

MRI data acquisition

Functional and structural brain imaging data were collected using a 3.0-Tesla Philips Achieva whole-body MRI scanner (Philips Healthcare, Best, the Netherlands). Functional imaging data was collected in a resting state, during which participants were instructed to rest with their eyes open, and fixate on a cross in the middle of a projected image inside the scanner and avoid engaging in any specific thoughts. A total of 180 T2-weighted functional image volumes were acquired using a 2D gradient echo-planar imaging (EPI) sequence with the following parameters: repetition time (TR) = 2,000 ms, echo time (TE) = 30s, flip angle = 90°, number of slices (Nslices) = 32, matrix = 64 x 64, slice thickness = 4 mm, field of view (FoV) =240 x 240 mm^2, ascending interleaved slice ordering. Following the EPI sequence, high resolution T1-weighted magnetisation-prepared rapid gradient-echo (MP-RAGE) imaging images were acquired for anatomic visualisation. Head motion was restricted using firm padding that surrounded the participants' head throughout the whole scanning process.

MRI data preprocessing

T1-weighted MP-RAGE images were preprocessed following the CAT12 protocol (Structural Brain Mapping group, Jena University Hospital, Jena, Germany), which was implemented as a toolbox in Statistical Parametric Mapping (SPM) 12 package (Institute of Neurology, London, UK). Images were corrected for bias-field inhomogeneities, then spatially normalised and segmented into grey matter, white matter, and cerebrospinal fluid (CSF) within the same generative model (Ashburner and Friston, 2005). A quality check was performed after the preprocessing, and according to the automated quality insurance protocol of CAT12, all scans included in this study passed the check. All grey matter images were then smoothed with an 8-mm, full width-at-half-maximum, isotropic Gaussian kernel to minimise cortical variation of the gyrus.

Functional images were preprocessed using the SPM 12 package. Dataset with excessive head movement (defined as > 3 mm maximum displacement in x, y, or z or >1.5° angular rotation in each axis) were discarded. Imaging data were then slice-time corrected and realigned. Functional volumes were co-registered and resliced to a voxel size of 2 mm^3, normalised to the Montreal Neurological Institute (MNI) template brain, and smoothed with an 8-mm, full width-at-half-maximum, isotropic Gaussian kernel.

Data analysis

Voxel-based morphometry (VBM) analysis

Structural images were analysed using the VBM technique, which provides comprehensive information of brain morphometric features while avoiding biases due to structural differences (Ashburner and Friston, 2000). The total intracranial volume (TIV) of each participant was calculated as the sum of the grey matter, white matter, and CSF volumes. To detect grey matter volume changes in subjects with dementia before and after CST intervention, paired sample *t*-tests were conducted on the processed images. Age and TIV were classified as nuisance covariates in the comparisons of grey matter volumes between baseline and follow-up conditions. Pearson's correlation coefficient was performed to assess bivariate correlations between brain volume and ADAS-Cog change. Statistical tests were corrected for multiple comparisons at a significance level of false-discovery rate (FRD) and family-wise error (FWE) rate at $p < 0.05$ significance level at peak and cluster levels.

Functional connectivity analysis

Functional connectivity of DMN and CEN were analysed using the Functional Connectivity toolbox (CONN) (Whitfield-Gabrieli and Nieto-Castanon, 2012) implemented in the MATLAB environment. In each participant, the CompCor method (Behzadi et al., 2007) in CONN was used to identify principal components associated with segmented white matter and CSF. The white matter, CSF, and realignment parameters were entered as confounds in a first-level analysis, and the data were band-pass filtered to 0.008 Hz – 0.09 Hz to reduce the effects of low-frequency drift and high-frequency noise. CompCor addresses the confounding effects of subject movement without affecting intrinsic functional connectivity (Chai et al., 2012), thus global signal was not regressed.

Previously defined regions of interest (ROIs) based on MNI coordinates were used in ROI-to-ROI analysis (Fox et al., 2005) for within-network connectivity. The four ROIs identified for the DMN were the MPFC (-1, 49, 15), PCC (-6, -52, 40), and left and right parietal cortices (lLP and rLP: -46, -70, 36/46, -70, 36). The four ROIs in CEN were left and right dorsolateral prefrontal cortex (ldlPFC and rdlPFC: -43, 18, 29/43, 18, 29), and left and right posterior parietal cortex (lPPC and rPPC: -32, -56, 42/35, -44, 37).

Behavioural data

Data was analysed using SPSS (version 23.0; IBM, Armonk, NY, United States). Participants were categorised into maintained/improved and declined subgroups according to predefined criteria (Spector et al., 2003). Independent sample *t*-tests were used to test for differences in baseline characteristics between clinical subgroups. Within-subject changes in ADAS-Cog, CSDD, and HCS were analysed using paired sample *t*-tests to identify areas of significant change after CST. Pearson's correlation coefficient was performed to assess bivariate correlations between demographics, brain and cognitive reserve proxies, and ADAS-Cog change. A multiple linear regression model was built to predict ADAS-Cog change with CST based on the bivariate correlations results.

Results

Among the 30 participants recruited into the study, 26 completed the follow-up neuropsychological assessment after CST (87% retention rate), with four lost to follow-up (change in care service), or withdrawn due to personal reasons. Mean attendance rate of the CST sessions was 92%. Among the 20 participants who were included in the MRI study, follow-up MRI data were available for 16 participants (80% retention rate), with four lost to follow up (hospitalised), or withdrawn due to personal reasons.

Demographics, cognitive reserve proxies, and neuropsychological profile

Baseline characteristics

Table 9.1 shows the baseline characteristics of the sample with complete follow-up behavioural data (n = 26). This sample is characterised by a female predominance with a mean age of 81.7 years. They had on average been diagnosed for 2.1 years. A small proportion (34.6%) had received any formal education, with an average of 3.5 years of education. The participants had worked for 35.1 years on average.

Using clinical criteria defined per changes in ADAS-Cog total score, 14 (53.8%) participants maintained/improved cognition, of which six (23.1%) showed improvement in cognitive performance. There were no significant differences in baseline behavioural characteristics that predicted clinical improvement subgroups, except that those who declined despite receiving CST showed a trend of worse baseline performance in the ADAS-Cog praxis subscale (Table 9.1). The two groups differed significantly on baseline normalised grey matter, white matter, and CSF (Table 9.2).

Table 9.1 Baseline demographic characteristics, cognitive reserve proxies, and cognition

Mean (SD)/n (%)	*All participants (n = 26)*	*Maintained/ improved (n = 14)*	*Declined (n = 12)*	t/χ^2
Female, *n*	20 (76.9)	12 (85.7)	8 (66.7)	0.25
Age, years	81.65 (5.79)	81.00 (6.13)	82.42 (5.53)	−0.61
Duration of diagnosis, years	2.11 (1.61)	2.08 (1.28)	2.16 (1.97)	−0.12
Education, years	3.46 (4.28)	3.36 (4.52)	3.58 (4.19)	−0.13
Any formal education, *n*	9 (34.6)	5 (35.7)	4 (33.3)	0.90
Work, years	35.05 (15.91)	38.11 (10.82)	32.55 (19.28)	0.77
ADAS-Cog total	20.37 (5.87)	20.48 (7.64)	20.25 (3.06)	0.10
Memory and learning	16.79 (4.84)	16.40 (6.00)	17.25 (3.21)	−0.44
Language	1.85 (1.85)	1.93 (2.02)	1.75 (1.71)	0.24
Praxis	1.73 (1.25)	2.14 (1.35)	1.25 (0.97)	1.91[a]
CSDD	3.46 (4.60)	3.86 (1.86)	3.00 (3.05)	0.47
HCS	7.50 (4.87)	6.86 (5.76)	8.25 (3.67)	−0.72

ADAS-Cog = Alzheimer's Disease Assessment Scale, Cognitive subscale; CSDD = Cornell Scale of Depression in Dementia; HCS = Holden Communication Scale

[a] Trend for significance (p = 0.07)

Table 9.2 Baseline brain structural characteristics and functional connectivity of DMN and CEN

Mean (SD)	*All participants (n = 16)*	*Maintained/ improved (n = 10)*	*Declined (n = 6)*	*t*
Absolute volume, cm^3				
Grey matter	499.06 (39.82)	504.80 (44.57)	489.50 (31.72)	0.34
White matter	392.00 (49.65)	396.00 (48.29)	385.33 (55.78)	0.44
CSF	502.00 (72.73)	481.40 (75.02)	536.33 (58.93)	−1.96[a]
TIV	1392.75 (141.86)	1381.90 (152.90)	1410.83 (132.91)	−0.70
Normalised volume, %				
Grey matter	35.94 (1.90)	36.64 (1.91)	34.78 (1.31)	2.12*
White matter	28.12 (1.54)	28.64 (0.10)	27.24 (1.96)	2.67*
CSF	35.96 (2.74)	34.74 (2.48)	38.00 (1.84)	−3.39**
DMN, beta	0.44 (0.21)	0.47 (0.25)	0.39 (0.13)	0.69
CEN, beta	0.33 (0.18)	0.32 (0.19)	0.33 (0.17)	−0.09

CSF = cerebrospinal fluid; TIV = total intracranial volume

*p < 0.05

[a] Trend for significance (p = 0.07)

Table 9.3 Within-subject changes in neuropsychological measurements after CST

Change in score from baseline[a]	*All participants (n = 26)*		*Maintained/improved (n = 14)*		*Declined (n = 12)*	
	Mean (SD)	*t*	*Mean (SD)*	*t*	*Mean (SD)*	*t*
ADAS-Cog total	+0.55 (4.49)	0.62	+3.85 (2.97)	4.84**	−3.31 (2.33)	−4.92**
Memory and learning	+0.74 (4.42)	0.85	+3.63 (3.65)	3.72**	−2.64 (2.36	−3.87**
Language	−0.12 (1.24)	−0.47	−0.29 (1.54)	−0.69	0.08 (0.79)	0.36
Praxis	−0.08 (1.44)	−0.27	0.50 (1.16)	1.61	−0.75 (1.48)	−1.75
CSDD	−0.38 (4.00)	0.49	−2.00 (3.96)	1.89[b]	1.50 (3.26)	−1.59
HCS	1.65 (6.64)	−1.27	0.14 (6.46)	−0.83	3.42 (6.69)	−1.77

ADAS-Cog = Alzheimer's Disease Assessment Scale, Cognitive subscale; CSDD = Cornell Scale of Depression in Dementia; HCS = Holden Communication Scale

**$p < 0.01$

[a]Positive values signify improvement.

[b]Trend for significance ($p = 0.08$)

Within-subject changes

Changes in ADAS-Cog, CSDD, and HCS from baseline in all participants and by clinical change subgroups were shown in Table 9.3. In the maintained/improved subgroup, significant within-subject improvement was observed in the memory and learning subscale of ADAS-Cog, with a trend of improvement in CSDD.

Amongst the 16 participants with complete baseline and follow-up MRI data, a trend of reduction of grey matter volume was observed. A cluster centred in the left temporal pole showed a reduction in grey matter volume (Figure 9.1). The reduction however became insignificant after controlling for TIV and age.

Table 9.4 shows the changes in grey matter volume, white matter volume, CSF, TIV, and functional connectivity in DMN and CEN before and after CST in all participants and by clinical change subgroups. Figure 9.2 shows the DMN connectivity before and after CST. There was an apparent decline, although the change was not significant. In the maintained/improved subgroup, significant within-subject reduction in grey matter volume and increase in CSF was observed, which remained significant after normalisation. In the declined subgroup, within-subject reduction in DMN connectivity was observed.

Bivariate correlates with ADAS-Cog change

Baseline cognitive reserve proxies and ADAS-Cog change

We investigated the bivariate correlation between age, cognitive reserve proxies (education, work), and change in score in ADAS-Cog. While the age of the participants was related to ADAS-Cog score at baseline and follow-up ($r = 0.38$

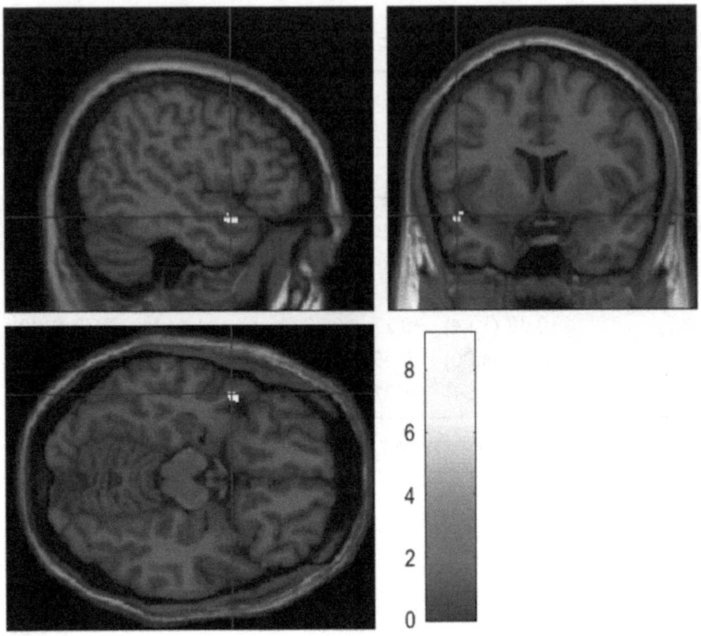

Figure 9.1 Absolute grey matter volume change in the left temporal pole (peak-level T = 9.16, size = 42; MNI (mm) −50, 8, −15, left BA38)

Table 9.4 Within-subject changes in brain structure and functional connectivity after CST

Change in score from baseline[a]	*All participants (n = 16)*		*Maintained/improved (n = 10)*		*Declined (n = 6)*	
	Mean (SD)	*t*	*Mean (SD)*	*t*	*Mean (SD)*	*t*
Absolute volume, cm^3						
Grey matter	3.94 (7.38)	2.13[b]	5.80 (6.25)	2.93*	0.83 (8.64)	0.24
White matter	−1.50 (7.99)	−0.75	−0.50 (5.46)	−0.29	−3.17 (11.51)	−0.67
CSF	−4.44 (23.62)	−0.75	−11.00 (14.94)	−2.33*	6.50 (32.28)	0.49
TIV	−2.44 (15.87)	−0.61	−6.00 (16.10)	−1.18	3.50 (14.88)	0.58
Normalised volume, %						
Grey matter	0.00 (0.01)	1.79	0.01 (0.01)	2.76*	−0.00 (0.01)	−0.05
White matter	−0.00 (0.01)	−0.28	0.00 (0.00)	1.05	−0.00 (0.01)	−0.65
CSF	−0.00 (0.01)	−0.87	−0.01 (0.01)	−2.71*	0.00 (0.02)	0.45
DMN, beta	0.06 (0.16)	1.40	0.04 (0.20)	0.66	0.08 (0.07)	2.86*
CEN, beta	−0.01 (0.16)	−0.28	−0.00 (0.19)	−0.07	−0.02 (0.10)	−0.56

CSF = cerebrospinal fluid; TIV = total intracranial volume

*$p < 0.05$

[a]Positive values signify decrease.

[b]Trend for significance ($p = 0.05$)

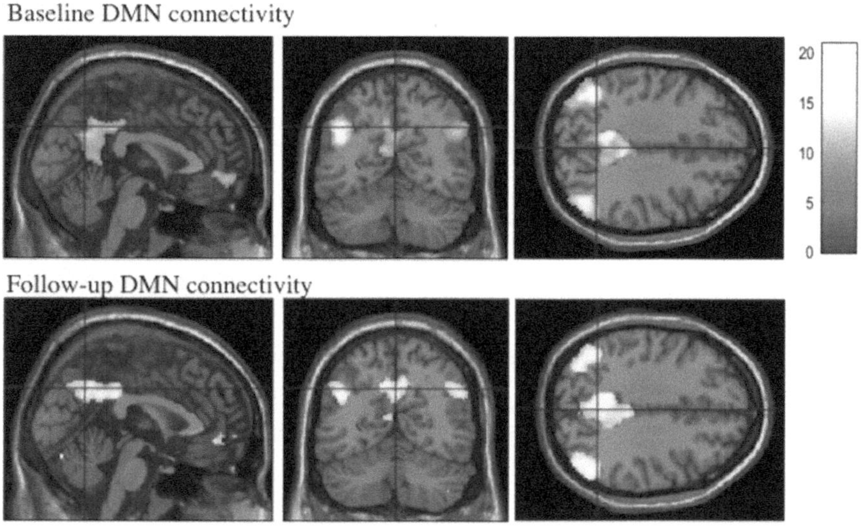

Figure 9.2 DMN connectivity before and after CST (n = 16). There was no significant decline in the group as a whole, although there appears to be some decline in the sub-group who have deteriorated in ADAS-Cog.

and 0.48, respectively, $p < 0.05$), it was unrelated to the change in ADAS-Cog score after CST. Years of education in our sample was not related to ADAS-Cog score at baseline or follow-up, or its changes after CST. We observed a significant positive correlation between years of work and improvements in the ADAS-Cog after CST ($r = 0.48$, $p < 0.05$) (Figure 9.3) which was not related to baseline or follow-up ADAS-Cog score.

Baseline brain reserve and ADAS-Cog change

We calculated the bivariate correlation between brain reserve (baseline grey matter volume, white matter volume, and TIV) and change in score in ADAS-Cog. Normalised baseline grey matter volume and white matter volume were correlated with improvements in ADAS-Cog score ($r = 0.47$ and 0.46, respectively, $p < 0.05$) (Figure 9.4).

Functional connectivity and ADAS-Cog change

We investigated the correlation between ADAS-Cog score changes and changes in DMN and CEN connectivity. Only changes in the language subscale was correlated with DMN connectivity ($r = -0.54$, $p = 0.03$).

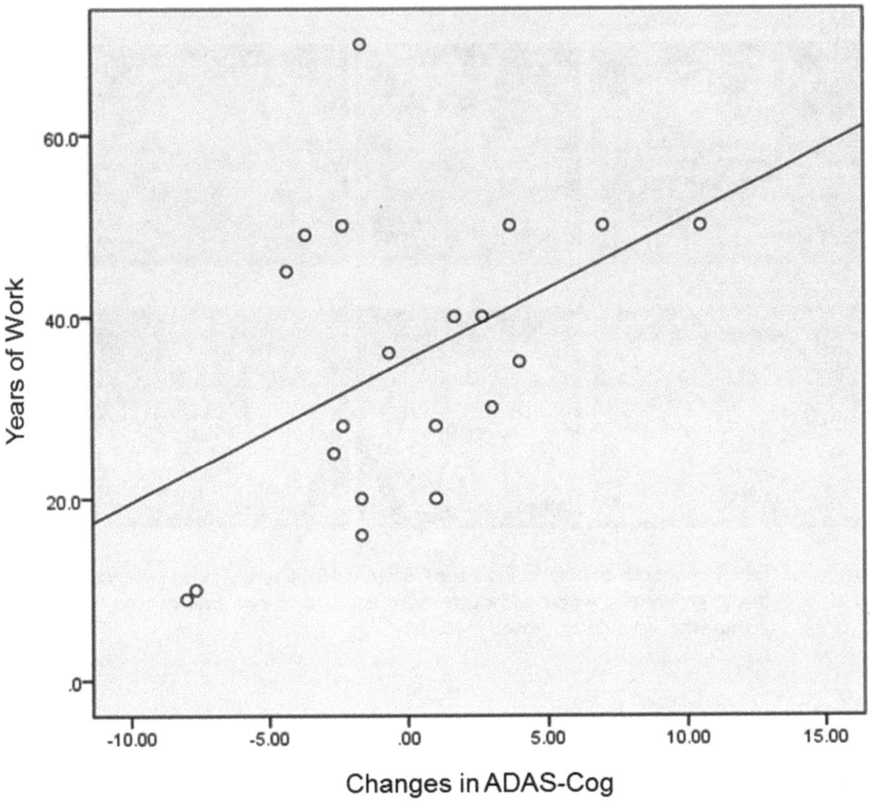

Figure 9.3 Correlation between years of work and ADAS-Cog changes[a]

[a]Positive values signify improvement on ADAS-Cog

Multiple linear regression

Based on the significant bivariate correlation between changes in ADAS-Cog score and years of work, baseline normalised grey matter, and baseline normalised white matter volume, we tested a multiple linear regression model to predict ADAS-Cog change with CST. The model explained 65% of the variance ($R^2 = 0.65$, $F(3,10) = 6.21$, $p = 0.01$). Years of work and baseline normalised grey matter volume significantly predicted ADAS-Cog change (β = 0.58 and 0.45, respectively, $p < 0.05$) (Table 9.5).

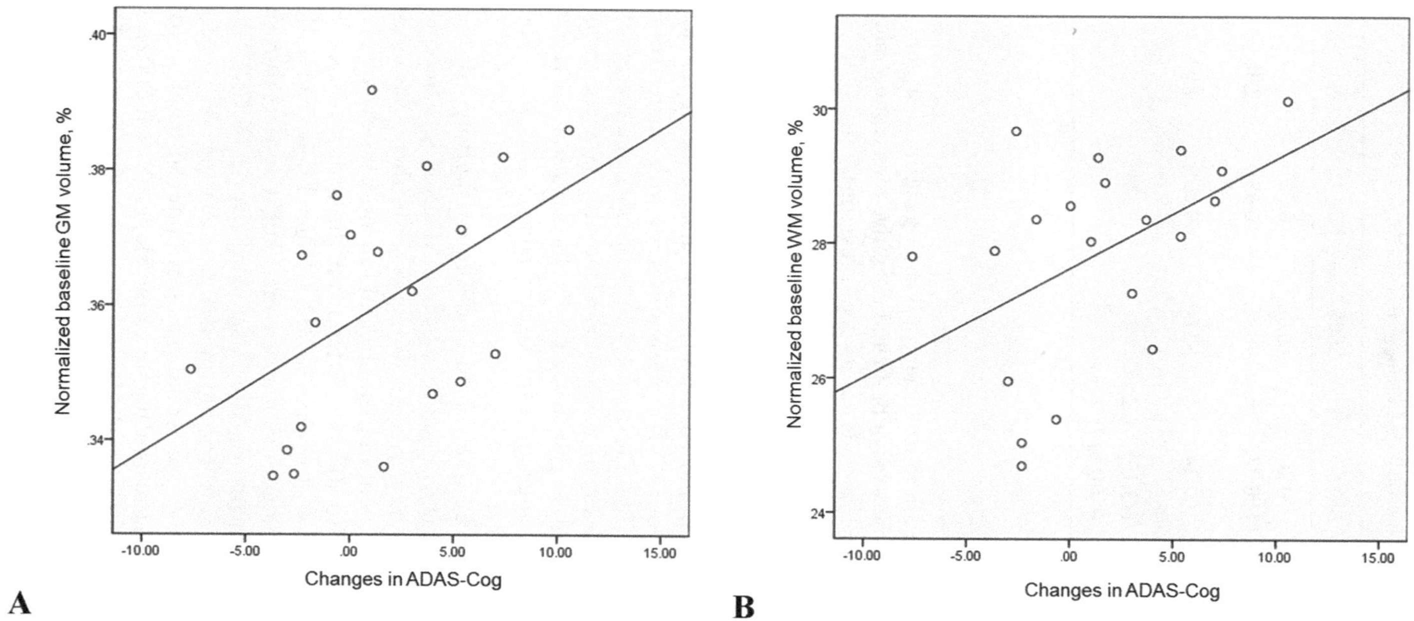

Figure 9.4 Correlation between normalised baseline (A) grey matter volume and (B) white matter volume and ADAS-Cog changes[a]

[a]Positive values signify improvement on ADAS-Cog

Table 9.5 Predictive model of ADAS-Cog change after CST

Predictor variable	B	SE(B)	β	t	*p*
Years of work	0.20	0.06	0.58	3.07	0.01
Baseline normalised grey matter volume	108.77	45.42	0.45	2.40	0.04
Baseline normalised white matter volume	102.34	52.68	0.36	1.94	0.81
$R^2 = 0.65$	$F(3,10) = 6.21$				
Adjusted $R^2 = 0.55$	P = 0.01				

Discussion

In this pilot study, we explored the neuropsychological mechanisms of CST under the theoretical framework of brain and cognitive reserve. Several observations can be drawn from this study for in-depth investigations.

Baseline brain and cognitive reserve predicts benefits

People with greater brain and cognitive reserve at baseline appear to be the ones who will benefit from CST, as measured using grey matter volume and white matter volume for brain reserve and years of work as a proxy for cognitive reserve. There is a linear dose-response relationship between these reserve measurements and cognitive gain from CST, which explains in combination 65% of variance of the changes in cognitive performance after CST. The higher the reserve, the better the intervention response.

This observation can be interpreted in the following ways. In the group of people who maintained or improved their ADAS-Cog score after CST, who also had a larger brain reserve to begin with, there was an absolute within-subject improvement in memory and learning, instead of a relatively slower decline. They also did not differ from the group that declined in their baseline ADAS-Cog. In other words, a larger brain reserve does not change the intercept of cognitive performance, but it appears to reverse the slope of cognitive performance, after a standard course of CST. This is in contradiction to a passive threshold model of reserve, which predicts that a person with a larger reserve would perform better at baseline (different intercept), but decline at a similar rate (same slope) (Stern, 2002). On the other hand, our data may support the active model of reserve, and a larger reserve may interact with CST to allow a person to cope more efficiently with cognitive tasks.

Cognitive benefits despite progression in brain damage

CST exerts its effect through a dissociation between neuropathology and cognitive performance. The above interpretation is consistent with our finding that cognitive improvement happened in the context of reducing grey matter volume and increasing CSF. In the entire sample, the observed absolute reduction in grey matter volume in the left temporal pole is in line with the known pathology of temporal lobe atrophy in AD (see Ballard et al., 2011 for a review). In the subgroup of people who have a larger brain reserve and improved memory and learning performance, the reduction in grey matter volume and increase in CSF was paradoxically more significant. These findings converge to suggest that the beneficial effects of CST are dissociated from the progression of neuropathology in dementia.

In our regression model of cognitive gains from CST, years of work independently predicted a change in ADAS-Cog in addition to baseline grey matter and white matter volume. Years of work is also not correlated with any of these brain reserve measures (results not shown). This appears to suggest contribution of active cognitive reserve in response to CST, again unrelated to brain pathology. Interestingly, we did not find any effect of education as a major cognitive reserve proxy in our sample. However, this should be evaluated against a background of very low education level and high illiteracy rate among older adults in Hong Kong due to the paucity of education opportunities in this cohort. In our study, less than 40% of the participants had any formal education, making it a less relevant cognitive reserve proxy compared with work experience.

Changes in brain network connectivity

We observed a non-significant decrease in DMN connectivity in the entire group, which is more apparent in the subgroup who deteriorated despite receiving CST. The decrease was not related to changes in ADAS-Cog total score, although there seems to be an association with changes in the language subscale of the ADAS-Cog. This observation should be interpreted with caution as the sample size with complete pre- and post-intervention fMRI data is small. Given the previous evidence that complex mental activities in healthy older adults increase functional connectivity in DMN and CEN (Chapman et al., 2013), it is plausible that similar changes would be observed in this study, although more data is needed to draw any concrete conclusion.

Study limitations, implications and future directions

This study has several major limitations. Firstly, the sample size is small with only 16 participants completing the post-intervention MRI scan, rendering it under-powered to detect smaller changes. Previous analysis suggests a minimum 12 participants, which doubles at 24 participants with correction for multiple comparisons (Desmond and Glover, 2002) as we have done in our analyses.

Despite the small sample, we were able to identify a model of brain and cognitive reserve for predicting cognitive benefits from CST, which appeared to have a large effect, although replication studies are needed. The key implication from this model is that CST appears to interact with brain and cognitive reserve to improve memory and learning function in a context of progression in structural brain damage. Further research should investigate with more refined design, such as by using the experimental method to systematically test the effect of CST in individuals with varying levels of baseline brain and cognitive reserve.

Secondly, we have included only years of education and work as proxies for cognitive reserve. Although years of work is found to be a significant predictor of cognitive gain from CST, more refined measurements of work attainment (e.g. any supervisory or managerial role, skilled work) may be a more relevant proxy. Other cognitive and brain reserve proxies such as engagement in social and leisure activities (Barulli and Stern, 2013), general intelligence factor *g*, hippocampal volume, and total white matter hyperintensity (Steffener and Stern, 2012; Murray et al., 2011) should be assessed in future studies to provide a more accurate reflection of a person's reserve.

This study has investigated brain network using only functional connectivity data from RS-fMRI. Theoretically, the neural basis of cognitive reserve can also be viewed as the efficiency and capacity of these brain networks in the face of varying levels of task demand (Steffener and Stern, 2012), which can be studied using a task-based fMRI design. More advanced analysis techniques based on graph theory should also be used to investigate network efficiency, such as global efficiency and path length (Bullmore and Sporns, 2012), which could provide insight into the brain functional changes that underlie cognitive improvements with CST. The use of diffusion tensor imaging (DTI) technique will also provide important information about synaptic changes that may explain the observed improvements in memory and learning.

Conclusion

This is the first study to explore the neuropsychological mechanisms of CST using MRI. Initial evidence supports the active cognitive reserve framework by suggesting that CST improves general cognition against the background of progressive neuropathology in people who have a larger brain reserve and cognitive reserve at the time of intervention. This exploratory research provided a proof of concept for more rigorous study of the mechanisms of CST under the reserve framework, with potential implication of early intervention before depletion of brain reserve in terms of grey matter and white matter volume.

References

Alexopoulos, G. S., Abrams, R. C., Young, R. C. and Shamoian, C. A. (1988). Cornell scale for depression in dementia. *Biol Psychiatry*, 23, 271–84.

Ashburner, J. and Friston, K. J. (2000). Voxel-based morphometry – the methods. *Neuroimage*, 11, 805–21.

Ashburner, J. and Friston, K. J. (2005). Unified segmentation. *Neuroimage*, 26, 839–51.

Ballard, C., Gauthier, S., Corbett, A., Brayne, C., Aarsland, D. and Jones, E. 2011. Alzheimer's disease. *Lancet*, 377, 1019–31.

Barulli, D. and Stern, Y. (2013). Efficiency, capacity, compensation, maintenance, plasticity: emerging concepts in cognitive reserve. *Trends Cogn Sci*, 17, 502–9.

Bassett, D. S., Wymbs, N. F., Porter, M. A., Mucha, P. J., Carlson, J. M. and Grafton, S. T. (2011). Dynamic reconfiguration of human brain networks during learning. *Proc Natl Acad Sci U S A*, 108, 7641–6.

Behzadi, Y., Restom, K., Liau, J. and Liu, T. T. (2007). A component based noise correction method (CompCor) for BOLD and perfusion based fMRI. *Neuroimage*, 37, 90–101.

Bressler, S. L. and Menon, V. (2010). Large-scale brain networks in cognition: emerging methods and principles. *Trends Cogn Sci*, 14, 277–90.

Breuil, V., De Rotrou, J., Forette, F., Tortrat, D., Ganansia-Ganem, A., Frambourt, A., Moulin, F. and Boller, F. (1994). Cognitive stimulation of patients with dementia: preliminary results. *Int J Geriatr Psychiatry*, 9, 211–17.

Buckner, R. L., Andrews-Hanna, J. R. and Schacter, D. L. (2008). The brain's default network: anatomy, function, and relevance to disease. *Ann N Y Acad Sci*, 1124, 1–38.

Buckner, R. L., Snyder, A. Z., Shannon, B. J., Larossa, G., Sachs, R., Fotenos, A. F., Sheline, Y. I., Klunk, W. E., Mathis, C. A., Morris, J. C. and Mintun, M. A. (2005). Molecular, structural, and functional characterization of Alzheimer's disease: evidence for a relationship between default activity, amyloid, and memory. *J Neurosci*, 25, 7709–17.

Bullmore, E. and Sporns, O. (2012). The economy of brain network organization. *Nat Rev Neurosci*, 13, 336–49.

Chai, X. J., Castanon, A. N., Ongur, D. and Whitfield-Gabrieli, S. (2012). Anticorrelations in resting state networks without global signal regression. *Neuroimage*, 59, 1420–8.

Chapman, S. B., Aslan, S., Spence, J. S., Hart, J. J., Jr., Bartz, E. K., Didehbani, N., Keebler, M. W., Gardner, C. M., Strain, J. F., Defina, L. F. and Lu, H. (2013). Neural mechanisms of brain plasticity with complex cognitive training in healthy seniors. *Cereb Cortex*.

Chiu, H. F. K., Lee, H. C., Chung, W. S. and Kwong, P. K. (1994). Reliability and validity of the Cantonese version of Mini-Mental State Examination – a preliminary study. *East Asian Arch Psych*, 4, 25–8.

Craig, P., Dieppe, P., Macintyre, S., Michie, S., Nazareth, I., Petticrew, M. and Medical Research Council, G. (2008). Developing and evaluating complex interventions: the new Medical Research Council guidance. *BMJ*, 337, a1655.

Desmond, J. E. and Glover, G. H. (2002). Estimating sample size in functional MRI (fMRI) neuroimaging studies: statistical power analyses. *J Neurosci Methods*, 118, 115–28.

Fox, M. D., Snyder, A. Z., Vincent, J. L., Corbetta, M., Van Essen, D. C., & Raichle, M. E. (2005). *The human brain is intrinsically organized into dynamic, anticorrelated functional networks.* Proc Natl Acad Sci U S A, 102(27), 9673–9678, doi: 10.1073/pnas.0504136102

Fox, M. D. and Raichle, M. E. (2007). Spontaneous fluctuations in brain activity observed with functional magnetic resonance imaging. *Nat Rev Neurosci*, 8, 700–11.

Ganguly, K. and Poo, M. M. (2013). Activity-dependent neural plasticity from bench to bedside. *Neuron*, 80, 729–41.

Grady, C. L., Mcintosh, A. R., Beig, S., Keightley, M. L., Burian, H. and Black, S. E. (2003). Evidence from functional neuroimaging of a compensatory prefrontal network in Alzheimer's disease. *J Neurosci*, 23, 986–93.

Greicius, M. D., Krasnow, B., Reiss, A. L. and Menon, V. (2003). Functional connectivity in the resting brain: a network analysis of the default mode hypothesis. *Proc Natl Acad Sci U S A*, 100, 253–8.

Greicius, M. D., Supekar, K., Menon, V. and Dougherty, R. F. (2009). Resting-state functional connectivity reflects structural connectivity in the default mode network. *Cereb Cortex*, 19, 72–8.

Hall, L., Orrell, M., Stott, J. and Spector, A. (2013). Cognitive stimulation therapy (CST): neuropsychological mechanisms of change. *Int Psychogeriatr*, 25, 479–89.

Holden, U. P. and Woods, R. T. (1995). *Positive Approaches to Dementia Care (3rd ed)*, Edinburgh, Churchill Livingstone.

Jones, D. T., Machulda, M. M., Vemuri, P., Mcdade, E. M., Zeng, G., Senjem, M. L., Gunter, J. L., Przybelski, S. A., Avula, R. T., Knopman, D. S., Boeve, B. F., Petersen, R. C. and Jack, C. R., Jr. (2011). Age-related changes in the default mode network are more advanced in Alzheimer disease. *Neurology*, 77, 1524–31.

Moreau, D. and Conway, A. R. (2014). The case for an ecological approach to cognitive training. *Trends Cogn Sci*, 18, 334–6.

Morris, J. C., Heyman, A., Mohs, R. C., Hughes, J. P., Van Belle, G., Fillenbaum, G., Mellits, E. D. and Clark, C. (1989). The Consortium to Establish a Registry for Alzheimer's Disease (CERAD). Part I. Clinical and neuropsychological assessment of Alzheimer's disease. *Neurology*, 39, 1159–65.

Murray, A. D., Staff, R. T., McNeil, C. J., Salarirad, S., Ahearn, T. S., Mustafa, N. and Whalley, L. J. (2011). The balance between cognitive reserve and brain imaging biomarkers of cerebrovascular and Alzheimer's diseases. *Brain*, 134, 3687–96.

NICE. (2011). *Dementia: A NICE-SCIE Guideline on Supporting People With Dementia and Their Carers in Health and Social Care (Revised ed)*, Leicester (UK), National Institute for Health and Clinical Excellence.

Oldfield, R. C. (1971). The assessment and analysis of handedness: the Edinburgh inventory. *Neuropsychologia*, 9, 97–113.

Pascual-Leone, A., Amedi, A., Fregni, F. and Merabet, L. B. (2005). The plastic human brain cortex. *Annu Rev Neurosci*, 28, 377–401.

Prince, M., Wimo, A., Guerchet, M., Ali, G.-C., Wu, Y.-T., Prina, M. and Alzheimer's Disease International. (2015). *World Alzheimer Report 2015: The Global Impact of Dementia*. London.

Raichle, M. E., Macleod, A. M., Snyder, A. Z., Powers, W. J., Gusnard, D. A. and Shulman, G. L. (2001). A default mode of brain function. *Proc Natl Acad Sci U S A*, 98, 676–82.

Rosen, W. G., Mohs, R. C. and Davis, K. L. (1984). A new rating scale for Alzheimer's disease. *Am J Psychiatry*, 141, 1356–64.

Seeley, W. W., Menon, V., Schatzberg, A. F., Keller, J., Glover, G. H., Kenna, H., Reiss, A. L. and Greicius, M. D. (2007). Dissociable intrinsic connectivity networks for salience processing and executive control. *J Neurosci*, 27, 2349–56.

Spector, A., Orrell, M. and Woods, B. (2010). Cognitive Stimulation Therapy (CST): effects on different areas of cognitive function for people with dementia. *Int J Geriatr Psychiatry*, 25, 1253–8.

Spector, A., Thorgrimsen, L., Woods, B. and Orrell, M. (2006). *Making a Difference: An Evidence-based Group Programme to Offer Cognitive Stimulation Therapy (CST) to People With Dementia*. London, Hawker Publications.

Spector, A., Thorgrimsen, L., Woods, B., Royan, L., Davies, S., Butterworth, M. and Orrell, M. (2003). Efficacy of an evidence-based Cognitive Stimulation Therapy programme for people with dementia: randomised controlled trial. *Br J Psychiatry*, 183, 248–54.

Steffener, J. and Stern, Y. (2012). Exploring the neural basis of cognitive reserve in aging. *Biochim Biophys Acta*, 1822, 467–73.

Stern, Y. (2002). What is cognitive reserve? Theory and research application of the reserve concept. *J Int Neuropsychol Soc*, 8, 448–60.

Stern, Y. (2012). Cognitive reserve in ageing and Alzheimer's disease. *Lancet Neurol*, 11, 1006–12.

Valenzuela, M. J. and Sachdev, P. (2006). Brain reserve and dementia: a systematic review. *Psychol Med*, 36, 441–54.

Whitfield-Gabrieli, S. and Nieto-Castanon, A. (2012). Conn: a functional connectivity toolbox for correlated and anticorrelated brain networks. *Brain Connect*, 2, 125–41.

Wong, G. H. Y. (2015). CST for Hong Kong Chinese: Cultural adaptation and mechanisms of change. In *Cognitive Stimulation Therapy (CST) for Dementia: An International Perspective*. London.

Woods, B., Aguirre, E., Spector, A. E. and Orrell, M. (2012). Cognitive stimulation to improve cognitive functioning in people with dementia. *Cochrane Database Syst Rev*, 2, CD005562.

Part IV

CST

An international perspective

Chapter 10

Guidelines for adapting cognitive stimulation therapy to other cultures

Elisa Aguirre and Katja Werheid

Background

Culture and cultural adaptation

Culture is a complex and multi-dimensional construct for which 164 definitions can be found (Cohen, 2009). In a review of the concept, Fiske (2002, p. 85) captured the points of consensus amongst these definitions:

> A culture is a socially transmitted or socially constructed constellation consisting of such things as practices, competencies, ideas, schemas, symbols, values, norms, institutions, goals, constitutive rules, artifacts, and modifications of the physical environment.

Cultural adaptation of evidence-based treatments (EBTs) or intervention protocols has been defined as 'the systematic modification of the treatment to consider language, culture, and context in such a way that it is compatible with the client's cultural patterns, meanings, and values' (Bernal et al., 2009, p. 362). Two contrasting positions to systematic modification of treatments can be found in the literature; (1) a universal "top-down" approach that views the original content of an intervention as applicable to all subcultural groups and not in need of alterations, and (2) a culture-specific 'bottom-up' approach that emphasises culturally grounded content consisting of the unique values, beliefs, traditions, and practices of a particular subcultural group (Falicov, 2009). Some purported 'cultural adaptations' were essentially 'top-down' intervention modifications lacking meaningful input from members of the particular culture.

Although theoretically driven frameworks and approaches to cultural adaptation provide a strong foundation for tailoring interventions, 'bottom' or 'ground-up' community-based approaches can provide invaluable information by confirming theory-related adaptations, generating ideas that more theory-driven approaches omit, or by providing greater specificity in the adaptations or examples offered. Community-based formative approaches to therapy adaptation can also serve as a powerful tool for cultural understanding because they involve consumers (therapists and clients), as well as community stakeholders and collaborators.

Theoretical methods for cross-cultural adaptations of psychological interventions

Different theoretical methods are available to develop 'cross-cultural adaptations' when preparing a questionnaire or therapy for use in other settings, including processes that consider language, such as translation, and processes that involve cultural adaptation issues. In recent years, a number of frameworks have been developed to guide cultural adaptations of therapies. There are four main frameworks available that have been used and tested in many evaluations of the adapted interventions.

The ecological validity model

The ecological validity model was developed by Bernal et al. (1995). This model was used to guide adaptations in cognitive-behavioural and interpersonal treatments for Puerto Rican adolescents with depression, with the resulting adapted treatment being shown to be efficacious in randomised controlled trials (RCTs) (Rosselló and Bernal, 1996; Rosselló and Bernal, 1999). The authors of this framework suggest that language and mere translation of the programme is only one aspect of adaptation, and other dimensions involving different elements need to be considered. This framework uses eight different dimensions to identify areas for adaptation, including language, people, metaphors, content, concepts, goals, methods, and context. For example, 'people' involves addressing cultural similarities and differences between the client and clinician; issues of 'content' refer to cultural knowledge and information about the values, traditions, and customs of the culture; 'context' involves consideration of changing circumstances that might increase risk to acculturative stress problems, disconnect from social supports and networks, and reduced social mobility (Bernal et al., 2009; Nicolas et al., 2009).

The cultural adaptation process model (Domenech-Rodriguez and Wieling 2005)

This model consists of a sequence of adaptation that involves three phases: (1) phase I focuses on the iterative and collaborative process that often includes the participation of persons from the targeted population for whom the adaptation is being developed, (2) phase II involves selection and adaptation of evaluation measures and continual exchange between the community and those creating the adaptations, and (3) phase III integrates the observations and data gathered in phase II to create a new intervention.

The psychotherapy adaptation and modification framework (PAMF) (Hwang et al.*, 2006)*

This model offers a three-tiered approach to making cultural adaptations and consists of 'domains', 'principles', and 'rationales'. 'Domains' identify general areas that practitioners should utilise when modifying therapeutic approaches for their clients; 'principles' provide more specific recommendations for adapting therapy for specific groups, and 'rationales' provide corresponding explanations for why these adaptations may be effective when used with the target population. This approach was created to help practitioners make the shift from abstract ideas of being culturally relevant to developing specific skills and strategies that can be effectively implemented when working with diverse clientele. In addition, it was designed to help practitioners thoroughly consider why certain adaptations were made, and to support these modifications with compelling justifications (Hwang et al., 2006). For example general domains for adaptations under this framework include: (1) understanding dynamic issues and cultural complexities, (2) orienting clients to psychotherapy and increasing mental health awareness, (3) understanding cultural beliefs about mental illness, its causes, and what constitutes appropriate treatment, (4) improving the client-therapist relationship, (5) understanding cultural differences in the expression and communication of distress, and (6) addressing cultural issues specific to the population.

Selective adaptation model (Lau et al.*, 2006)*

This framework recommends sequences for developing culturally adapted interventions using an evidence-based approach that; (1) prioritises selectively targeting problems and identifying communities that would derive the most benefit, and (2) uses direct data outcomes to justify adaptations.

Dementia and the use of the formative method for adapting psychotherapy (FMAP) for the development of CST guidelines

Dementia is a major public health problem, which is acknowledged worldwide (World Health Organization, 2012). Criteria outlined in the Diagnostic and Statistical Manual of Mental Disorders Fourth Edition (DSM-IV) (American Psychiatric Association, 2000), which is widely used all over the world, take a biomedical definition of dementia. However, different communities and cultures understand dementia in different ways (Pollitt et al., 1996; Poveda et al., 2003; Enjolras et al., 2005; Werner et al., 2005; Whitehouse et al., 2005; Blay et al., 2010). Social relationships with people living with dementia may be influenced by tolerance or stigmatisation (Goffman et al., 1963), leading to either social support or discrimination, which in turn can impact the quality of life (QoL) of people living with dementia. However, few studies have been carried out to ascertain perceptions and representations of dementia throughout the world, especially in non-western countries (Jeste et al., 1999).

To date, the majority of frameworks that have been used to adapt therapies to different cultures have taken a 'top-down' theoretical approach (Hwang et al., 2009), which involves beginning with theoretical ideas of how best to culturally adapt the programme. However, frameworks for adaptation of interventions that focus on people living with dementia need to first reflect on how dementia is perceived in the culture in which the intervention will be used. As a result, in order to develop the presented guidelines, it was decided that a community-based developmental approach taking into account how users from different cultures understand dementia was the most suitable approach. This approach for adapting Cognitive Stimulation Therapy (CST) was expected to maximise the ecological validity of the adaptation. The framework chosen to develop the guidelines for the CST adaptation was based on the Formative Method for Adapting Psychotherapy (FMAP), a 'bottom-up' approach that involves collaborating with service users as a first step to generate and support ideas for therapy adaptation (Hwang et al., 2009).

Using this framework allowed for exploration of the different cultural representations of dementia and the social influences of these representations. This information was then used to: (1) generate ideas for therapy adaptation, (2) provide additional support for theoretically identified modifications, and (3) provide more specific and refined recommendations for increasing therapeutic responsiveness. As the chosen model and framework selected to be used for CST adaptation was generated in parallel to other adaptation models, it contributes to the growing body of literature on culturally responsive treatment development. In order to develop the guidelines, we combined the community-based FMAP approach alongside evidence from international groups already established and running. The aim of the guidelines was to facilitate the creation of new culturally adapted CST programmes around the world.

The FMAP approach consists of five phases (Figure 10.1) that target developing, testing, and reformulating therapy modifications; (a) generating knowledge

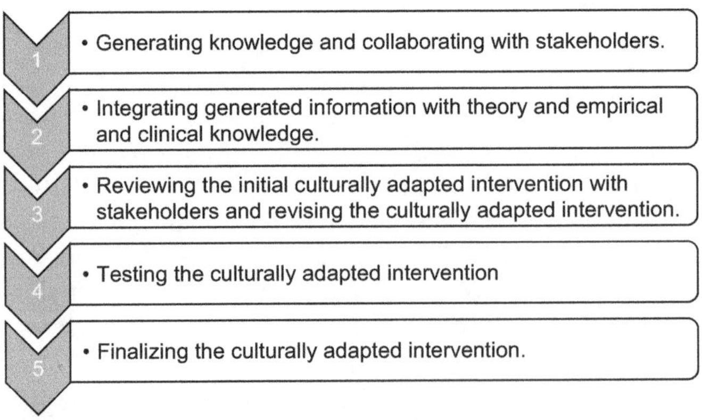

Figure 10.1 The five steps of the FMAP to other cultures (Hwang, 2006)

and collaborating with stakeholders, (b) integrating generated information with theory and empirical and clinical knowledge, (c) reviewing the initial culturally adapted clinical intervention with stakeholders and revising the culturally adapted intervention, (d) testing the culturally adapted intervention, and (e) finalising the culturally adapted intervention.

Each of the phases of the FMAP model can be tailored to meet the individual needs of different projects. Moreover, application of the FMAP is illustrated through ongoing and past examples.

Step by step guide for CST adaptation

Phase 1: generating knowledge and collaborating with stakeholders

The first step to take when adapting CST to a different culture is to decide which stakeholders to involve in the adaptation process and when to involve them. According to the FMAP, stakeholders may include; (1) participants, (2) mainstream health and mental healthcare providers, (3) community-based organisations and agencies, (4) traditional and indigenous healers, and (5) spiritual and religious organisations. For the purposes of adapting CST, it is recommended that the following stakeholders relevant to each culture are approached:

1 participants and family caregivers
2 community health workers such as village health workers
3 mental healthcare staff (psychiatrists, psychologists, social workers, therapists, and healthcare assistants)
4 other older people with knowledge of relevant historical, cultural, and religious issues.

It is essential that local health workers and staff are included because they have hands on experience, expertise, and knowledge in directly working with and providing services to people with dementia in the particular culture and context. Included stakeholders will be able to provide direct feedback on developing, adapting, and improving CST. Eliciting participants' feedback is also very important; however, it is recommended to do this at a later stage in Phases 4 and 5 of the process.

A good way of consulting at this stage is through focus groups. Each focus group might consist of around four to six health workers with a range of clinical and working experiences, which will help to facilitate both breadth and depth of discussions. The first part of the focus group can include general discussions of cultural adaptation and review the treatment manual and intervention as described in 'Making a Difference' (Spector et al., 2006) and 'Making a Difference 2' (Aguirre et al., 2011). Specifically, this could include their impressions of CST, whether different aspects of CST would work in their particular culture, and how best to modify CST for their community. It is important to hold consultations across multiple community settings because they will each possess different characteristics, biases, and different perceptions in relation to what best practice is. This will allow the collection of a range of feedback that can be used to produce a more ecologically valid adaptation of the programme (see Box 10.1).

Focus groups can also be complemented with individual interviews with other key practitioners in each culture who are not part of a particular setting. For example healers or priests if they are prominent and influential figures in the particular culture. This will also provide an opportunity to exchange ideas, build a sense of community, and strengthen referral networks.

Box 10.1 Example of the development of a culture-specific CST programme from South Asian adaptation

A South Asian version of the CST programme was developed in London, UK. Adaptation of most activities took place within each theme, using cultural and ethnic issues relevant to the Indian subcontinent. The programme was run by two bilingual doctors in their first language along with a support worker. It was decided that the discussion of the day, time, and place that takes part at the beginning of each session was going to be around events and issues relevant to localities in group members' countries of origin, including news of their local community, about their own families and friends, or from the daily TV programmes they were following. Adapted activities included games such as a 'Carom board' for the number games session, familiar sounds from their past such as Rickshaw and Tonga (horse cart) for the sounds session, discussion around the immigration process, routes, and difficulties for the orientation session, and famous historical personalities from the Indian subcontinent for the faces session.

Phase 2: integrating generated information with theory, empirical, and clinical knowledge

At this stage information generated from the community-based focus groups will be synthesised, and a new culturally adapted version of the manual will be developed and produced. Focus group collaborations and feedback will help to reduce personal and clinician specific biases, and collaborating with local health workers will help to ensure that cultural adaptations are grounded in the relevant cultural belief systems (see Boxes 10.2 and 10.3).

Box 10.2 Example of phase 2 community generated information from developing countries

For the adaptation process for cultures in developing countries, the structure of sessions as described in the manuals had to be modified due to logistical issues. For example, distances between villages, transport arrangements, carer commitments depending on the season, harvesting or planting crops, and access of villages during rainy season.

Another element for consideration in this phase was the use of materials that had to be locally available and, most importantly, familiar to the group and culture (see Boxes 10.4 and 10.5).

Box 10.3 Example from Tanzanian adaptation

At this phase for some culturally adapted programmes, such as the Tanzanian adaptation, it was decided that the setting to run the programme should be somewhere local where children could not watch; avoiding churches, mosques, or hospitals in order for participants to feel comfortable regardless of their religion, and to avoid feeling treated as being sick.

Phase 3: review of the culturally adapted CST intervention by stakeholders and further revision

After developing a draft of the culturally adapted CST manual, it is recommended that a further focus group is organised and conducted with the planned CST group facilitators. At this focus group, initial impressions of the adapted intervention and feedback for improvement should be elicited, paying special attention to the activities included in the revised and adapted manual. This feedback will then be used to finalise the manual prior to implementation. Manuals developed at this phase will then be written and translated from the original English text into the required language. It is best practice to follow a standardised forward and back translation method whereby the manual is translated into the local language, then translated back into English. It is recommended that the back translation at this point is reviewed by the UK CST team.

Box 10.4 Example of phase 3 consultations from Tanzanian and Nigerian adaptation

For the Tanzanian and Nigerian versions, three sessions were allocated to each member of the group for consideration and then discussed in the focus group. The main issues considered were: important local events for the centres and villages, how people become aware of current affairs (e.g. sermon on the radio, TV, ceremonies), consideration of local materials for maps, food, sweets, games, and expansion to other areas in the country. The Sub-Saharan Africa adaptation is described in Chapter 16.

Box 10.5 Example of activities featured in South Asian adaptation

For the adaptation of the programme to South Asian groups, materials were made culturally relevant by including topics that are popular in India and Pakistan, such as cricket. Other adapted activities included: preparing two different curry dishes for the 'being creative' session, and sharing the dishes with the day centre staff. An Urdu drama was shown and discussed as part of the 'visual clips discussion' session. As most participants' level of literacy was expected to be low (based on advice from family members), the programme was designed to maximise the use of materials and equipment that incorporated visual (images) and auditory content and minimise the use of reading and writing.

Phase 4: pilot testing the culturally adapted intervention

The developed CST manual from phase 3, should then be piloted in phase 4 in different settings in order to test the adapted programme. This could involve running a full programme in two carefully selected settings and using minimal outcomes to test its efficacy, such as cognitive and QoL measures.

Ideally the pilot would be run in community centres, which normally provide services for people with dementia, to ensure sustainability and feasibility (e.g. the frequency of sessions, number of participants, number of staff, duration of the sessions, transport, and financial limitations). In addition, consulting with other staff and managers within the selected centres to gather feedback at this stage will help to facilitate their support and adaptation of the CST programme (see Box 10.6).

Box 10.6 Example of activities featuring in the Japanese adaptation

The pilot study conducted as part of the adaptation of CST to Japanese culture revealed it was necessary to modify the content of eight sessions. For example, crossword puzzles were not a suitable activity for the word games session, therefore 'Shiritori,' a Japanese traditional word-chain game was included instead. Based on the results from the first pilot, the content of eight sessions out of the 14 was amended and subsequently validated by a second pilot as described below in phase 5. The Japanese adaptation is described in Chapter 11.

Phase 5: synthesising stakeholder (participants and facilitators) feedback from pilot studies and finalising the culturally adapted intervention

For this phase it is recommended that facilitators and participants involved in the culturally adapted pilot in phase 4 are asked to take part in interviews or focus groups to elicit feedback regarding their experiences. For instance what they found useful, what they did not like, and their recommendations for programme improvement (see Box 10.7). Additional recommendations can be integrated in the adapted programme manual. The workgroup developing the adaptation can use this information along with their own experiences and produce the final version of the adapted CST manual.

Box 10.7 Example of addressing logistical considerations from the Tanzanian and Nigerian adaptation

For the Tanzanian and Nigerian adaptation it was noted that questions posed to participants had to be culturally sensitive and consider how much information the group would be comfortable sharing. An important element was to avoid asking for personal information in the discussion, particularly names or numbers of children they had, unless participants decided to share this information themselves. Logistical considerations such as access to a comfortable table and chairs, refreshments, and bathroom facilities were considered very important. Most participants were expecting a small gift after the sessions, so a token such as a sweet, was given at the end of every session for group members to give to their grandchildren.

Step by step case example of adapting CST using the guidelines: the German adaptation of CST

Phase 1: generating knowledge and collaborating with stakeholders

Issues related to the development of the culturally appropriate German intervention for people with dementia were discussed at two different events. Discussions were facilitated by the lead for the CST adaptation in Germany.

1 A workshop at the International CST Conference in London, July 2015: participants at this stage were psychologists and occupational therapists from Germany, the Netherlands, and Denmark. The topics discussed in this workshop included; (i) the dementia healthcare system in Germany, and (ii) the ways in which education of health professionals in Germany differs from other European countries, and how these general conditions affect delivery and distribution of CST.
2 A meeting at the National Dementia Guidelines Committee in Berlin, January 2016: all delegates attending this meeting worked in dementia-related health professions, such as neurologists, psychiatrists, geriatricians, occupational therapists, speech therapists, physiotherapists, nurses, clinical psychologists, and neuropsychologists. The topics included for discussion in this meeting were the evidence-based recommendations of CST for specific outcomes. The Committee decided to recommend CST as a psychosocial intervention for improvement of cognition. Improvement of QoL and depression in some randomised controlled trials (RCTs) should be mentioned in the guidelines, however, without recommending CST as a specific intervention for these outcomes.

Results from the two events indicated that for successful implementation of the adapted programme in Germany, detailed materials would be needed in order to enable health professionals without scheduled preparation time, or nursing staff educated with a focus on a biomedical rather than psychosocial care approach, to prepare CST sessions quickly. For example, printable worksheets with word games, family tree, thinking card questions, photographs of artwork, or advertisements should be provided.

Regarding the German Guidelines, CST received a strong recommendation as the only manual-based (and therefore, standardised and replicable) psychosocial intervention. Outcome measures were discussed for use in research as well as therapy evaluation. It was suggested that the Alzheimer's Disease Assessment Scale (ADAS-Cog; Mohs et al., 1997) should be replaced by the more commonly used CERAD-NP (Consortium to Establish a Registry for Alzheimer's Disease, www.memoryclinic.ch) battery, the latter having the advantage of being a more appropriate measure of verbal episodic memory (word list delayed recall). It was recommended that the equivalence of both measures should be tested in the pilot study. QoL was considered as a possible secondary outcome. The severity of depressive symptoms, but not a Diagnostic and Statistical Manual of Mental Disorders (DSM) diagnosis of major depression, was considered as a further suitable secondary outcome as many patients suffer from depressive symptoms without fulfilling the full range of diagnostic criteria. However, on a single case level, CST may act like a 'pleasant activities' programme. Self-efficacy scales, which are also suitable for non-depressed populations and shown to be sensitive to other types of psychosocial interventions, (Kurz et al., 2012; Fankhauser et al., 2017) were also considered as outcome measures in the pilot study.

Phase 2: integrating generated information with theory and empirical and clinical knowledge

The CST translation and adaptation project was presented at the German Annual Meeting Neuropsychologists' conference in September 2016, which was attended by both clinicians and scientists. In this meeting, the activities included in the CST programme were linked to separate cognitive functions: the utility of the regular repeated structure of the sessions in addressing the prevailing procedural memory capacities of people with dementia (which are usually better preserved as episodic memory) was acknowledged. In addition, the CST key principle of presenting different options and encouraging group members to make choices was linked to the fact that recognition memory is better preserved than free recall. Executive functions, although exercised in every session, were considered to be specifically addressed in sessions such as Categorising Objects and Thinking Cards.

Moreover, CST was compared to other types of interventions available in the country shown in Table 10.1.

The RO component and possible tensions with a humanistic, person-centred approach was specifically discussed. Compared to other countries, German age cohorts from the 1930s and 1940s may have experienced a more authoritarian teaching style, including physical violence, in their childhood within the

Table 10.1 Interventions for people with dementia available in Germany

Intervention	*Summary description*
Neurotransmitter stimulation	Acetylcholinesterase inhibitors (AChEI), pharmacological treatment
Reality Orientation (RO)	Use of a whiteboard as RO board, introductory part of each session, reading and discussing actual newspaper headlines
Person-centred, validating dementia care approach	Focus on individual preferences and opinions and discussions around these
Cognitive-behavioural therapy (CBT)	Pleasant Activities and Cognitive Reframing.

context of growing up in a dictatorial regime. It was agreed that in order to avoid unpleasant associations or memory blockades, questions about the current date and location, as well as certain word games or number games, should be presented in a pleasant and humorous manner, as a group quiz rather than as an individual test or enquiry.

Phase 3: reviewing and revising the initial culturally adapted intervention with stakeholders

After the workshop and meetings, the manual was translated into German using the forward and back translation method suggested in the CST guidelines. In addition, the German team adapting the intervention discussed the adaptation with the developers of the original CST manual in the UK to confirm that the adapted programme remained true to CST key principles. Professionals working in dementia care were invited to attend a focus group to further discuss the adapted version and advise on whether the intervention could be easily accepted amongst their clients and in their particular settings. An initial review of the translated manual was done by two neuropsychologists, one psychology student, and a social worker from two settings: a community setting and a residential home. The focus group recommended the following points:

- The manual title should contain the term 'stimulation', similar to the English version, instead of another German synonym used in previous translations, to be recognisable, and easily associated to research reports.
- The title 'Making a Difference', was in this context considered to be confusing. Instead, Vol. 1 and 2 of the manual should be distinguished by the terms 'Basic course' and 'Advanced course'.
- To facilitate a '2 in 1' use of the two manuals, the overview of corresponding sessions should be provided in a prominent place, and corresponding sessions of the Basic and Advanced course should be highlighted throughout the manual.
- The titles of the sessions should focus on the topic (Words, Numbers, Money) rather than on the aspect of 'gaming', which is synonymous with 'playing' in the German language, and might be associated with children's games.
- Some of the suggested games, like 'hangman' or skittles are also common in Germany. However, others, such as 'thinking cards', were replaced by common games such as 'Denk fix', which also involves cards with short person-related or knowledge-related questions, e.g.: 'Things that can fly' or 'What decorates a person'. A small turntable determines the first letter of the answer, or the colour of a box from which the card is drawn. Bingo, which is less popular in Germany than in other European countries, was replaced by the popular 'memory' game (searching for pairs of cards) in different variants, with famous faces, artwork, or household objects, which were either presented openly or face down.

Phase 4: testing the culturally adapted intervention

A feasibility assessment of the adapted CST intervention was held at both study sites using the adapted manual. The basic course of CST sessions took place from May to July 2016. Sessions were led by a neuropsychologist assisted by a research assistant. Patients were included if they had mild to moderate dementia (diagnosed according to the DSM-IV criteria; American Psychiatric Association [APA], 1994), were aged 65 years or over, were able to engage in group activity for up to an hour, were able to understand simple instructions, communicate verbally, and had no agitation or psychosis. The CST basic course was tested in a community setting as well as residential home setting.

Phase V: finalising the culturally adapted intervention

After the feasibility pilot study, the CST manual was further adapted based on the findings. The main aims of the feasibility study were: (1) to assess the feasibility of conducting CST sessions in settings in Germany, (2) to assess the acceptability of the adapted CST sessions for people with dementia and their carers, and (3) to identify any areas for further adaptation.

Once all sessions were completed, the clinicians, patients, and carers were asked to give feedback. Key outcome measures for the pilot study were administered including the ADAS-Cog, the CERAD-NP, which also involves the Mini-Mental State Examination (MMSE) (Folstein et al., 1975), the Quality of Life-Alzheimer's Disease Scale (QoL-AD; Logsdon et al., 1999), the Center of Epidemiological Studies depression questionnaire (CES-D; Eaton et al., 2004), and the General Self-efficacy scale (GSE; Schwarzer and Jerusalem, 1995). Despite the small number of participants, significant improvements were found in the ADAS-Cog and the GSE scale.

Commentary and reflections

CST impact worldwide

National and international policy makers are now starting to pay attention to the huge potential of CST. In 2011, the NHS Institute for Innovations concluded that CST can save the NHS £54.9 million a year through reduced use of antipsychotic medication. In 2012, the Memory Services National Accreditation Programme (MSNAP) (run by the Royal College of Psychiatrists) included CST as one of their key standards for accreditation. They now report that, consequently CST is used in 66% of memory clinics. Worldwide, CST is now used; the manual has been adapted and translated into Japanese, Spanish, Italian, German, Portuguese, Dutch, and Swahili. Since 2008 CST has been used in numerous developed and developing countries including Australia, Nepal, Tanzania, Brazil, China, and Nigeria. As a result, an international CST centre has recently been established at University College London (UCL) that includes 24 countries in which CST is available.

The guidelines presented in this chapter prove a useful framework for the adaption of CST and ensure that the adapted programme retains the same principles, effectiveness, and impact on clinical outcomes for people with dementia as the original CST programme (Spector et al., 2003; Orrell et al., 2014). The guidelines allow a structured approach to ensuring cultural acceptability. In the UK, CST techniques have been applied successfully as an intervention within South Asian ethnic groups who did not have English as their first language (Mahmood et al., 2012). This suggests that, provided that it is modified to be culturally specific, CST can be used effectively in a variety of populations, retaining its effectiveness in clinical outcomes.

The World Alzheimer's Report 2014 recommends that CST should routinely be given to people with early stage dementia around the world. It advocates using CST especially in developing countries in order to provide an effective low-cost intervention to help improve cognition and QoL. Therefore, these guidelines are very valuable and will support future CST adaptations worldwide.

Final remarks and future CST adaptations

These practical recommendations provide guidance on how to culturally adapt the content and structure of CST to make it suitable for other cultures, without compromising on its effectiveness. The recommendations were based on clinical and practical experience plus evidence from a review of the most common frameworks that have been used to adapt therapy to other cultures. In particular, the guidelines have been grounded in the FMAP framework and its five phases. The available evidence from small studies of the adapted programmes indicates that they are also of benefit (Yamanaka et al., 2013; Mkenda et al., 2016).

Although guidelines were developed and CST continues to be adapted for different cultures, further studies will need to explore the cultural influences as a critical point. As previous literature shows, culture affects the understanding of dementia, utilisation of services, and caring experiences for family members and formal caregivers (Janevic et al., 2001; Mahmood et al., 2013; Yamanaka et al., 2013). Therefore, it is expected that interventions that are developed with culturally and linguistically well-defined community-based methods may best fit the standards, needs, and expectations of that culture and beliefs system, that we know influence beliefs and attitudes (Mukadam et al., 2011). Therefore, further research should pay attention to how culturally explained definitions of old age and dementia in the different societal contexts where the intervention occurs, will shape and influence the effectiveness of CST.

Despite European consensus on outcome measures for psychosocial intervention research in dementia care (Moniz-Cook et al., 2008), worldwide there is little evidence available in relation to which outcome measures to use to evaluate effectiveness, preventing meaningful comparisons between different studies and interventions. Further studies will need to explore this and reach consensus in order to better understand the effectiveness of adapted interventions such as CST.

References

Aguirre E, Spector A, Streater A, Hoe J, Woods B and Orrell M. (2012). (2011). *Making A Difference 2: an evidence based group program to offer maintenance Cognitive Stimulation Therapy (CST) to people with dementia.* UK: Hawker Publications.

American Psychiatric Association. (2000). *Diagnostic criteria from DSM-IV-TR.* American Psychiatric Pub.

Bernal G, Bonilla J, Bellido C. (1995). Ecological validity and cultural sensitivity for outcome research: Issues for the cultural adaptation and development of psychosocial treatments with Hispanics. *Journal of Abnormal Child Psychology.* 23(1):67–82.

Bernal G, Jiménez-Chafey M, Domenech Rodríguez M. (2009). Cultural adaptation of evidence-based treatments for ethno-cultural youth. *Professional Psychology: Research and Practice.* 40.

Blay, SL, Toledo, P, Peluso, E. (2010). 'Public stigma: the community's tolerance of Alzheimer disease'. *American Journal of Geriatric Psychiatry.* 18:163–171.

Cohen AB. (2009). Many forms of culture. *American Psychologist.* Apr;64(3):194.

Domenech-Rodriguez M, Wieling E. (2005). Developing culturally appropriate, evidenced-based treatments for interventions with ethnic minority populations. In: Rastogi M, Wieling E, editors. *Voices of color: First-person accounts of ethnic minority therapists.* Thousand Oaks, CA: Sage Publications. 313–34.

Eaton WW, Smith C, Ybarra M, Muntaner C, Tien A. (2004). Center for Epidemiologic Studies Depression Scale: review and revision (CESD and CESD-R). In: Maruish ME, editor. *The use of psychological testing for treatment planning and outcomes assessment: Instruments for adults.* 3rd ed. Mahwah, NJ: Lawrence Erlbaum. 363–77.

Enjolras, F. (2005). 'Incidence du pronostic sur la construction des modèles explicatifs de la maladie d'Alzheimer à l'île de la Réunion'. *Sci Soc Santé;* 23:69–94.

Falicov CJ. (2009). Commentary: On the wisdom and challenges of culturally attuned treatments for Latinos. *Family Process.* 48:292–309.

Fiske AP. (2002). Using individualism and collectivism to compare cultures – A critique of the validity and measurement of the constructs: Comment on Oyserman et al. (2002). *Psychological Bulletin.* 128:78–88.

Folstein MF, Robins LN, Helzer JE. (1975). The mini-mental state examination. *Archives of General Psychiatry.* Jul 1;40(7):812.

Goffman E. (1963). *Stigma: Notes on the Management of Spoiled Identity.* New York: Simon & Schuster.

Hwang WC. (2006). The psychotherapy adaptation and modification framework: Application to Asian Americans. *American Psychologist.* Oct;61(7):702.

Hwang WC. (2009). The formative method for adapting psychotherapy (FMAP): A community-based developmental approach to culturally adapting therapy. *Professional Psychology: Research and Practice.* Aug;40(4):369.

Janevic MR, Connell CM. (2001). Racial, ethnic, and cultural differences in the dementia caregiving experience recent findings. *The Gerontologist.* Jun 1;41(3):334–47.

Jeste, DV, Alexopoulos, GS, Bartels, SJ, et al. (1999). *Consensus statement on the upcoming crisis in geriatric mental health: research agenda for the next two decades. Archives of General Psychiatry.* 56:848–853.

Kurz A, Thöne-Otto AIT, Cramer B, Egert S, Frölich L, Gertz HJ, Knorr C, Kehl V, Wagenpfeil S, Werheid K (2012). CORDIAL: Cognitive rehabilitation and cognitive-behavioural treatment for early dementia in Alzheimer's disease. A multi-centre, randomized, controlled trial. *Alzheimer's Disease and Associated Disorders,* 26, 246-253.

Lau A. (2006). Making the case for selective and directed cultural adaptations of evidence-based treatments: Examples from parent training. *Clinical Psychology: Science and Practice.* 13(4):295–310.

Logsdon RG, Gibbons LE, McCurry SM, Teri L. (1999). Quality of life in Alzheimer's disease: Patient and caregiver reports. *Journal of Mental Health and Aging.* Jan 1;5:21–32.

Mahmood S, Ahmed S, Orrell M, Kinsler H. (2012). Developing Cognitive Stimulation Therapy (CST) for dementia with South Asian ethnic groups. In *27th International Conference of Alzheimer's Disease International.* 7–10.

Mkenda S, Olakehinde O, Mbowe G, Siwoku A, Kisoli A, Paddick SM, Adediran B, Gray WK, Dotchin CL, Adebiyi A, Walker RW. (2016). Cognitive stimulation therapy as a low-resource intervention for dementia in sub-Saharan Africa (CST-SSA): Adaptation for rural Tanzania and Nigeria. *Dementia.* Jun 21:1471301216649272.

Mohs RC, Knopman D, Petersen RC, Ferris SH, Ernesto C, Grundman M, Sano M, Bieliauskas L, Geldmacher D, Clark C, Thai LJ. (1997). Development of cognitive instruments for use in clinical trials of antidementia drugs: Additions to the Alzheimer's Disease Assessment Scale that broaden its scope. *Alzheimer Disease & Associated Disorders.* Jan 1;11:13–21.

Moniz-Cook E, Vernooij-Dassen M, Woods R, Verhey F, Chattat R, Vugt MD, Mountain G, O'Connell M, Harrison J, Vasse E, Dröes RM. (2008). A European consensus on outcome measures for psychosocial intervention research in dementia care. *Aging and Mental Health.* Jan 1;12(1):14–29.

Mukadam N, Cooper C, Livingston G. (2011). A systematic review of ethnicity and pathways to care in dementia. *International Journal of Geriatric Psychiatry.* Jan 1;26(1):12–20.

NHS Institute for Innovation and Improvement. *An economic evaluation of alternatives to antipsychotic drugs for individuals living with dementia.* Matrix Evidence. 2011 Oct.

Nicolas G, Arntz DL, Hirsch B, Schmiedigen A. (2009). Cultural adaptation of a group treatment for Haitian American adolescents. *Professional Psychology: Research and Practice.* 40.

Orrell M, Aguirre E, Spector A, Hoare Z, Woods RT, Streater A, Donovan H, Hoe J, Knapp M, Whitaker C, Russell I. (2014). Maintenance Cognitive Stimulation Therapy for dementia: Single-blind, multicentre, pragmatic randomised controlled trial. *The British Journal of Psychiatry.* Jun 1;204(6):454–61.

Pollitt PA. (1996). Dementia in old age: An anthropological perspective. *Psychological Medicine.* Sep 1;26(5):1061–74.

Poveda AM. (2003). An anthropological perspective of Alzheimer disease. *Geriatric Nursing.* Feb 28;24(1):26–31.

Rosselló J, Bernal G. (1996). Adapting cognitive-behavioral and interpersonal treatments for depressed Puerto Rican adolescents. In: Hibbs and Jensen PS, editors. *Psychosocial treatments for child and adolescent disorders: Empirically based strategies for clinical practice.* 157–85.

Rosselló J, Bernal G. (1999). The efficacy of cognitive-behavioral and interpersonal treatments for depression in Puerto Rican adolescents. *Journal of Consulting and Clinical Psychology.* 67(5):734–45.

Schwarzer, R., & Jerusalem, M. (1995). *Generalized Self-Efficacy scale. Measures in health psychology: A user's portfolio. Causal and control beliefs,* S. 35–37.

Spector A, Thorgrimsen L, Woods B, Orrell M. (2006). *Making a difference: An evidence based group programme to offer Cognitive Stimulation Therapy (CST) to people with dementia: Manual for group leaders*. UK: Hawker Publications.

Spector A, Thorgrimsen L, Woods BO, Royan L, Davies S, Butterworth M, Orrell M. (2003). Efficacy of an evidence-based Cognitive Stimulation Therapy programme for people with dementia. *The British Journal of Psychiatry*. Sep 1;183(3):248–54.

Werner, P. (2005). 'Social distance towards a person with Alzheimer's disease'. *International Journal of Geriatric Psychiatry,* 20:182–188.

Whitehouse, PJ, Gaines, AD, Lindstrom, H, Graham, JE. (2005). 'Anthropological contributions to the understanding of age-related cognitive impairment'. *Lancet Neurology.* 4:320–326.

World Health Organization. *Dementia: a public health priority*. (2012). World Health Organization.

Yamanaka K, Kawano Y, Noguchi D, Nakaaki S, Watanabe N, Amano T, Spector A. (2013). Effects of Cognitive Stimulation Therapy Japanese version (CST-J) for people with dementia: A single-blind, controlled clinical trial. *Aging & Mental Health*. Jul 1;17(5):579–86.

Chapter 11

Japan

Katsuo Yamanaka, Yugo Ueda, and Chihiro Matsuda

Need to develop a Japanese version of CST (CST-J)

Japan already has an ageing population which continues to grow rapidly. The proportion of the population over 65 years old was 26.7% in 2015, and the proportion of people over 75 years old was 13.6%, which is the highest figure worldwide (Ministry of Health, Labour and Welfare: MHLW, 2016a). Moreover, there were 65,692 centenarians in Japan (MHLW, 2016b). In line with increasing numbers of older people, the number of people with dementia is also increasing; the most recent government estimate was approximately 4.62 million in 2012 (MHLW, 2014), which is about 15% of the Japanese population over 65 years old. This means that one-tenth of the worldwide population with dementia is Japanese, as estimated by Alzheimer's Disease International (2015).

Elderly care, including dementia care, is currently one of the most pressing political issues in Japan. In an effort to tackle the problem, a long-term care system began in 2000 with reviews taking place approximately every five years. The system is based on social insurance and consists of many types of services including conventional institutional care and various types of home-style care. In addition, many kinds of 'day care' services are available. In 2011, the long-term care system law was revised (Health and Welfare Bureau for the Elderly in MHLW, 2011) to create a community-based integrated care system, which has been in place since 2012. The priority of the social service system is to enable people, especially the elderly, to live a life of quality in their own familiar community until the end. Under this principle, 'community-based integrated care centres' were created in each local area. For the elderly, these centres provide care services and activities to maintain their health and prevent disabilities, solutions and safeguards against problems such as elderly abuse, and for developing their social resources.

In terms of care methods for elderly people with dementia, many psychosocial approaches aiming to improve function and QoL have been imported from other countries and implemented, including Reminiscence Therapy (Butler, 1963), Reality Orientation (Holden and Woods, 1982), Validation (Feil, 1993), and Humanitude (Gineste and Marescotti, 2007). Learning Therapy, which is expected to improve the cognitive function of people with dementia, was developed by a Japanese research group (Kawashima et al., 2005). However, in general Japanese specialists seem to pay less attention to evidence-based approaches compared to other developed countries. For example, Cognitive Stimulation Therapy (CST) and Behavioural Management Technique (BMT), based on applied behavioural analysis, have consistently obtained a higher grade of recommendation compared to other psychosocial approaches for people with dementia (Livingston et al., 2005; Olazarán et al., 2010). However, for BMT in Japan, only a preliminary study without a control group was implemented (Sato et al., 2013). There have been some studies of other cognitive-stimulation-based approaches with small samples and no blinding or randomisation (Matsuda, 2007; Matsuda et al., 2010). Group CST is a well-structured programme which has acquired the highest grade of recommendation for impact on QoL (Cooper et al., 2012). Yet, despite evidence suggesting CST warranted investigation, CST had not been fully implemented in Japan. As such, our research group identified the need to develop a Japanese version of the intervention. One of the most important reasons for pursuing the development of CST was that it is a manual-based approach, which allows for easy administration of sessions. Many psychosocial approaches have not been disseminated in Japanese care settings for this reason. In addition, it is particularly important that basic training in CST is concise and takes only one day (Cognitive Stimulation Therapy, 2017). Our research group also acknowledged that cultural adaptation is necessary for programmes originally developed in other counties, noting there were no studies for adaptations of geriatric psychosocial programmes imported from other countries in Japan. As a result, our work on adapting the original UK version of CST to create CST-J, suitable for use in Japanese culture, is innovative.

Development of CST-J

CST has been translated and adapted, and is used in care and health service settings in many countries. It is recommended that the development of versions of CST for other cultures should be based on 'Guidelines for adapting cognitive stimulation therapy to other cultures' (Aguirre et al., 2014). These guidelines emphasise a community-based developmental approach for adapting CST, outlining the five phases of the formative method for adapting psychotherapy (FMAP) by the Medical Research Council (MRC) (Campbell et al., 2000). However, our research group developed CST-J before the publication of these guidelines, and in the absence of well-known frameworks for cultural adaptation of psychosocial interventions. Instead, we were able to use a reference for adaptations of assessment scales (Steis and Schrauf, 2009).

In the adaptation of assessment scales, it is essential to use the same tasks as the original versions and confirm if the instructions and questions are translated precisely. However, this framework was limited for adaptations of activity-based interventions such as CST. Most of the activities (games and quizzes) featuring in the original CST programme depend heavily on British culture. Essentially, the activities are examples based on the theme of each session. Therefore, we decided that if the activities did not exist in Japanese culture, we would find comparable activities retaining the cognitive characteristics of each original activity. The development of CST-J followed a four-stage process (Yamanaka et al., 2013):

1 Directly translate the original programme to Japanese (translation by three experts)
2 Administer a pilot study to Japanese people with dementia using the translated version
3 Amend sections of the programme, which were found to be unfamiliar and unsuitable for Japanese culture according to the results of the pilot study. Create samples of alternative activities similar to the original ones, according to the theme and purpose of each session
4 Re-administer a second pilot study. Adopt alternative activities which appear to fit to Japanese culture based on the results

Based on a manual translated into Japanese according to the process outlined above, a pilot study was administered. We found it was necessary to modify much of the content which seemed unsuitable for Japanese culture. For instance, crossword puzzles which feature in the word games session are not familiar in Japanese culture, therefore 'Shiritori', a Japanese word-chain game, was introduced as a replacement. In a similar way, the contents of eight sessions ('Sounds, Food', 'Faces/Scenes', 'Word associations', 'Being creative', 'Categorising objects', 'Using money', 'Number games', and 'Word games') were modified by the translators including the first author of this chapter (KY). Subsequently, the suitability of the modified contents (e.g. that participants could understand and play 'Shiritori' more easily than crossword puzzles) was confirmed through a second pilot study before we finalised the CST-J programme.

In the process we followed, we did not have a phase of consultation with participants, family carers, and care staff members as is recommended in the guidelines for cultural adaptation of CST (Aguirre et al., 2014). Other than this, the process was very similar.

In addition, we adapted the way in which sessions were conducted. For instance, when meeting someone for the first time, Japanese people tend to worry about whether their words and behaviour are out of place or not. For this reason, it is traditionally thought that Japanese people do not like to be seen as different or distinguished from other members as a behavioural norm. Moreover, some participants with dementia experience executive dysfunction, such as having difficulty planning how to introduce themselves. Therefore, in the first part of the first session, and also again in the first half of all sessions, facilitators show the format of a simple introduction on a whiteboard, such as giving their full name, or nickname, and place of birth, etc. After that, facilitators guide each member to introduce themselves, prompting them by pointing and explaining each process shown on the whiteboard where necessary. Facilitators help the participants bond with each other, using techniques such as repeating the information after individuals introduce themselves and applauding.

In all sessions, we consciously took time to administer each part of 'Introductions' including self-introduction, ice-breaking activities, singing a theme song, and discussing topics about orientation to time and place so that people would feel comfortable. In addition, we used a whiteboard to show themes and quizzes rather than distributing papers amongst the group, so that all participants could concentrate on the same point, focus more, and communicate more with the group.

CST-J studies

Controlled clinical trial (Yamanaka et al., *2013)*

Here, we briefly introduce the findings of a controlled clinical trial of the adapted intervention (Yamanaka et al., 2013). Readers may access details of the trial in an article provided at the URL given in the reference list.

Method

We compared a treatment group (n = 26) in which members participated in CST-J sessions, and a control group (n = 30) who didn't participate in any treatment outside of usual activities (e.g. short stretching exercises, annual events).

Outcomes

Blind assessments were conducted for cognition, QOL, and self-reported mood. Additionally, proxy ratings of QOL and mood of participants were made by care workers who were not blinded to group allocation. The outcomes were:

1 Cognition measured by COGNISTAT (Neurobehavioral Cognitive Status Examination, Northern California Neurobehavioral Group, 1995) and MMSE (Mini-Mental State Examination, Folstein et al., 1975)];
2 QOL measured by Quality of Life-Alzheimer's Disease Scale (QoL-AD, Logsdon et al., 1999) and EQ-5D (EuroQol Group, 1990)];
3 Mood measured by a face scale developed by Lorish and Maisiak (1986), and later modified by Tabira et al. (2002).

Analyses

Based on the intention-to-treat (ITT) principle, a linear mixed model was used for analyses of cognition and QOL. The Mann-Whitney U test was used for the face scale of mood rated by five ranks.

Results

Cognition was significantly improved in the CST-J treatment group compared to the control group (COGNISTAT, $p < .0017$; MMSE, $p = .003$). Regarding QOL, EQ-5D was significant ($p = .019$) and QoL-AD showed a positive trend ($p = .060$) when rated by care workers, although not when rated by the participants themselves. The results of the Mann-Whitney test showed significant improvements in the face scale for mood, rated both by the participants ($p = .009$) and the care workers ($p = .017$).

Conclusion

In Japanese care settings, CST-J may improve cognition, mood, and aspects of QOL for people with dementia.

Impact to the specific areas of cognitive function

In order to further understand the functions of CST, we felt it would be important to investigate the specific cognitive areas on which the CST-J impacts. This was not possible in the study described above (Yamanaka et al., 2013). However, in a second study, we re-analysed data to examine these outcomes again in more depth.

Analysis

We used MMSE and COGNISTAT data from our previous study (Yamanaka et al., 2013). Changes from the baseline of scores of each subscale in these tests were compared between the treatment group and the control group. The Mann-Whitney U test was used for the analysis, since the ranges in subscales were limited. For the nonparametric test, we used data without missing values. Regarding analysis of the MMSE, we had complete data from 25 of the 26 participants in the treatment group, and all 30 participants of the control group. We had complete data for analysis of the COGNISTAT from 24 of the 26 participants in the treatment group, and 29 of the 30 participants in the control group. Using this data, we calculated the effect sizes (Cliff, 1993) of the differences between the groups in each subscale.

Results

Table 11.1 shows the results of the analysis of cognitive subscales. In the MMSE, 'orientation', and 'attention & calculation' were significantly improved in the treatment group compared to the control group. In addition, a trend towards significant improvement in the 'language' subscale was observed in the treatment group. As for COGNISTAT, 'orientation', 'construction', 'calculation', and

Table 11.1 Change from baseline of treatment group and control group

	Change from baseline Treatment group		*Change from baseline Control group*		*Mean difference (Mann-Whitney test)*		*Effect size (cliffs d)*
MMSE	mean	(sd)	mean	(sd)	Z	p	
Orientation	0.60	1.66	−0.43	2.01	−2.03	0.034	0.32
Registration	0.00	0.00	−0.07	0.25	−1.30	0.193	0.07
Attention & Calculation	0.44	1.53	−0.13	1.04	−2.10	0.035	0.29
Recall	−0.12	0.83	0.17	0.95	1.03	0.304	0.15
Language	0.68	1.63	0.03	1.22	−1.83	0.067	0.28
COGNISTAT							
Orientation	1.04	2.69	−0.41	1.80	−2.13	0.033	0.32
Attention	0.75	3.40	0.28	2.42	−1.05	0.294	0.14
Comprehension	1.38	2.93	0.31	2.21	−1.13	0.261	0.17
Repetition	−0.42	1.64	0.38	1.95	0.93	0.352	0.15
Naming	0.50	1.62	0.28	2.05	−0.18	0.854	0.03
Constructions	0.63	0.92	−0.21	1.68	−2.14	0.032	0.32
Memory	0.17	1.34	0.00	1.54	−0.22	0.829	0.03
Calculations	1.00	1.77	−0.62	1.21	−3.53	0.001	0.50
Similarities	0.46	1.06	0.38	1.24	−0.50	0.620	0.07
Judgement	0.50	0.98	−0.07	0.75	−2.24	0.025	0.34

'judgement' improved significantly more in the treatment group than in the control group.

Discussion

It was common in both the MMSE and COGNISTAT tests that the score in subscales for orientation was improved. Thus, it could be said that CST-J improves orientation. Taking time to administer the 'introduction' part of CST-J sessions including topics about orientation to time and place may contribute to this positive effect. Moreover, improvements in the calculation subscales of both cognitive measures were observed. This skill is measured by asking the person to perform mental calculations, which are thought to be related to attention span and working memory. Frequent opportunities to concentrate on the same point using a whiteboard might activate those cognitive functions. 'Attention' in COGNISTAT was measured in a similar way to attention span, but did not improve significantly. The subscale consisted of simple digit span tasks, which were comparatively easy for all members with mild or moderate dementia in both groups. As a result, a significant difference between the two groups could not be detected. Regarding 'construction' and 'judgement' in COGNISTAT, completing activities such as puzzles and quizzes in CST-J may account for the positive effects on these subscales. 'Language' in MMSE showed a trend for significant improvement. Although COGNISTAT includes subscales which directly evaluate language function, these are different from those evaluated using the ADAS-Cog, which is the measure used in the original CST trial (Spector et al., 2010). Therefore, CST-J may also be able to improve language in a similar way to the original trial, but this could not be detected with the measures used.

Conclusion

CST-J may impact on several cognitive skills including orientation, calculation, construction, and judgement.

Training

Procedure

The development of a system of staff training is vital in order to provide high quality CST-J to participants. As a basic study before constructing the system, we examined the development of 14 care workers in a group home, who were trained as co-facilitators. They attended a one-day training session in which CST-J was explained to them including the aim, the principles, structure, and procedure, contents of the sessions, and roles of co-facilitators. Subsequently, three care workers rotated as co-facilitators in each session of CST-J. The leaders were clinical psychologists (YU and CM).

Qualitative results

During the initial sessions (one to four), the co-facilitators often did not understand how they should interact with participants with dementia, and were confused. For example, they often responded to instructions from the group leader in the same way as the participants, rather than as co-facilitators, and sometimes pointed out mistakes made by the participants, making comments such as 'Funny. I definitely said so, but she didn't remember that'. During middle sessions (five to ten), they were more able to wait for responses from the participants, prompting them in a timely way, and talking with them naturally and gently according to the theme of the session and the guidance of the leader. Moreover, interactions with co-facilitators and participants often continued after the session. In this way, co-facilitators' skills were improved, yet it still appeared difficult for them to share participants' comments or ideas and improve relationships between group members. However, during later sessions (11–14), they were more able to do so.

Quantitative results

Co-facilitators' (n = 8) scores on the general self-efficacy scale (GSES, Sakano and Tojo, 1986) improved significantly between the pre and post-intervention periods (Wilcoxon signed rank test; $Z = 2.12$, $p = .034$). The effect size for paired nonparametric data (Hand, 1992), labelled as 'PS_{dep}' (Grissom and Kim, 2012) was .75.

Conclusion

Our study indicated that carers were able to gradually develop in their role as co-facilitators, and improve their self-efficacy in the delivery of CST-J.

Benefits and challenges of implementing CST in Japan

The CST-J manual was published in 2015 (Yamanaka et al., 2015) and is very useful for Japanese practitioners who wish to implement CST-J. In the manual, we described basic technical points of group work, for example, recommending seating layouts for staff members and group members to cater for cases in which group members have special needs such as hearing loss. The manual also includes guidance to help practitioners implement CST-J easily including the preparation of standard sheets of procedures for 'introductions', and techniques for therapists and carers to help participants with mild to moderate dementia and other needs to enjoy the games and quizzes in each session. The contents of the manual were approved by the original authors of CST in the UK. Additionally, a series of tips for administering CST-J written by the first author (KY) was featured in a Japanese popular magazine targeting staff members in care settings. It is hoped that these tips will also be useful references for implementation of CST-J in real care settings.

A challenge which may affect the widespread implementation of CST-J in Japan is the lack of supervisors to administer training of CST-J. Another is the difficulty of choosing people with mild and moderate dementia who are appropriate targets for CST-J, as almost all Japanese care settings are mixed so there are people with varying levels of severity of dementia as well as older people without dementia who have other care needs. As a consequence, it could be a challenge for administrators not to hurt the residents' feelings by dividing them into groups – those who may participate in CST-J and those who may not. It would be preferable to create activities for people without dementia to enjoy in another place while CST-J is held. However, there is typically a lack of staff members available to hold additional activities since they are engaged in other work including physical care of people with severe disabilities and coping with severe behavioural and psychological symptoms of dementia. Other challenging points are difficulties of making appropriate size groups for CST-J and finding spaces for activities in most care settings.

Future directions for CST-J

In order to disseminate CST-J further, it is necessary to educate and train new supervisors. Moreover, we should administer more training seminars of CST-J. After that, it would be preferable to establish a clear, standardised, training and supervision system. It would also be useful to create a casebook for supervisors and members of staff containing case studies and frequently asked questions resources as an additional tool alongside training. The uptake of CST-J countrywide could be increased by encouraging national organisations to recommend the intervention.

References

Aguirre, E., Spector, A. and Orrell, M. (2014). Guidelines for adapting Cognitive Stimulation Therapy to other cultures. *Clinical Interventions in Aging*, 9, pp. 1003–1007. doi:10.2147/CIA.S61849.

Alzheimer's Disease International. (2015). *World Alzheimer Report 2015, Alzheimer's Disease International*. Available at: www.worldalzreport2015.org/ (Accessed: 23 November 2016).

Butler, R. N. (1963). The life review: an interpretation of reminiscence in the aged. *Psychiatry*, 26, pp. 65–76. Available at: www.ncbi.nlm.nih.gov/pubmed/14017386 (Accessed: 23 November 2016).

Campbell, M., Fitzpatrick, R., Haines, A., Kinmonth, A. L., Sandercock, P., Spiegelhalter, D. and Tyrer, P. (2000). Framework for design and evaluation of complex interventions to improve health. *BMJ (Clinical Research ed.)*, 321(7262), pp. 694–696. Available at: www.ncbi.nlm.nih.gov/pubmed/10987780 (Accessed: 23 November 2016).

Cliff, N. (1993). Dominance statistics: ordinal analyses to answer ordinal questions. *Psychological Bulletin*, 114(3), pp. 494–509. doi:10.1037/0033-2909.114.3.494.

Cognitive Stimulation Therapy, 2017. *Training and Events*. Available at: http://www.cstdementia.com/page/training-and-events [Accessed 28 February 2017].

Cooper, C., Mukadam, N., Katona, C., Lyketsos, C. G., Ames, D., Rabins, P., Engedal, K., de Mendonça Lima, C., Blazer, D., Teri, L., Brodaty, H. and Livingston, G. (2012). Systematic review of the effectiveness of non-pharmacological interventions to improve quality of life of people with dementia. *International Psychogeriatrics*, 24(6), pp. 856–870. doi:10.1017/S1041610211002614.

EuroQol Group. (1990). EuroQol – a new facility for the measurement of health-related quality of life. *Health Policy (Amsterdam, Netherlands)*, 16(3), pp. 199–208. Available at: www.ncbi.nlm.nih.gov/pubmed/10109801 (Accessed: 23 November 2016).

Feil, F., 1993. *The Validation Breakthrough: Simple Techniques for Communicating with People with Alzheimer's and Other Dementias*. Baltimore: Health Professions Press.

Folstein, M. F., Folstein, S. E. and McHugh, P. R. (1975). Mini-mental state; A practical method for grading the cognitive state of patients for the clinician. *Journal of Psychiatric Research*, 12(3), pp. 189–198. Available at: www.ncbi.nlm.nih.gov/pubmed/1202204 (Accessed: 23 November 2016).

Gineste, Y. and Marescotti, R. (2007). *Humanitude: Understanding aging and caring for the elderly.* Paris: Armand Colin.

Grissom, R. J. and Kim, J. K. (2011). *Effect Sizes for Research: Univariate and Multivariate Applications, 2nd ed.* New York: Routledge.

Hand, D. J. (1992). On comparing two treatments. *The American Statistician*, 46(3), pp. 190–193. doi:10.2307/2685211.

Health and Welfare Bureau for the Elderly in Ministry of Health, Labor and Welfare. (2011). *Act for Partial Revision of the Long-Term Care Insurance Act, Etc., in Order to Strengthen Long-Term Care Service Infrastructure.* Tokyo: Health and Welfare Bureau for the Elderly in Ministry of Health, Labor and Welfare.

Holden, U. and Woods, R. (1982). *Reality Orientation: psychological approaches to the 'confused' elderly.* second edition. London: Churchill Livingstone.

Kawashima, R., Okita, K., Yamazaki, R., Tajima, N., Yoshida, H., Taira, M., Iwata, K., Sasaki, T., Maeyama, K., Usui, N. and Sugimoto, K. (2005). Reading aloud and arithmetic calculation improve frontal function of people with dementia. *The Journals of Gerontology: Series A, Biological Sciences and Medical Sciences.* Oxford University Press, 60(3), pp. 380–384. doi:10.1093/GERONA/60.3.380.

Livingston, G., Johnston, K., Katona, C., Paton, J. and Lyketsos, C. G. (2005). Systematic review of psychological approaches to the management of neuropsychiatric symptoms of dementia. *American Journal of Psychiatry*, 162(11), pp. 1996–2021. doi:10.1176/appi.ajp.162.11.1996.

Logsdon, R. G., Gibbons, L. E., McCurry, S. M. and Teri, L. (1999). Quality of life in Alzheimer's disease: patient and caregiver reports. *Journal of Mental Health and Aging*, 5(1), pp. 21–32.

Lorish, C. D. and Maisiak, R. (1986). The Face Scale: a brief, nonverbal method for assessing patient mood. *Arthritis and Rheumatism*, 29(7), pp. 906–909. Available at: www.ncbi.nlm.nih.gov/pubmed/3741503 (Accessed: 23 November 2016).

Matsuda, O. (2007). Cognitive stimulation therapy for Alzheimer's disease: the effect of Cognitive Stimulation Therapy on the progression of mild Alzheimer's disease in patients treated with donepezil. *International Psychogeriatrics*, 19(2), pp. 241–252. doi:10.1017/S1041610206004194.

Matsuda, O., Shido, E., Hashikai, A., Shibuya, H., Kouno, M., Hara, C. and Saito, M. (2010). Short-term effect of combined drug therapy and Cognitive Stimulation Therapy on the cognitive function of Alzheimer's disease. *Psychogeriatrics*, 10(4), pp. 167–172. doi:10.1111/j.1479-8301.2010.00335.x.

Ministry of Health, Labour and Welfare. (2014). *Current policy issues for dementia care in Japan.* [pdf] Tokyo: Ministry of Health, Labour and Welfare. Available at: http://www.mhlw.go.jp/file/05-Shingikai-12601000-Seisakutoukatsukan-Sanjikanshitsu_Shakaihoshoutantou/0000065682.pdf [Accessed: 23 November 2016].

Ministry of Health, Labour and Welfare (2016a). *Annual Health, Labour and Welfare Report 2016.* Tokyo: Ministry of Health, Labour and Welfare.

Ministry of Health, Labour and Welfare. (2016b). *About celebration letter and gifts to new centenarians (press release on September 13, 2016).* [pdf] Tokyo: Ministry of Health, Labour and Welfare. Available at: http://www.mhlw.go.jp/file/04-Houdouhappyou-12304250-Roukenkyoku-Koureishashienka/0000136883.pdf [Accessed: 23 November 2016].

Northern California Neurobehavioral Group. (1995). *Neurobehavioral Cognitive Status Examination (COGNISTAT).* California: The Northern California Neurobehavioral Group Inc.

Olazarán, J., Reisberg, B., Clare, L., Cruz, I., Peña-Casanova, J., Del Ser, T., Woods, B., Beck, C., Auer, S., Lai, C., Spector, A., Fazio, S., Bond, J., Kivipelto, M., Brodaty, H., Rojo, J. M., Collins, H., Teri, L., Mittelman, M., Orrell, M., Feldman, H. H. and Muñiz, R. (2010). Nonpharmacological therapies in Alzheimer's disease: a systematic review of efficacy. Dementia and Geriatric Cognitive Disorders, 30(2), pp. 161–178. doi:10.1159/000316119.

Sakano, Y. and Tojo, M. (1986). The general self-efficacy scale (GSES): Scale development and validation. *Japanese Journal of Behavior Therapy*, 12(1), pp. 73-82.

Sato, J., Nakaaki, S., Torii, K., Oka, M., Negi, A., Tatsumi, H., Narumoto, J., Furukawa, T. A. and Mimura, M. (2013). Behavior management approach for agitated behavior in Japanese patients with dementia: a pilot study. *Neuropsychiatric Disease and Treatment*, 9, pp. 9–14. doi:10.2147/NDT.S38943.

Spector, A., Orrell, M. and Woods, B. (2010). Cognitive Stimulation Therapy (CST): effects on different areas of cognitive function for people with dementia. *International Journal of Geriatric Psychiatry*, 25(12), pp. 1253–1258. doi:10.1002/gps.2464.

Steis, M. R. and Schrauf, R. W. (2009). A review of translations and adaptations of the Mini-Mental State Examination in languages other than English and Spanish. *Research in Gerontological Nursing*, 2(3), pp. 214–224. doi:10.3928/19404921-20090421-06.

Tabira, Y., Yasunaga, M., Nagamoto, N., Matsushita, H., Fukunaga, Y., Ihara, T. and Kawasuji, M. (2002). Quality of life after esophagectomy for cancer: an assessment using the questionnaire with the Face Scale. *Surgery Today*, 32(3), pp. 213–219. doi:10.1007/s005950200023.

Yamanaka, K., Kawano, Y., Noguchi, D., Nakaaki, S., Watanabe, N., Amano, T. and Spector, A. (2013). Effects of Cognitive Stimulation Therapy Japanese version (CST-J) for people with dementia: a single-blind, controlled clinical trial, *Aging & Mental Health*, 17(5), pp. 579–586. doi:10.1080/13607863.2013.777395.

Yamanaka, K., Kawano, Y., Spector, A., Thorgrimsen, L., Wood, B. and Orrell, M. (2015). *A Manual of Cognitive Stimulation Therapy Japanese Version (CST-J)*. Tokyo: Chuo-Hoki.

Chapter 12

New Zealand

Gary Cheung and Kathryn Peri

Dementia and ageing

Current healthcare services for people with dementia in New Zealand

In New Zealand (NZ) approximately 14% of the population is over the age of 65 (Statistics NZ, 2013). By 2051 this number will increase to 25%, and by 2035 the first post-war baby boomers will be reaching the age of 85. With this increase in the ageing population, by 2050 NZ will have 41,008 new cases of dementia each year and over 147,000 New Zealanders will have a diagnosis of dementia (Alzheimer NZ, 2012). This follows the worldwide trend, where dementia is doubling every 20 years. The total financial cost of dementia in New Zealand in 2008 was estimated at $712.9 million (Alzheimer NZ, 2012).

Development of dementia care pathways in New Zealand

NZ health services are primarily funded by the central government based on a community-oriented model. There are 20 District Health Boards (DHBs) of varying sizes. In 2012 the NZ Ministry of Health published a National Dementia Care Framework (Ministry of Health, 2013) to provide guidance for DHBs to plan their dementia services and develop dementia care pathways for a better coordination of dementia services. The framework aims to provide people with dementia and their families with the services they need, from diagnosis to the end of life stage, encouraging different health and social services to work together to provide people with integrated care. In this framework, Cognitive Stimulation Therapy (CST) is one of two specific treatments recommended as good practice for dementia.

Adaption and feasibility of CST in New Zealand

Little was known about the implementation of CST programmes in NZ, so a dementia sector survey was developed and conducted through the National Dementia Cooperative (NDC) in 2013. At the time of the survey, the NDC had approximately 600 members from a wide range of occupations and backgrounds including medical, nursing, allied health, carers, managers, and academics in NZ who would have knowledge of current programmes being delivered to people with mild to moderate dementia in their area. The results of the survey found only one DHB[1] was delivering CST to people with mild to moderate dementia, while a number cited financial constraints as the main barrier for non-implementation .

CST research project

Establishing that CST had had very little uptake in NZ, a feasibility study was conducted in 2014 with the aim of establishing acceptability of CST in both community and aged residential care settings (Cheung and Peri, 2015).

CST feasibility study design

This feasibility study utilised a mixed methods approach, and employed a blinded research assistant to collect data on demographics, diagnosis, and outcome measures from participants. Within-subject outcome measures included quality of life (QoL), cognitive function, self-reported depressive symptoms, and family outcomes (for example, carer burden, and self-reported health status). Informant interviews using a semi-structured interview guide were undertaken to assess perceptions of CST from participants receiving CST, their families, and practitioners delivering the programme in both the community and aged residential care settings.

Three CST groups, two in the community and one in an aged residential care facility, were tested. A total of 18 participants completed the programme. The two community groups consisted of participants recruited from Alzheimer's Auckland. Twelve participants completed the 14 CST sessions. The aged residential care facility replicated the study entry criteria that participants: (1) had a diagnosis of mild to moderate dementia, (2) had the ability to have a 'meaningful' conversation, (3) were able to see and hear well enough to participate in a small group discussion, and (4) were likely to remain in a group for 45 minutes. Six participants completed the 14 CST sessions. The study demonstrated that very few modifications were required to deliver CST programmes in NZ in either community or aged residential care settings (Cheung and Peri, 2015).

Main outcomes

This feasibility study showed similar results to other international studies. Table 12.1 shows the combined results in community and aged residential care settings at baseline and following 14 sessions of CST. Notably, there was a reduction in depressive symptoms amongst older people in the aged residential care facility. The mean Geriatric Depression Scale (GDS)-15 (Sheikh and Yesavage, 1986) score was 12 (indicating a high level of depressive symptoms)

Table 12.1 Outcome Measures at Baseline and Post-CST (Cheung and Peri, 2015)

Outcome measures	*n*	*Baseline*	*Post-CST*	*Change from baseline*	*Standard deviation*	*p-value*
ADAS-Cog	18	33.2	31.2	−2.0	5.5	0.158
MMSE	18	22.6	22.9	+0.3	2.2	0.602
QOL-AD (self-reported)	18	36.8	34.8	−2.0	5.8	0.163
QOL-AD (Family/staff-reported)[1]	17	31.7	35.2	+3.5	9.3	0.137
SF12[2]	11	94.6	93.1	−1.5	16.4	0.761
CBI[2]	11	34.0	35.3	+1.3	17.2	0.811
GDS-15[3]	6	12.2	6.7	−5.5	4.1	0.022*

[1] One participant lived alone and a family member is not available to complete this part of QOL-AD
[2] Completed only by families of participants living in the community
[3] Completed only by participants living in the aged residential care facility
* Significant at 5% level.

at baseline, and 6.7 post-CST. Across both groups there was an improvement in memory with an average increase of 0.3 points on the Mini-Mental State Examination (MMSE) (Folstein et al., 1983) and 2.0 points on the Alzheimer's Disease Assessment Scale-Cognitive subscale (ADAS-Cog) (Rosen et al., 1984). Although these results were not statistically significant (due to small sample size and lack of a control group), the amount of change was comparable to the results identified in the recent Cochrane review of CST (Woods et al., 2012). Finally, while participants receiving treatment did not report improved QoL, there was a positive trend towards this among participants as reported by their families and caregivers (Cheung and Peri, 2015).

Acceptability of CST

Qualitatively, the participants found the social engagement aspect of the group was as important as the CST activities undertaken. Being in the company of others with similar memory problems provided not only a supportive environment, but a place where they felt relaxed and comfortable.

From the perspectives of family members, benefits outside the group context were noted within two to three sessions. It was this group that coined the term 'switch on' phenomenon, arriving at this notion as they saw changes in their loved ones who had been disengaged, and at times aggressive and socially inept. Following the initial CST sessions they noticed new-found confidence, capabilities, and vastly improved communication skills (see Box 12.1).

From the CST facilitators perspectives, improving the uptake of CST in the future requires financial consideration in relation to transport and access to information technology (IT). Providing transport for CST attendees living in the community would alleviate some of the burden that families experienced in this study. Access to technological aids would allow both facilitators and participants a 'vehicle' to access resources during sessions (Cheung and Peri, 2015).

Box 12.1 Aroha's* story

Aroha is a Maori woman in her early fifties. She shares her home with her partner and several grandchildren for whom they provide support and care. This case study describes Aroha's engagement and progress while attending a community run CST programme in Auckland, New Zealand. Aroha was diagnosed with vascular dementia in her mid-forties. Her behaviour had been quite unsettling for some time. She was loath to engage in social activities, and experienced separation anxiety when her partner went out. For example, she repeatedly phoned her partner to find out where she was and when she would come home. In the last year Aroha had become increasingly unhappy and despondent. She didn't get any benefit from taking an antidepressant medication started by her family doctor six months earlier. Eventually her distress became aggression. There were several episodes of verbal aggression and the grandchildren became cautious of their Nana.

When her partner first heard of the CST programme offered by Alzheimer's Auckland Charity Trust and suggested this to Aroha, she was very distressed and said she was being forced into this activity. However, from the first CST session Aroha has been a loyal attendee. In anticipation of attending the group, she gets her clothes ready the night before so she is ready the next day for the session. Her low mood appears to have resolved. She enjoys the socialisation in the group and is spontaneous and effusive in her interactions. The episodes of aggression and separation anxiety also resolved. Aroha and her partner relate this to the enrichment provided in the group. Aroha is very happy, as are her partner and family, that she is involved in the CST programme (Cheung and Peri, 2015).

*Name changed

CST facilitator training and evaluation

While the benefits of CST have been well described, there has been a paucity of information about CST facilitator's role and competencies in the implementation of a CST programme. Spector et al. (2006) suggested that CST could be administered by a range of health professionals working in dementia care, for example nurses, psychologists, care workers, and occupational therapists.

There was not a recognised CST training programme in NZ prior to 2015. However, on the CST developer's recommendations a one-day training workshop was developed by Cheung and Peri that involves didactic teaching, group discussion, exercises, video observation, and role-play. In NZ, as CST was likely to be delivered by a range of health professionals and volunteers who have different prior learning and experience, a generic set of competencies was developed to ensure consistency in the delivery of CST.

CST competencies

We believed that mapping the CST competencies was a priority as part of the dissemination of this evidence-based treatment, and these competencies fall into three categories:

1 Knowledge – e.g. the content and principles of CST (Competency 1–4)
2 Skills – e.g. small group facilitation (Competency 5–9)
3 Attitudes – e.g. person-centred approach in dementia care (Competency 10–11)

Table 12.2 shows the 11 CST competencies and self-evaluation of facilitator's pre- and post-attendance of the one-day CST training.[2]

Table 12.2 Evaluation of the one-day CST training workshops

CST Competencies	*Pre-workshop self- evaluation*	*n*	*Post-workshop self- evaluation*	*n*	*p-value*
	1=Strongly disagree 2=Disagree 3=Neither 4=Agree 5=Strongly agree		*1=Strongly disagree 2=Disagree 3=Neither 4=Agree 5=Strongly agree*		
1. I had a good understanding of the etiologies of mild to moderate dementia, including the pathophysiology of Alzheimer's disease.	3.70	150	4.12	153	0.000
2. I had a good understanding of the clinical features of mild to moderate dementia.	3.80	148	4.20	154	0.000
3. I had a good understanding of the neuroanatomy and impact of communication and language deficits for people with dementia.	3.53	149	4.09	152	0.000

(*Continued*)

Table 12.2 (Continued)

CST Competencies	*Pre-workshop self- evaluation* *1=Strongly disagree* *2=Disagree* *3=Neither* *4=Agree* *5=Strongly agree*	*n*	*Post-workshop self- evaluation* *1=Strongly disagree* *2=Disagree* *3=Neither* *4=Agree* *5=Strongly agree*	*n*	*p-value*
4. I was confident in describing the key principles and evidence base of CST and Maintenance CST (MCST).	2.73	148	4.19	154	0.000
5. I was confident in describing the role of a CST facilitator.	2.73	148	4.32	153	0.000
6. I had a good understanding of how to apply the principles of person-centred care to CST.	3.05	150	4.32	154	0.000
7. I was confident in conducting a CST session according to the structure.	2.61	147	4.18	154	0.000
8. I was confident in facilitating group participation.	3.40	150	4.28	152	0.000
9. I have a good understanding of how to set up and implement treatment programme.	2.91	146	4.25	154	0.000
10. I have a good understanding of how to involve families and friends in treatment.	3.37	150	4.17	153	0.000
11. I am confident in evaluating clinical practice and treatment modalities, and providing feedback.	3.23	150	4.14	152	0.000

CST implementation: the current picture

In order to fully understand how trained CST facilitators were maintaining their competencies, a stock take of CST programme implementation was conducted to identify the number of CST programmes that have commenced since the training workshops as well as the barriers and challenges that trained facilitators had experienced across the country.

A questionnaire was developed and sent via email in April 2016 to 84 trained CST facilitators who attended one of the first four workshops. Fifteen CST

Table 12.3 Summary of enablers and barriers in community and aged residential care settings

	Enablers	*Barriers*
Community	• Buy-in from senior management and DHB (district health board) • Passion and vision drives the implementation of CST • People already attending day-care makes it easier to recruit and identify suitable participants • DHB professionals engaged and engaging others in the service to set and run CST • Having collaborative relationships with other NGO and DHB groups	• Finding time to train staff • Transport • Financial support • Not having enough participants to start up a group • People with more severe dementia not suitable for CST • Lack of engagement with primary health organisations • No real platform to embed CST into practice
Aged residential care	• Extra credits from Health Cert auditors recently when an accreditation audit was conducted in the facility • Having trained staff who are motivated • Improvements in residents provides a powerful message to staff • Having health undergraduate students to act as co-facilitators and a great way for them to learn about older people with dementia in an enriched environment	• Lack of staff and time • Lack of resources; financial and activity props • Not able to provide co-facilitator role with resources • CST not accepted as a routine treatment by health professionals • Unable to change the work culture; 'the way we do things around here'

facilitators from DHBs, dementia day-care centres, aged residential care facilities and the Alzheimer's Society completed the questionnaire. A summary of the enablers and barriers in both community and aged residential care settings is presented in Table 12.3.

Adaption of CST to New Zealand culture

NZ is an ethnically diverse country. With the projected increase in the incidence of dementia in coming years, a greater proportion of those with dementia in NZ will be made up of those with non-European backgrounds. The Māori

Table 12.4 Adaptation CST sessions to Māori culture

1	Physical games	Stick games, poi, creative in teamwork (e.g. taiha), Kapa Haka
2	Childhood	Pictures of marae, draw a plan of marae, mountains, rivers, Pepeha, toys made by group, knuckle bones, sweets (blackballs and barley sugars)
3	Food	Rotten corn, crayfish
4	Current affairs	Community newsletter, Māori politics
5	Faces/scenes	Pictures of maraes

Kapa Haka: Māori cultural group
Marae: Meeting House
Pepeha: Māori introductions that include places and events relating to where ancestors came from
Taiha: Weapon

population (the indigenous people of NZ) with dementia will increase from 4.0% of the total of people in 2011 to 5.7% in 2026 (New Zealand Census 2013). Adapting non-pharmacological interventions such as CST to this ethnic culture will be important.

Members of the Ngāti Whātua Ōrākei whanua group were engaged with CST key stakeholders to translate and adapt CST to the Māori culture using the evidence-based guidelines for adapting CST to other cultures (Aguirre et al., 2014). These practical guidelines ensured that the content and structure of the adapted CST programme was suitable for Māori culture without compromising its effectiveness. The adaption process followed the five phases of the formative process for adapting psychotherapy (FMAP), which included involving family caregivers, community health workers, and individuals with knowledge and expertise in Māori culture in focus groups. Information from these focus groups generated the adaptation of activities within each session and some of the specifics are detailed in Table 12.4. Currently, the Māori CST adapted version is being developed in manual form and will be piloted in the near future with a group of Māori participants with a diagnosis of mild to moderate dementia.

Future direction of CST in New Zealand

Individual cognitive stimulation therapy (iCST) project

Studies have shown and acknowledged that a number of people with dementia are often reluctant or unwilling to participate in group activities including CST (Orrell et al., 2012). As a consequence a home-based CST programme known as individual CST (iCST) was developed (Yates et al., 2015). However, the first iCST trial in the UK found no significant improvement in the primary outcomes of cognition, and QoL for people with dementia or their carers (Orgeta et al., 2015). The researchers suggested future research should investigate the efficacy of iCST when delivered by others including healthcare professionals. Internationally there has been a keen interest in continuing research to explore iCST and one such organisation in New Zealand has been Dementia Auckland.[3] This organisation in conjunction with researchers[4] from the University of Auckland is currently conducting a feasibility study to compare the efficacy of iCST (in terms of cognition and QoL) delivered by health professionals and trained volunteers with treatment as usual (TAU) for people with mild to moderate dementia.

Integrating CST with physical exercises (CogEX)

In older people it is possible to strengthen muscles, improve balance, and promote brain neuroplasticity (Petzinger et al., 2013). The idiom 'use it or lose it' applies to the brain, muscles, and systems involved in balance. There is a growing interest internationally to understand more fully the complex interaction between cognition and physical function. For example, dementia increases the risk of falling by impairing judgement, walking ability, visual-spatial perception, and the ability to recognise and avoid hazards, whereas exercise benefits those with dementia in improving behaviour and may slow the progression of functional decline (Jensen and Padilla, 2011).

Therefore, an intervention called CogEx that uses a top-down (cognitive stimulation) and bottom-up (strength and balance exercises) approach was developed by a group of Auckland researchers to address some of the modifiable falls risk factors. CogEx aims to integrate the UpRight progressive muscle strengthening and balancing programme with CST. A study testing the feasibility and acceptability of CogEx in people with dementia in Auckland is planned for 2017.

Concluding comments

We are excited about the ongoing progression of CST programmes within NZ. We believe ongoing strength will come when DHB dementia care pathways fund CST as an early treatment option for people with a diagnosis of mild to moderate dementia, and provide resources for CST facilitators to maintain their competencies, continuing education, and professional development.

Notes

1 Hawke's Bay District Health Board
2 Six workshops were conducted between May 2015 and Dec 2016. Approximately 150 facilitators have been trained in CST.
3 Previously known as Alzheimer Auckland Inc
4 Drs Kathy Peri and Gary Cheung

References

Aguirre E, Spector, A., and Orrell, M. (2014). Guidelines for adapting Cognitive Stimulation Therapy to other cultures. *Clinical Interventions in Aging*. Jun 26;9:1003–7. Available at doi:10.2147/CIA.S61849.

Alzheimer, N. Z. (2012). *Updated dementia economic impact report 2011*. Report for Alzheimer's New Zealand, Canberra, January.

Cheung, G., and Peri, K. (2015). *Cognitive stimulation therapy: A New Zealand pilot*. Auckland: Te Pou o Te Whakaaro Nui.

Dyall, L. (2014). Dementia: Continuation of health and ethnic inequalities in New Zealand. *The New Zealand Medical Journal* (Online). 127:1389.

Folstein, M. F. Robins, L. N., and Helzer, J. E. (1983). The Mini-Mental State Examination. *Archives of General Psychiatry*. 40:812.

Jensen, L. and Padilla, R. (2011). Effectiveness of interventions to prevent falls in people with Alzheimer's disease and related dementias. *American Journal of Occupational Therapy*. September/October; 65:532–40. doi:10.5014/ajot.2011.002626.

Ministry of Health. (2013). *New Zealand framework for dementia care*. Wellington: Ministry of Health. Available at:www.alz.kudosweb.com/news/dementa-a-strategic-framework-launched. [Accessed January 2017].

New Zealand Census. (2013). *Quick stats about people aged 65 and over*. Available at:www.stats.govt.nz/Census/2013-census/profile-and-summary-reports/quickstats-65-plus/population-overview.aspx [Accessed January 2017].

Orgeta, V., Leung P., Yates, L., Kang, S., Hoare, Z., Henderson, C. et. al. (2015). Individual Cognitive Stimulation Therapy for dementia: A clinical effectiveness and cost-effectiveness pragmatic, multicentre, randomised controlled trial. *Health Technology Assessment*. 19(64).

Orrell, M., Yates, L. A., Burns, A., Russell, I., Woods, R. T., Hoare, Z., Moniz-Cook, E., Henderson, C., Knapp, M., Spector, A. and Orgeta, V. (2012). Individual Cognitive Stimulation Therapy for dementia (iCST): Study protocol for a randomized controlled trial. *Trials*. 13(1):172. ISSN 1745-6215.

Petzinger, G. M., Fisher, B., McEwen, S., Beeler, J., Walsh, J. P., Jakowec, M. W. (2013). Exercise-enhanced neuroplasticity targeting motor and cognitive circuitry in Parkinson's disease. *Lancet Neurology*. Jul;12(7):716–26. doi:10.1016/S1474-4422(13)70123-6.

Rosen, W. G., Mohs, R. C. and Davis, K. L. (1984). A new rating scale for Alzheimer's disease. *American Journal of Psychiatry*. 141:1356–64.

Sheikh, J. I. and Yesavage, J. A. (1986). Geriatric Depression Scale (GDS): Recent evidence and development of a shorter version. In TL Brink (Ed.), *Clinical gerontology: A guide to assessment and intervention* (pp. 165–173). New York: The Haworth Press.

Spector A, Thorgrimsen L, Woods B, Royan L, Davies S, Butterworth M, Orrell M. (2003) Efficacy of an evidence-based cognitive stimulation therapy programme for people with dementia: randomised controlled trial. *Br J Psychiatry. Sep; 183:*248–54.

Statistics New Zealand. (2013). *Census*. Available at: www.stats.govt.nz/Census/2013-census/profile-and-summary-reports/quickstats-about-national-highlights/age-and-sex.aspx. [Accessed January 2017].

Woods, B., Aguirre, E., Spector, A. E., Orrell, M. (2012). Cognitive stimulation to improve cognitive functioning in people with dementia. *Cochrane Database of Systematic Reviews*. Issue 2;Art. No.: CD005562. doi:10.1002/14651858.

Yates, L. A., Leung, P., Orgeta, V., Spector, A., Orrell, M. (2015). The development of individual Cognitive Stimulation Therapy (iCST) for dementia. *Clinical Interventions in Aging*. 10:95–104.

Chapter 13

United States

Janice Lundy, Deborah Hayden, Marla Berg-Weger, Daniel B. Stewart, and John E. Morley

CST implementation in the United States

Currently, 5.4 million Americans live with dementia, and this number is expected to increase dramatically in coming decades (Alzheimer's Association, 2016). Alzheimer's disease is the sixth leading cause of US deaths, costing 180+ billion dollars per year; a figure that is expected to top a trillion dollars per year by 2050 (Alzheimer's Association, 2017). Available drug treatments for dementia are costly, have proven unsuccessful in altering disease course, and show varying temporary effectiveness in treating symptoms (Alzheimer's Association, 2016). US government regulations aim to reduce the use of psychotropic medication and promote first-line use of non-pharmacological interventions (Centers for Medicare and Medicaid Services, 2014).

Use of non-pharmacological dementia interventions in the United States is inconsistent and not routinely prescribed by healthcare providers. Though American providers favour use of non-pharmacological interventions for their patients, there is a lack of knowledge of evidence-based cost-effective interventions (Cohen-Mansfield and Jensen, 2008; Specht and Beattie, 2016). Resources tend to be regionally-based, including the Staff Training in Assisted Living Residences (STAR) programme in Seattle, Washington which uses Cognitive Behavioural Therapy (CBT) approaches to reduce behavioural disturbances in dementia (Karlin, Visnic, McGee and Teri, 2014; Teri, McCurry, Logsdon and Gibbons, 2005). In Missouri, building on the Scottish-based Football Reminiscence League (Tolson and Schofield, 2012), a baseball-themed reminiscence league programme was developed by Saint Louis University and the St Louis Alzheimer's Association which has now launched the creation of a number of baseball-focused reminiscence groups (Wingbermuehle et al., 2014). While evidence suggests that non-pharmacological approaches can improve cognitive function, social engagement, and quality of life (QoL), while decreasing depression symptoms, few interventions have strong evidence-based data required to justify widespread implementation.

Quantitative and qualitative evaluations show CST is an effective intervention for dementia (Spector, Gardner and Orrell, 2011; Spector et al., 2003), meeting key goals of a successful intervention as described by US healthcare professionals (Schaber and Lieberman, 2010) and the Alzheimer's Association (2016). Although the United States trails others in implementing CST, successful integration exists in the Midwest with outcomes similar to other countries. With increasingly strong evidence supporting CST as a promising dementia intervention, the authors formed a CST-focused team leading the effort to expand CST across the nation.

Interest in CST in the United States was stimulated by a visit from Professor Martin Orrell, (University College of London) in 2013 to Saint Louis University to provide CST training in St Louis and Kansas City, Missouri. Dr Amy Streater also of UCL provided in-depth training in both St Louis and at the NHC Maryland Heights skilled-care nursing facility. This led two of the authors (Lundy and Hayden) to travel to the UK and complete CST training with Dr Aimee Spector and colleagues. In 2016, Dr Spector delivered the James Flood Endowed Lecture at the Saint Louis University Summer Geriatric Institute. Dissemination of CST information, training, and resources has been primarily initiated by professionals in the US Midwest.

Adaption of CST in the United States

Development of a CST programme at a suburban skilled-care facility

In 2013, three groups of 6–10 residents received CST coupled with walking therapy at NHC Maryland Heights skilled-care facility. This 12-week programme increased Saint Louis University Mental Status Exam scores (Cummings-Vaughn et al., 2014) from 10.2 to 14.3 ($p < 0.05$) (Loraine, Taylor and McAllister, 2014). A video of this popular programme, now in its fifth year of continuous operation, is available at ageing.slu.edu.

Development of a CST programme at a rural American hospital

Perry County Memorial Hospital (PCMH), a small rural American hospital in southeastern Missouri, is the only healthcare facility in this rural county, serving a population of approximately 19,000 people, with its population of older adults (17%) significantly above state (15.7%) and national averages (14.7%) (U.S Census, 2015), and was the setting for the development of the first comprehensive CST programme. Upon introduction to CST at SLU GEC, hospital professionals now lead the CST training effort in the United States with colleagues at SLU GEC. The programme has expanded from one, six-member community-dwelling CST group to currently providing 10 CST groups per week for over 90 community and has assisted living facility residents, integrated exercise into sessions, taught caregivers to provide individual CST (iCST), and implemented CST with hospitalised patients.

Pre-programme development stage

Funding

During planning for CST, funding possibilities were explored and selection of facilitators was partially determined by funding options. In the United States, multiple heath care professionals (e. g. occupational therapists (OT), speech therapists, social workers, and psychologists) treating persons with dementia receive reimbursement from Medicare Insurance (federal health insurance programme for older adults and persons with disabilities) if clinical guidelines for treatment and time-framed goals are determined to be appropriate for each profession. Medicare guidelines for group size and time vary by profession (e.g. OT, psychologists, and clinical social workers may bill for four individuals in a one-hour session, while speech therapists have a two-person limit). Limited reimbursement for six to eight participants in an hour session is possible by two professions co-facilitating, billing for the participants with treatment goals most suitable per profession.

Considering the expertise of individual healthcare professionals within the hospital, a geriatric social worker with programme administration skills and an OT with skills in memory and cognitive processing were identified to lead the CST initiative. Speech therapists evaluated cognitive impairment as they can be reimbursed by Medicare for individual evaluation.

As only a small portion of the cost of the programme could be generated from Medicare participant billing (usually, limited to the initial 14 sessions), other funding was required. Unique to certain US counties is a Senior Tax Commission, which allocates funds from local county retail sales tax to programmes that improve health and QoL of older residents. Funding is accessed through a grant application process offered to non-profit organisations that show evidence of meeting the Commission's objectives for older adults. In 2014, the hospital was awarded the first of several grants which now provides primary funding for CST with additional support from the hospital, including space, partial programme administration, and additional resources. There is no cost to participants.

Marketing and recruitment

Initial CST marketing began by educating the medical community, specifically targeting primary care physicians. Presentation of the evidence was critical in gaining medical staff support. Additional marketing included local news publications, public radio (featuring an interview with Dr Aimee Spector (UCL), and the PCMH website (Perry County Hospital, 2016), which includes information and videos.

Physicians are the primary referral source. The integration of rapid cognitive screening (Malmstrom et al., 2015) and CST referral into primary care practice has facilitated early identification to referral. Other referrals result from CST participants, families, community marketing, and healthcare professionals.

Transportation

Due to lack of public transportation (commonplace in most rural communities) and caregiver stressors, transportation is often a barrier to healthcare. In programme planning, CST transportation was included in funding requests and now funds all transportation for participants. The hospital's private car service, along with a public transportation system and individuals/families provides transportation.

Adapting CST manuals to American culture

CST manuals are a pivotal resource for new facilitators. The English language manuals were easily adaptable for sessions focused on universal topics such as faces and scenes or favourite foods, allowing for cultural adaptation. In Perry County, the older population is primarily white, with most participants having lived only in this community. Older US adults are increasingly racially and ethnically diverse, requiring CST facilitators attend to the need for cultural competence when delivering CST. Pre-CST, comprehensive social histories, including cultural preferences, are needed to adapt CST in a culturally competent manner.

Barriers to implementation

Having established funding and staffing to support the essential elements (e.g. space, transportation, and session materials), the barriers were the unanticipated amount of time required for session development, participant screenings, and psychosocial assessments, and data collection and evaluation.

Maintenance CST (MCST) and individual CST (iCST)

Upon competition of the 14-session group intervention, all participants are offered the opportunity to participate in ongoing weekly maintenance MCST. Approximately 70% transition to MCST with nearly 50% continuing at 12 months. CST is now integrated into two assisted living facilities and one skilled nursing home in the community. To manage programme growth, additional facilitators are trained to deliver MCST with support and oversight (e.g. OT assistants, teachers, college students, and nursing aides). This transition has been successful with original facilitators assisting trainees in their early MCST sessions.

iCST training is now provided to community-dwelling participants/caregivers if the person with dementia is too frail or not appropriate for group CST. OT,

ST, nursing, and nursing aides are trained in CST key principles to deliver iCST for delirium treatment and prevention of older hospitalised patients.

Studies of CST in the rural American hospital

Comparing pre- and post-CST data, participants were evaluated for cognition, depression, QoL, and mobility with the following measures:

1 Saint Louis University Mental Status Exam (SLUMS) (Tariq, Tumosa, Chibnall, Perry and Morley, 2006)
2 Cornell Scale for Depression in Dementia (Alexopoulos, Abrams, Young and Shamoian, 1988)
3 Quality of Life-AD (Logsdon, Gibbons, McCurry and Teri, 2002)

Seventy-nine participants attended CST sessions over the span of seven weeks. Approximately 75% were female, averaging 80.35 years (SD = ± 8.39), 43% took dementia medication, and 29% resided in a care facility while 71% were community-based (Table 13.1). A paired sample *t*-test compared scores pre- and post-CST (Table 13.2). For community-based groups, SLUMS scores (cognition) were statistically significantly higher post-intervention (M = 2.85, SD = 3.73), depression was statistically lower (M = 2.66, SD = 3.28), and quality of life was statistically higher (M = 3.25, SD = 4.24). For long-term care groups, there was a statistically significant difference in SLUMS scores (cognition) (M = 1.91, SD = 3.50), depression scores (M = -2.15, SD = 3.09), and QoL scores (M = 3.52, SD = 3.20).

Table 13.1 Characteristics of participants

Characteristics	*CST Group (n = 79)*
Age (years): mean (SD)	80.35 (8.39)
Female: male ratio	3:1
Dementia Medication	43%
Community dwelling	71%

Table 13.2 Paired sample *t*-test compared scores pre- and post-CST

Measure	*CST Group (community-based)*	*CST Group (residential)*
SLUMS score: mean (SD)	2.85 (3.73)	1.91 (3.50)
CSDD score: mean (SD)	2.66 (3.28)	2.15 (3.09)
QoL-AD score: mean (SD)	3.25 (4.24)	3.52 (3.20)

Table 13.3 Paired sample *t*-test compared scores in maintenance of residential participants

Measure	*12 Months*
SLUMS score: mean (SD)	3.50 (3.75)
CSDD score: mean (SD)	2.70 (3.06)
QoL-AD score: mean (SD)	3.10 (4.15)

Table 13.4 Paired sample *t*-test compared scores in maintenance of community-based participants

Measure	*12 Month*	*24 Month*	*32 Month*
SLUMS score: mean (SD)	2.44 (3.94)	nss	4.17 (2.71)
CSDD score: mean (SD)	2.11 (3.55)	3.89 (4.83)	nss
QoL-AD score: mean (SD)	4.22 (5.73)	4.56 (5.73)	nss

nss=no statistical significance

Of the 79 participants, 32 remained in maintenance CST at 12 months (10 in long-term care and 22 in community-based group). For those in long-term care, there was a statistically significant difference in SLUMS score (cognition) (M = 3.50, SD = 3.75), depression score (M = -2.70, SD = 3.06), and QoL (M = 3.10, SD = 4.15) (Table 13.3). For those in community-based groups, there was significant difference in SLUMS score (cognition) (M = 2.44, SD = 3.94) at 12 months (Table 13.4). There was no statistically significant difference at 24 months but there was at 32 months (M = 4.17, SD = 2.71). There was a statistically significant difference in depression score at 12 months (M = -2.11, SD = 3.55), at 24 months (M = -3.89, SD = 4.83), and at 21 months (M = -4.83, SD = 2.93). Statistically significant differences in QoL scores were observed at 12 months (M = 4.22, SD = 5.73) and at 24 months (M = 4.56, SD = 5.73) but not in 32-month QoL scores.

Further innovation: incorporating exercise into CST

Research suggests exercise improves cognitive functioning and assists in improving and maintaining functional status (Lam, Chau and Wong, 2012; Yamada, Arai, Sonda and Aoyama, 2012; Herzog, Kremer, Wilson and Lindenburger, 2008). Integrating exercise into CST should then benefit cognition and functional status. Using the US Centers for Disease Control and Prevention guidelines (2014) 'Growing Stronger' with modifications for population diversity in cognition and physical levels, a 25-minute exercise component was added.

For participants in Perry County, a small subset of MCST participants (n = 18) experienced CST with exercise. Additional function-related measures were administered prior to adding exercise and at six months. A statistically significant difference in function occurred at six months for Functional Reach (M = .8 inches, SD = .45 inches) and Five Time Sit to Stand time (M = -2.82 seconds, SD = 3.45). There was no statistically significant difference in Timed Up and Go score. Participants maintained their previous change scores in all other measures, but no additional statistically significant differences were found in cognition, depression, or QoL measures. Future research should involve an exercise protocol as our initial results show promise in not only improving participant's emotional and cognitive well-being but functional health as well.

CST and yoga

The Saint Louis University CST team has investigated the efficacy of CST within institutionalised and community-dwelling older US adult populations. One study was conducted at four Missouri locations (three sites in St Louis, Missouri (urban) and one site in Perryville, Missouri (rural)). Over seven weeks, 84 older adults participated in CST with a subset (n = 21) experiencing CST with a 15-minute yoga protocol. Among all participants, there was a statistically significant improvement in cognition, depression, and QoL but no significant effect due to yoga was found (Stewart et al., 2016).

Saint Louis University CST education, training, and research

Through funding from the US Department of Health and Human Services, Health Resources Service Administration, Geriatric Education Center and Geriatric Workforce Enhancement Programme, an interprofessional team of faculty and students including medicine, social work, OT, medical family therapy, and gerontology was formed to develop and disseminate CST education and training. Utilising the 'Making a Difference' materials (Aguirre et al., 2011; Spector, Thorgrimsen, Woods, and Orrell, 2006), the team developed training, including an online information toolkit (Saint Louis University Geriatric Education Center, 2016) to support professionals and students. Currently, over 1,000 students, faculty, and professionals have been educated in CST including staff at Alzheimer's San Diego, California; Medical Psychological Associates, Tennessee; and Missouri Long Term Care Association Activity Directors.

The team's efforts have resulted in groups launching in multiple settings and populations, including: outpatient hospitals; skilled nursing and assisted living with memory support facilities; Programme for All-Inclusive Care for the Elderly (PACE – a day programme for persons who meet criteria for skilled nursing care; community-based (e.g. social service agencies) and university-based (e.g. faculty-supervised, student-facilitated groups); and home care organisations. CST training is incorporated into curricula of graduate-level OT, speech therapy, and social work programmes. While most CST training and service delivery has focused on group-based interventions, training in iCST has been conducted and iCST services are currently being offered by the university team in rural and urban locations in eastern Missouri. Research continues to assess the effects of CST and iCST within diverse populations of older adults with dementia and their caregivers.

Challenges and benefits of implementing CST in the United States

CST-related challenges include assuring appropriate group placement based on dementia severity which can be difficult due to brief assessment interactions. Realising a participant's strengths and needs can require multiple sessions. Furthermore, finding a balance of engagement and stimulation, particularly for those participants with mild cognitive impairment, is challenging; assuring that all participants are engaged. Caregivers need support and providing for group members and caregivers presents challenges. Caregivers often request professional guidance in managing fluctuating and challenging behaviours from facilitators and require support, education, and guidance in providing iCST at home. With staff turnover during programme growth, training, supporting, and monitoring facilitators can prove difficult. With long-term MCST, keeping sessions stimulating and interesting requires diligence and creativity.

Many areas of the United States have diverse populations making cultural adaption imperative to success. A particular challenge is facilitating groups whose members represent diverse cultures and ethnicities. Other challenges for broad implementation in the United States include; attaining funding for programme implementation and sustainability, particularly for ongoing MCST (e.g. transportation, staffing, training, session materials, programme space, and administration); a need for widespread dissemination supporting CST as a cost-effective, evidence-based intervention to gain physician and organisational support for programme implementation; caregiver support and education of CST benefits; and adapting CST to provide a greater challenge for those individuals with higher intellect/education and/or early dementia.

Participants and caregivers tend to respond positively to CST, comments regarding their experiences and the benefits of taking part include:

- After one year of CST participation, one group member offered: 'I look forward to coming' while her daughter shared 'Mom is more social and seems less anxious about not remembering'.
- A participant who has been involved for two and a half years declared that CST is 'Best part of my week, I am surer of myself' and her husband reports that 'Doctors said I would have to put her in a home a year ago, now it is down the road aways. She thinks more and does more now, instead of sitting in a corner crying. Changed her entire life, brought her out of her shell'.
- A caregiver whose family member is engaged in both CST and exercise comments that 'The exercise has been a great addition, she is stronger and is very faithful in doing exercises you send home'.

- Staff members reap benefits as well as one facilitator comments: 'I love seeing the positive changes in the participants'; 'I love being a part of the programme'; 'This is a wonderful programme, it is amazing to see how much it helps them.'

Future direction for CST in the United States

The US CST team continues to promote and offer training in group and iCST throughout the country and are aware of groups being formed and offered in multiple states from coast-to-coast. We are committed to continuing our efforts to enhance research, increase CST training and support, promote widespread use, and advocate for policy changes in an effort for all Americans living with dementia to have access to CST.

References

Aguirre, E., Spector, A., Streater, A., Hoe, J., Woods, B. and Orrell, M. (2011). *Making a Difference 2.* UK: Hawker Publications.

Alexopoulos, G. A., Abrams, R. C., Young, R. C. and Shamoian, C. A. (1988). Cornell scale for depression in dementia. *Biological Psychology, 23*, 271–284.

Alzheimer's Association. (2017). Alzheimer's disease facts and figures. *Alzheimer's and Dementia.* [Online] Available at: http://www.alz.org/documents_custom/2017-facts-and-figures.pdf [Accessed 17 July 2017].

Centers for Medicare and Medicaid Services. (2014). *National Partnership to Improve Dementia Care Exceeds Goal to Reduce Use of Antipsychotic Medications in Nursing Homes: CMS Announces New Goal.* [Online] Available at: www.cms.gov/newsroom/medicareleasesdatabase/Press-releases-item/2014-09-19.html [Accessed 1 November 2016].

Cohen-Mansfield, J. and Jensen, B. (2008). Nursing home physicians knowledge of and attitudes towards nonpharmacological intervention for treatment of behavioural disturbances associated with dementia. *Journal of the American Medical Directors Association, 9*, 491–498.

Cummings-Vaughn, L. A., Chavakula, N. N., Malmstrom, T. K., Tumosa, N., Morley, J. E. and Cruz-Oliver, D. M. (2014). Veterans Affairs Saint Louis University Mental Status examination compared with the Montreal Cognitive Assessment and the Short Test of Mental Status. *Journal of the American Geriatrics Society, 62*(7), 1341–1346.

Herzog, C., Kremer, A. F., Wilson, R. S. and Lindenburger, U. (2008). Enrichment effects on adult cognitive development: Can the functional capacity of older adults be preserved and enhanced. *Psychological Science in the Public Interest, 9*, 1–65.

Karlin, B. E., Visnic, S., McGee, J. S. and Teri, L. (2014). Results from the multisite implementation of STAR-VA: A multicomponent psychosocial intervention for managing challenging dementia-related behaviors of veterans. *Psychological Services, 11*(2), 200–208.

Lam, L. C., Chau, R. C. and Wong, B. M. (2012). A 1-year randomized controlled trial comparing mind body exercise (Tai Chi) with stretching and toning exercise on cognitive function in older Chinese adults at risk of cognitive decline. *Journal of the American Medical Director Association, 13*(568), 15–20.

Logsdon, R. G., Gibbons, L. E., McCurry, S. M. and Teri, L. (2002). Assessing quality of life in older adults with cognitive impairment. *Psychosomatic Medicine, 64*, 510–519.

Loraine, J., Taylor, S. and McAllister, M. (2014). Cognitive and physical stimulation therapy. *Journal of the American Medical Directors Association, 15*, 140–149.

Malmstrom, T. K., Voss, V. B., Cruz-Oliver, D. M., Cummings-Vaughn, L. A., Tumosa, N., Grossberg, G. T. and Morley, J. E. (2015). The Rapid Cognitive Screen (RCS): A point-of-care screening for dementia and mild cognitive impairment. *Journal of Nutrition and Health Aging, 19*(7), 741–744.

Perry County Memorial Hospital. (2016). *Cognitive Stimulation Therapy.* [Online] Available at: www.pchmo.org/services-CST.aspx [Accessed 15 November 2016].

Saint Louis University Geriatric Education Center. (2016). *Cognitive Stimulation Therapy.* [Online] Available at: http://aging.slu.edu/index.php?page=cognitive-stimulation-therapy-cst-project [Accessed 20 November 2016].

Schaber, P. and Lieberman, D. (2010). *Occupational Therapy Guidelines for Adults With Alzheimer's Disease and Related Disorders.* Bethesda: AOTA Press.

Specht, J. and Beattie, E. (2016). Effective nonpharmacological interventions needed now. *Journal of Gerontological* Nursing, *3*(March), 3–5.

Spector, A., Gardner, C. and Orrell, M. (2011). The impact of Cognitive Stimulation Therapy groups on people with dementia: Views from participants their carers and group facilitators. *Aging and Mental Health, 15*(8), 945–949.

Spector, A., Thorgrimsen, L., Woods, B. and Orrell M. (2006). *Making a Difference: An Evidence-based Group Programme to Offer Cognitive Stimulation Therapy (CST) to People With Dementia.* UK: Hawker Publications.

Spector, A., Thorgrimsen, L., Woods, B., Royan, L., Davies, S., Butterworth, M. and Orrell, M. (2003). Efficacy of evidence-based Cognitive Stimulation Therapy progamme for people with dementia. *British Journal of Psychiatry, 183*(3), 248–254.

Stewart, D. B., Berg-Weger, M., Tebb, S. S., Sakamoto, M., Roselle, K., Downing, L., Lundy, J. and Hayden, D. (2016). *Making a Difference: A Quasi-Experimental Study of Cognitive Stimulation Therapy (CST) for Persons With Dementia With and Without Yoga.* Unpublished manuscript.

Tariq, S. H., Tumosa N., Chibnall, J. T., Perry, H. M. and Morley, J. E. (2006). Comparison of the Saint Louis University Mental Status examination and the Mini-Mental State Examination for detecting dementia and mild neurocognitive disorder – A pilot study. *American Journal of Geriatric Psychiatry, 14*, 900–910.

Teri, L., McCurry, S.M., Logsdon, R. and Gibbons, L.E. (2005). Training community consultants to help family members improve dementia care: A randomized controlled trial. *Gerontologist, 45*(6), 802–811.

Tolson, D. and Schofield, I. (2012). Football reminiscence for men with dementia: Lessons from a realistic evaluation. *Nursing Inquiry, 19*, 63–70.

United States Census Bureau. (2015). *Quick Facts United States.* [Online] Available at: www.census.gov/quickfacts/table/PST045215/00,29157,29 [Accessed 3 November 2016].

Wingbermuehle, C., Bryer, D., Berg-Weger, M., Tumosa, N., McGillic, J., Rodriguez, C., Gill, D., Wilson, N., Leonard, K. and Tolson, D. (2014). Baseball reminiscence league: A model for supporting persons with dementia. *Journal of American Medical Directors Association, 15*(2), 85–89.

Yamada, M., Arai, H., Sonda, T. and Aoyama, T. (2012). Community-based exercise programme is cost-effective by preventing care and disability in Japanese frail older adults. *Journal of the American Medical Directors Association, 13*, 507–511.

Chapter 14

China

Zhaorui Liu, Yueqin Huang, Tao Li, and Guangming Xu

Urgent need for the implementation of cognitive stimulation therapy (CST) in China

In China, the prevalence of dementia is increasing with an unprecedented rate of ageing (Zhang et al., 2005), and as a result it has become an important public health issue.

Compared with other countries in the world, the ageing problem and care burden are more challenging in China because of the Family Planning Policy. In recent decades, this has resulted in a situation whereby relatively fewer numbers of younger children are required to take care of a larger amount of older family members. The care needs of the older population are a serious problem that cannot be ignored. Based on the Chinese Longitudinal Healthy Longevity Survey (CLHLS) (Zeng, 2010) report, 17.5% of persons aged 65 years and over needed help for their activities of daily life. Pension coverage was less than 20% in 2005, and less than 30% in 2012 (Zeng, 2013a). Financial support from children constitutes an important contribution to the daily life of older people. The percentage of people relying on financial support from their children raised from 30% for persons aged 65 to 69 years old, to 70% for persons aged 95 years and over (Zeng, 2013b). Most older people live with their children and/or spouses (Zeng, 2013b) and family members are still the main carers in China. Less than 2% of older people receive care in social care institutions (Zeng, 2013b). Similarly to the general older population, most dementia patients live at home and are cared for by unpaid family members. Professional social care institutions are very limited, even in metropolitan areas.

Current treatment of dementia in Chinese clinical practice consists mainly of pharmacologic treatment, and behavioural and psychological interventions. The aims of pharmacologic treatments are symptomatic therapy, or disease-modifying therapy. The most popular pharmacologic treatments for Alzheimer's disease are Cholinesterase inhibitor drugs (such as Donepezil or Rivastigmine), or Anti-N-methyl-D-aspartate receptor encephalitis (such as Memantine) (Li et al., 2014). There are also some reports on treatments based on the theory of Chinese traditional medicine, such as using herbs to activate bold circulation, or nourish the kidney (Wang, 2013). However, in China, compared with pharmacological strategies, the use of non-pharmacological interventions is limited. Behavioural, or psychological intervention packages are not well developed due to the lack of evidence-based information.

Although medication may slow the progression of dementia, there is no effective treatment or intervention that can prevent or cure the disease. The importance of early intervention for dementia is clear because of the features of the disease, i.e. unclear cause, no prevention, no effective treatment and fatal outcome. Current evidence already indicates Cognitive Stimulation Therapy (CST) for people with early and middle stage dementia can benefit cognition and improve quality of life (QoL) (NICE, 2006). This kind of treatment is urgently required for both older people and their family members in China in order to decrease caregiver strain and improve QoL. CST is not included in the Chinese Treatment Guidelines for Dementia, but it is not difficult to implement, and can be carried out by trained psychologists or social workers. Therefore, it would be feasible to use the intervention in clinical practice, after undergoing culture adaption.

Supported by funding from the Capital Health Research and Development of Special,[1] a research team at the Institute of Mental Health, Peking University introduced CST to China in 2012 and 2013. The CST manual was translated into Chinese and underwent cultural adaptation. Subsequently, a single-blinded randomised control trial (RCT) was carried out among Chinese dementia patients. In this chapter, we will introduce the development process of the Chinese version of CST, discuss the effectiveness and feasibility of CST in China, and provide suggestions for future directions of CST in this setting.

Development of the Chinese version of CST

The most essential step to implement CST in China was to translate the English manual of CST into Chinese, and make adaptions based on Chinese culture. The standard CST package contains 14 sessions with different themes and each theme contains several ideas for activities. The Chinese version of CST manual retains the main design of the original, but provides detailed examples, and adds some new activities.

Adaptations session by session

Adaptations to each session theme are described here; however. sessions with the same content or design as the English version are not explained here.

Session 1: physical games

This is the first session in the original CST programme, and the group is required to decide upon a name and a theme song. A selection of names is provided in the Chinese manual as examples. Words containing two Chinese characters, such as *Jian Kang* (healthy), *Kuai Le* (happy), or *Yang Guang* (sunshine) are designed for more severe dementia patients, while words including four Chinese characters, such as *Qi Cai Wan Xia* (the colourful sunset), *Gao Shan Liu Shui* (lofty mountains and flowing water), *Chun Nuan Hua Kai* (warm spring and flowers bloom) are generally used for mild dementia patients, or those with higher education levels. Similar to the group name, theme songs are also suggested in the Chinese manual. To replace playing skittles or indoor bowls, or boules, a magnetic darts game is recommended (darts with points are not suggested for health and safety reasons).

Session 2: sound

Detailed examples are provided in the Chinese manual. Indoor sounds include crashes, bangs, the sound of pots and pans, clapping, coughing, or children's laughter. Outdoor sounds include animal noises (e.g. cat, pig, dog, tiger, or bird), or the sound of vehicles (e.g. car, plane, ship, or train). Similar to the sound activity suggested in the UK version of CST, names of popular songs or singers are recommended. Questions are asked after listening to songs, such as 'which songs do you like, and why?' to encourage discussions in the group.

Session 3: childhood

Some Chinese old-fashioned childhood toys are listed in this session, such as spinning tops, a catching game played with small stones or sheep bone joints, rolling a hoop, quoits, and Kaleidoscope.

Session 4: food

A mini market with food models (e.g. food items made of plastic) is recommended in this session. It is suggested that group members use a basket to 'buy' food from the mini market. They then plan meals and calculate the price. Special dishes starting with the name of a place are provided, such as *Fu Ling* X, *Wu Chang* X, *Dong Po* X, *Xi Hu* X. For the name of a food beginning with a particular letter, *Xi* is recommended to be used, as it can generate several names of foods, such as *Xi Hong Shi* (tomato), *Xi Lan Hua* (broccoli), *Xi Gua* (watermelon), *Xi Qin* (celery), *Xi You* (grapefruit), or *Xi Hu Lu* (courgette).

Session 5: current affairs

The main idea of this session is to encourage group members to talk, and in particular to give reasons for their opinions. Some examples, which are provided in the English manual, such as gay weddings, the royal family, and favourite charity are not used in the Chinese manual, because Chinese people are not familiar with them.

Session 6: faces/scenes

Famous people, such as *Mao Ze Dong*, *Deng Xiao Ping*, *Zhou En Lai* are listed in the manual. Important sightseeing places, such as the Great Wall, the Forbidden City, and the Olympic Park are recommended for use. Moreover, discussions about the same feature of two sightseeing places are suggested. For example, there are lakes in the Summer Palace, as well as in the Bei Hai Park.

Session 7: word association

This session is more related to language and culture compared to other sessions in the CST programme. Some famous couples in Chinese culture, such as Premier *Zhou En Lai* and his wife Ms *Deng Ying Chao*, Chairman *Xi Jin Ping* and his wife Ms *Peng Li Yuan* are listed as examples. All the words of places are those of famous sites, such as *Tian An Men*, or *Wang Fu Jing*. Some Chinese well-known proverbs and idioms are listed as resources. However, these proverbs or idioms might be highly related to the education background of group members.

Session 8: being creative

In this session, the main activity is to draw pictures on eggs, which is typically an Easter-time activity in western countries. Egg models, watercolour brushes, and shining decoration pieces are provided to group members. Group members have a photo with their painted eggs to record a good memory of CST.

Session 9: categorising objects

The 'odd one out' game features in the Chinese version of the manual. Group members are asked to find one object which belongs in a different category amongst three objects. For example, in a selection of an apple, a cucumber and an onion, the apple is the odd one out as it is a type of fruit, whereas the other two objects are vegetables.

Session 10: orientation

This session retains the original idea of the English version of CST, except that magnet dots are recommended to be used to indicate places of interest on maps rather than pins.

Session 11: using money

This session also keeps the idea of the English version of CST. However, the idea of categorising objects is added in this session. Group members are asked to categorise objects first, and calculate the total price of each category afterwards.

Session 12: number games

In China, bingo and dominoes are not popular. Therefore, the point to point game (drawing lines based on the order of the numbers), and a simple matching card game named are played by group members.

Session 13: word games

In our experience, this session is the most difficult one for dementia patients. It is highly related to the education level and the stage of the disease. In this session, all activities are designed based on Chinese writing. For example, one task is to generate at least three words based on one Chinese character. Another example is to finish phrases according to special rules, such as AAB, ABB, AABB, ABAB or ABAC.

Session 14: team quiz

Word Solitaire is used in the final session. The idea is to generate a new word based on the final character of the former word. To decrease the difficulty, there is no need to keep the same character, but only to follow the pronunciation of the character.

There are key differences in the structure of each session between the original CST programme and in Chinese CST. In English CST, each session begins with an introduction (see Figure 14.1), followed by main activities, and ends in a conclusion. In the Chinese version, this main structure is retained, but the refreshments component is not used in accordance with Chinese culture. Instead, a thank-you gift is provided to each member before each session ends. Homework,

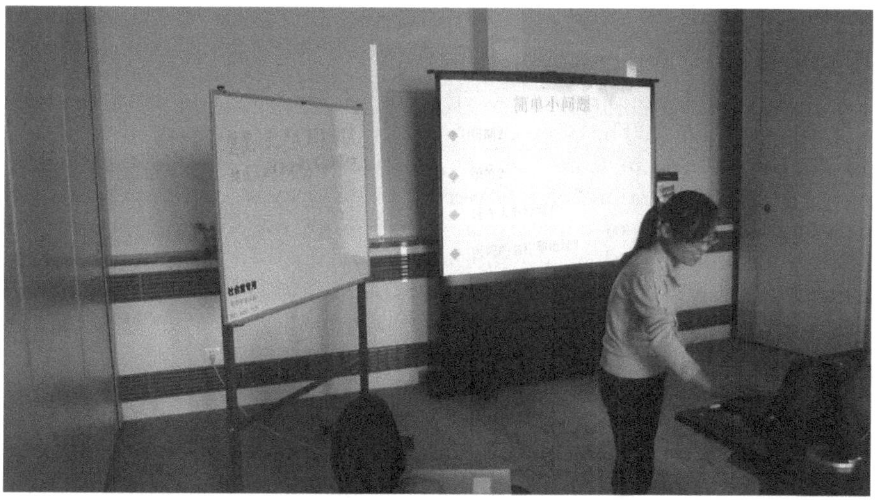

Figure 14.1 The CST group facilitator discussing location and time at the beginning of the CST session

such as writing down news or finding a poem including something specific such as a flower or season, is compulsory for each member, and it is shared within the group during the next session. Each group member has their own treatment recording book, to write their homework, or record their thoughts during or after the session, and to collect all the materials they have used in the sessions. Moreover, group members are usually divided into two small subgroups to have competitions. Each group receives a paper prize, which can be kept in their treatment recording books. A final CST certificate is given to all group members and group photos are taken and printed for each person to keep.

Effectiveness and feasibility of CST in China: findings from a trial

Method

Participants and inclusion criteria

A single-blind RCT of CST among mild or moderate dementia patients was carried out in Beijing, China from 2014 to 2016. Patients were eligible for recruitment into the trial if they met the DSM-IV criteria for a dementia diagnosis (APA, 1994), had a Mini-Mental State Examination (MMSE) (Cockrell and Folstein, 1988) score of 10 to 23, were able to see or hear well enough to participate in an activity, and were without major illness or disability which could affect their participation. Patients were divided into the intervention group and control group using a stratified randomised sampling strategy based on the severity of dementia.

Intervention

The intervention group received CST, while the control group received treatment as usual (TAU). The carers of those in the intervention group also received the 'Helping Carers to Care' (Dias et al., 2008; Gavrilova et al., 2009; Guerra et al., 2011) intervention for five weeks, which focused on health education regarding knowledge of dementia, and suggestions on how to deal with the behavioural and psychological symptoms of dementia (BPSD). All carers were requested to stay in the same room with patients during the CST sessions, but they were not allowed to provide help or talk with the patients.

Outcomes

Outcome evaluations were conducted at baseline, three weeks, seven weeks, and three months by medical professionals blind to treatment allocation. Outcomes for patients included: cognitive function assessed by the MMSE, quality of life (QoL) from the person with dementia's perspective based on Dementia Quality of Life Questionnaire (DEMQoL) (Smith et al., 2007), and behavioural and psychological symptoms of dementia evaluated by Neuropsychiatric Inventory Questionnaire (NPI) (Kaufer et al., 2000). Outcomes for caregivers include care burden measured by the Zarit Caregiver Burden Interview (Zarit et al., 1980), QoL judged by World Health Organisation Quality of Life-Brief (WHO, 1998), and physical and mental health collected by Self-Report Questionnaire-20 (Livianos Aldana et al., 1990).

Results

Preliminary findings suggest evidence of delayed deterioration of cognitive function during CST. Caregiver strain also decreased in carers of those receiving CST. However, at the three-month follow-up, these improvements were not detected. In addition to the quantitative evaluation of the intervention, qualitative interviews were conducted with a sample of patients and their caregivers to gather feedback on their experience of CST. Most caregivers were spouses of the patients and were familiar with the CST sessions. Many carers reported they thought CST could be used to prevent cognitive impairment, and taking part in similar stimulating activities might be beneficial for their own memory problems. They also learned ways to communicate more effectively with the patients. For example, they said they followed the ideas and principles of CST outside sessions at home. In addition, they encouraged the patients to have discussions, focusing on the emotional needs of the patients, rather than the answers. Carers also suggested that the research group should carry out CST in the community, rather than in hospitals, which they felt would be more convenient. Most carers and patients were satisfied with the arrangement of the CST sessions, and they said they felt very happy after finishing them. Indeed they said they would like to attend more, if further CST sessions were provided.

Interpretation

The findings of the trial suggest the current Chinese version CST is effective during the treatment period, and it is feasible and acceptable. However, our findings show the seven-week duration of treatment may not be enough to maintain cognitive benefits, and as such more sessions may be required. We also experienced several challenges in implementation. Firstly, participant retention was an issue. Patients tended to drop out if they lived far away from the hospital where the groups were run, or their carers were too busy to help them travel to the groups. Secondly, although the manual recommends that patients with same level of cognitive status or education backgrounds should be included in the same group, it is difficult to organise groups in this way, as patients usually come to see doctor individually. Therefore, it could take a long time to recruit enough patients for a particular group. The interactions between patients and their carers might be important to the outcome of the CST, particularly the understanding and use of the key principles of CST (e.g. respect, fun, opinions rather than facts, and building/strengthening relationships).

Current application of CST and future directions

After the Chinese version of CST was developed in Beijing at the Institute of Mental Health, Peking University, psychiatric hospitals in other cities, including Tianjin, Wuxi (in Jiangsu Province) and Hangzhou (in Zhejiang Province) showed an interest in the programme. Recently, a group of psychiatrists and psychotherapists at the Department of Rehabilitation in Tianjin Anding Hospital began CST sessions for people with dementia and patients with mild cognitive impairment. A psychiatrist was trained by the Beijing team to carry out CST in a geriatric ward at Wuxi Mental Health Centre, and a research team at the Seventh Hospital in Hangzhou also has plans to carry out CST in communities.

The next step for CST in China is to carry out culture adaptation of maintenance CST (MCST) (Orrell et al., 2014) and individual CST (iCST) (Yates et al., 2015), and conduct RCTs to test the effectiveness of the adapted programmes. An RCT to investigate the effectiveness of MCST supported by Beijing Municipal Science and Technology Commission will be conducted from 2017 to 2020. Furthermore, based on the experiences from the hospital-based treatment, community-based CST should be developed and more CST therapists should be trained to provide services in the community, in order to increase accessibility of CST amongst the older population. Although it has been reported that the iCST might not improve cognitive function (Orgeta et al., 2015), it is still worth examining the effectiveness of iCST in Chinese settings because most patients live with their family members, therefore home-based iCST could be delivered easily. Caution may need to be taken regarding the compliance and self-motivation of the carers when implementing iCST. Similar to the idea of electronic mental health (E-mental health) (NHS, 2014) programmes and services, electronic CST (E-CST) based on the use of information and communication technologies might also be the future direction of CST in China. The availability of iCST would be valuable as human resources of mental health professionals is limited.

Note

1 Grant number: Shou Fa 2011–4024–05

References

APA. (1994). *Diagnostic and Statistical Manual of Mental Disorders*, fourth version (DSM-IV), Washington, DC, Ameican Psychiatric Association.

Cockrell, J. R. and Folstein, M. F. (1988). Mini-Mental State Examination (MMSE). *Psychopharmacol Bull*, 24, 689–92.

Dias, A., Dewey, M. E., D'souza, J., Dhume, R., Motghare, D. D., Shaji, K. S., Menon, R., Prince, M. and Patel, V. (2008). The effectiveness of a home care program for supporting caregivers of persons with dementia in developing countries: A randomised controlled trial from Goa, India. *PLoS ONE*, 3, e2333.

Gavrilova, S. I., Ferri, C. P., Mikhaylova, N., Sokolova, O., Banerjee, S. and Prince, M. (2009). Helping carers to care – The 10/66 dementia research group's randomized control trial of a caregiver intervention in Russia. *Int J Geriatr Psychiatry*, 24, 347–54.

Guerra, M., Ferri, C. P., Fonseca, M., Banerjee, S. and Prince, M. (2011). Helping carers to care: The 10/66 dementia research group's randomized control trial of a caregiver intervention in Peru. *Rev Bras Psiquiatr*, 33, 47–54.

Kaufer, D. I., Cummings, J. L., Ketchel, P., Smith, V., Macmillan, A., Shelley, T., Lopez, O. L. and Dekosky, S. T. (2000). Validation of the NPI-Q, a brief clinical form of the Neuropsychiatric Inventory. *J Neuropsychiatry Clin Neurosci*, 12, 233–9.

Li, M., Zhang, W., Chen, T. and Liu, L. (2014). Evaluation of medication treatment for Alzheimer's disease on clinical evidence. *Chin J Contemp Neurol Neurosurg*, 14, 192–7.

Livianos Aldana, L., Rojo Moreno, L., Dominguez Carabantes, A. and Bofill Moscardo, I. (1990). Validation of the SRQ in mental health examinations of the general public. *Actas Luso Esp Neurol Psiquiatr Cienc Afines*, 18, 286–9.

NHS. (2014). *E-mental Health: What's All the Fuss About?* Available: www.nhsconfed.org/~/media/Confederation/Files/Publications/Documents/E-mental-health.pdf.

NICE. (2006). *Improving Health and Social Care Through Evidence-based Guidance*. Available: www.nice.org.uk/guidance.

Orgeta, V., Leung, P., Yates, L., Kang, S., Hoare, Z., Henderson, C., Whitaker, C., Burns, A., Knapp, M., Leroi, I., Moniz-Cook, E. D., Pearson, S., Simpson, S., Spector, A., Roberts, S., Russell, I. T., De Waal, H., Woods, R. T. and Orrell, M. (2015). Individual Cognitive Stimulation Therapy for dementia: A clinical effectiveness and cost-effectiveness pragmatic, multicentre, randomised controlled trial. *Health Technol Assess*, 19, 1–108.

Orrell, M., Aguirre, E., Spector, A., Hoare, Z., Woods, R. T., Streater, A., Donovan, H., Hoe, J., Knapp, M., Whitaker, C. and Russell, I. (2014). Maintenance Cognitive Stimulation Therapy for dementia: Single-blind, multicentre, pragmatic randomised controlled trial. *Br J Psychiatry*, 204, 454–61.

Smith, S. C., Lamping, D. L., Banerjee, S., Harwood, R. H., Foley, B., Smith, P., Cook, J. C., Murray, J., Prince, M., Levin, E., Mann, A. and Knapp, M. (2007). Development of a new measure of health-related quality of life for people with dementia: DEMQOL. *Psychol Med*, 37, 737–46.

Wang, E. (2013). Using herbs of reinforcing kidney and activating blood to treat AD. *Liao Ning J Chin Med*, 40, 1867–8.

WHO. (1998). The World Health Organization Quality of Life Assessment (WHOQOL): Development and general psychometric properties. *Soc Sci Med*, 46, 1569–85.

Yates, L. A., Leung, P., Orgeta, V., Spector, A. and Orrell, M. (2015). The development of individual Cognitive Stimulation Therapy (iCST) for dementia. *Clin Interv Aging*, 10, 95–104.

Zarit, S. H., Reever, K. E. and Bach-Peterson, J. (1980). Relatives of the impaired elderly: Correlates of feelings of burden. *Gerontologist*, 20, 649–55.

Zeng, Y. (2010). *Research on Elderly Population, Family, Health and Care Needs/Costs*, Beijing, Science Press.

Zeng, Y. (2013a). Chinese longitudinal healthy longevity survey and related policy research review: Part I. *Sci Res Aging*, 1, 67–72.

Zeng, Y. (2013b). Chinese longitudinal healthy longevity survey and related policy research review: Part II. *Sci Res Aging*, 1, 63–71.

Zhang, Z. X., Zahner, G. E., Roman, G. C., Liu, J., Hong, Z., Qu, Q. M., Liu, X. H., Zhang, X. J., Zhou, B., Wu, C. B., Tang, M. N., Hong, X. and Li, H. (2005). Dementia subtypes in China: Prevalence in Beijing, Xian, Shanghai, and Chengdu. *Arch Neurol*, 62, 447–53.

Chapter 15

India

Sridhar Vaitheswaran, Monisha Lakshminarayanan, and Shruti Raghuraman

Introduction

The number of older people in India has increased to over 100 million (8.6%), and is expected to grow further. Consequently, India is facing many health and social issues associated with older people (Central Statistics Office – Ministry of Statistics and Programme Implementation, Government of India, 2016). A rising public health concern is that of increased prevalence of dementia, which has a devastating impact on those living with the illness, as well as their families. It is estimated that there are 4.4 million people with dementia in India currently, and by 2040 this number is expected to reach over 10 million (Alzheimer's and Related Disorders Society of India, 2010).

To cope with this rising prevalence of dementia, it is important to strengthen protocols of effective management. Drug interventions (e.g. cognitive enhancers) have been beneficial in helping those with dementia (NICE, 2011). However, it is important for drug therapies to be supplemented with non-pharmacological interventions to improve clinical outcomes and delay the progression of the illness. There is a general consensus among experts in the field regarding the importance of non-pharmacological interventions in dementia management (Yamaguchi, Maki, and Yamagami, 2010; Takeda et al., 2012).

Cognitive Stimulation Therapy (CST) has been shown to be effective in improving cognition and quality of life (QoL) in persons with dementia. Data from randomised control trials (RCTs) (Spector et al., 2003; Knapp et al., 2006) have demonstrated the efficacy and cost-effectiveness of CST. Moreover, this data is supporting by findings from qualitative examination of the subjective experiences of CST, wherein participants perceived emotional and cognitive benefits following the programme (Spector, Gardner, and Orrell, 2011).

CST has thus far not reliably been tested for efficacy in India. In order to apply the programme to the local sociocultural setting, it is imperative to culturally adapt and test the programme for acceptability and feasibility. This chapter describes the adaptation of CST for use in Chennai, India.

Chennai is the capital city of the state of Tamil Nadu in India. It is located in the southeast coast of the Indian peninsula. The Chennai metropolitan area has a population of about 8.6 million (Census of India, 2011). It has a diverse and eclectic population, as it is an important economic, cultural, and educational centre in South India. It has retained a traditional and conventional image, despite being quite modern. The region has a rich cultural heritage that is reflected in its unique forms of music, dance, food, and architecture. The predominant language spoken is Tamil, although many residents are bilingual and also speak English. The literacy rate of the city is around 90% (Census of India, 2011).

Researchers at the Schizophrenia Research Foundation (SCARF) conducted a feasibility study to assess the adaptability of Cognitive Stimulation therapy (CST) for persons with dementia in Chennai, India, under the Dementia Care in SCARF (DEMCARES) project. In addition, preliminary data on outcome measures was collected to assess the direction of change post-intervention.

Method

A mixed-methods model involving qualitative methods and a non-randomised unblind approach was conducted to assess the acceptability and feasibility of CST. Limited efficacy data was also collected to determine whether the programme showed promise of having a positive impact on participants in line with other studies of CST (Aguirre, Woods, Spector, and Orrell, 2013) (Spector et al., 2003).

The five-phase adaptation process adhered to the published guidelines for the adaptation of CST to other cultures (Aguirre, Spector, and Orrell, 2014), which utilise the formative method for adaptation psychotherapy (FMAP).

Phase I: generating knowledge and collaborating with stakeholders

A focus group discussion was conducted with key stakeholders who work closely with persons with dementia. This group of participants was comprised of a general physician, a geriatric psychiatrist, two formally trained nurse practitioners, a psychologist, the centre manager of a local dementia day centre, a senior research coordinator, and a caregiver of a person with dementia. These individuals were contacted and invited to participate for their individual expertise in the field of dementia care and research. The group was first given a brief presentation on CST and the adaptation process by the moderator of the session.

Activities

Participants were invited to examine the CST manual closely to initiate discussions around each session. They were asked to share their thoughts on the feasibility and relevance of all CST activities in the local setting. If certain items were not considered applicable in our cultural setting, suitable alternatives were identified by the group.

Some activities were viewed as culturally inappropriate by participants, and were replaced with suitable alternatives.

1 'Childhood Memories' – Recreating a childhood bedroom was the original activity suggested. However, the concept of a separate bedroom for a child is foreign to people from this cultural upbringing. Therefore, it was modified to recreating festivals, celebrations, and memories of group members' childhood homes.
2 'Food' – Meal planning and cooking activities suggested were considered problematic because Indian meals are complex and involve a lot of ingredients, even if it is only breakfast. Moreover, it is uncommon for men from the older generation to be involved in household chores, such as cooking. For this session, it was suggested that participants be asked to plan and budget for a meal for a predetermined number of guests, which is a gender-neutral activity that is suitable for the specific theme.

New, culturally relevant items were generated for some sessions to replace the UK equivalents in the manual. For example –

1 'Word Associations' – Associations involving measurements were replaced with culturally relevant terms. One 'mozham' is a measurement commonly used in Chennai to measure flowers by the length of one's forearm. Participants were required to match the term with 'flowers'.
2 'Faces and Scenes' – Famous personalities were also used for associating them with iconic movies or other celebrities. Comedian 'Goundaṃani' is usually associated with his famous sidekick 'Senthil' which paralleled 'Laurel and Hardy' in the manual.
3 'Team Quiz' – 'Antakshari' which is a very popular game all over India was suggested. It is usually played with two or more teams. The first team sings a song (usually from a regional film) and stops abruptly. The next team must start another song with the letter/sound that the previous team ended with immediately. It is a very fast-paced game where all members are on edge to quickly think of a song as soon as the previous team stops singing.

Activities that were found to be culturally appropriate for a particular theme were added. For example, a traditional counting game called 'Pallanguzhi' was added as an option to the Number Games session. Pallanghuzi, is a traditional mancala game played in South India. The game is played by two players, with a wooden board that has 14 pits, each of which contain five or seven cowry shells/seeds/small pebbles used as counters. Pallanguzhi is popular among children and older people (Kandasamy, 1999).

Phase 2: integrating generated information with existing theoretical frameworks

Apart from session-wise discussions, the structure of the programme, scheduling, and logistics were also discussed in detail and key changes were made where appropriate.

Scheduling

The experts in the group found the recommended schedule of 45-minute sessions, twice a week to be suitable for this setting. However, it was also thought that caregivers using their own transport would find it hard to pick up clients within an hour of dropping them off for the sessions. Chennai is a big city, and participants may be spread out across its length and breadth. In order to justify the travel time for session attendance, it was recommended that clients spend at least 2–3 hours at the centre overall. Moreover, due to lack of respite facilities in India for caregivers of persons with dementia, it was discussed that a programme such as this could serve as a source of respite for family caregivers.

As to the timings, it was agreed that late morning to early afternoon would be the best time to hold the sessions because it would enable informal caregivers, who are mostly women with other family responsibilities, to arrange for the client to be brought to the centre on time. Thus, it was scheduled such that groups would meet by 11 AM, for the start of the CST session at 11.30 AM. This buffer period of half an hour would help ensure that if any of the participants were delayed (due to traffic or other unforeseen circumstances), they would not miss too much of the session.

Following the CST activity, it was suggested that participants should have lunch together with the facilitators and then return home. Eating is a social activity in India, and including the lunch element as part of the programme was believed to increase the chances of bonding and fostering familiarity among the group and with the facilitators.

Logistics

Transport was discussed as a crucial point of concern. Clients participating in the programme hail from different sections of society, and not all of them will be able to arrange for transport on their own. The logistics of organising transport was discussed, and experts were of the opinion that the availability of transport could potentially ensure regular attendance as well as punctuality for the sessions.

Structure of sessions

It is customary to provide tea and snacks upon the arrival of guests in Indian culture. This resulted in scheduling tea time just as clients arrive at the centre, before the start of the CST activity. During this half hour period, it was anticipated that clients could interact and socialise when one another, which was seen as crucial for the success of the group session format. This also ensured that participants wouldn't feel rushed into the activity upon arrival, allowing them time to relax before the start of the session.

An induction period of two weeks was incorporated into the programme to help the participants familiarise themselves with the setting and the group. Participants were encouraged to get to know one another by taking part in informal activities such as board games such as chess or carom board. Facilitators were also encouraged to engage the participants actively in discussions about current affairs, international news, and other topics of relevance to the participants. This period of induction was deliberately unstructured, as it was necessary for the staff to establish rapport with the participants. Eight participants were invited to attend this period of induction along with their caregivers to determine who would be best suited for participation in the programme. During this period, some participants dropped out for personal reasons, or because they were not well suited to the group environment. For example, during the induction it became clear that some clients required more individualised attention than it was possible to provide in the group. Others were unable to participate fully because of communication difficulties or other symptoms suggestive of stress and distress in dementia, such as agitation that were not obvious initially in the outpatient setting. Having an induction period such as this can be a useful means of finding a cohesive group, which is crucial for the success of CST.

Phase 3: review of the culturally adapted CST intervention by stakeholders, and further revision

Following the focus groups with key stakeholders, the manual was modified. It was not possible to schedule a second focus group due to unavailability of experts. Instead, the amended manual was emailed to the first group of experts who reviewed the changes and provided further feedback. Upon implementation of this feedback, the final manual was then reviewed with the CST group facilitators who were going to implement the programme. Materials and items that were to be part of the programme were individually assessed, and further changes to resources were made to make the activities more culturally relevant. For example, in the faces and scenes activity, the UK resources were replaced with equivalents that would be familiar to Indians and Tamilians, including popular movie actors from the past such as M. G. Ramachandiran (popularly known as MGR) and 'Sivaji' Ganeshan; political figures such as Indira Gandhi and Jawaharlal Nehru; and places such as the well-recognised steps of bathing ghats in Varanasi or the Taj Mahal. A list of all modifications, additions, and deletions completed before the implementation of the activities described in the 'Making a Difference' CST manual is shown below (Table 15.1).

Table 15.1 Modifications made before pilot study

Session	*Theme*	*Reasons for modifications based on data from focus groups*	*Modifications*
3	My Life	The concept of personal bedroom is not familiar to Indian participants and indigenous festivals and religious customs during occasions would be more relevant and easily recreated.	Activity involving drawing on memories of festivals and celebrations were added to the forms that they were required to complete
4	Food	Planning and preparing a meal is not equally familiar to both genders. Most men of the generation participating in the CST would not have traditionally cooked. Local recipes are complex and it might not be feasible to obtain all the ingredients required to prepare a single dish.	Participants were asked to budget and plan tea and snacks from the items that were displayed for a predetermined number of guests.
9	Categorising objects	Using familiar and culturally relevant activities would increase participation.	The activities in the manual were relevant but some categorising games that were familiar to the participants were added like 'Name, place, animals, things'
12	Number games	Participants may not be familiar with the concept of dominoes.	Playing dominoes was removed while bingo (also locally known as 'housie') was retained. Other culturally relevant number games like 'Pallanguzhi' were added.

Phase 4: testing the culturally adapted intervention

Once the manual was adapted based on the recommendations from key stakeholders and group facilitators, the programme was tested on two subsequent groups of participants. The first pilot (P1) took place at the DEMCARES Resources and Training Centre. The main facilitator for P1 was a psychologist and the co-facilitator was a nursing assistant.

The second pilot (P2) took place at the Centre for Active Ageing, which is a dementia day-care centre located in SCARF. The centre has the capacity to host up to eight participants, with enough space to carry out activities that ranged from table games to indoor physical activities. A nurse practitioner trained in CST led the group and a nursing assistant was the co-facilitator. All the staff facilitating P1 and P2 programmes were trained to deliver the programme using the 'Making a Difference' manual and the training videos.

Participants

Participants were selected from the DEMCARES outpatient register, and their diagnosis was confirmed by an experienced consultant psychiatrist based on the Diagnostic and Statistical Manual of Mental Disorders – Fifth Edition (DSM-V) criteria for major neurocognitive disorder (American Psychiatric Association [APA], 2013). The main inclusion criteria were: that participants must be living with mild-to-moderate dementia, must be mobile, and must not face severe communication difficulties. An assessment of functional ability was conducted using the Instrumental Activities of Daily Living in the Elderly scale (Mathuranath, George, Cherian, Mathew, and Sarma, 2005) to ensure that participants were suitable for the programme. In addition, participants were required to be living in Chennai for the entire length of the programme and able to speak Tamil. Consent to participate was obtained from both the person with dementia and their families.

In P1, following the two-week induction, two participants withdrew from the programme, primarily due to behavioural difficulties such as agitation and inability to participate in group activities. One participant could not be included in the study as she was going to relocate to another country and would not be able to complete the programme. Five clients consented to participate in the study, of whom three participants completed the full programme.

In P2, seven potential participants were identified, four of whom agreed to participate for the entire duration of the programme. At the end of the programme, one participant dropped out for personal reasons, and three participants completed the programme.

Procedure

Assessments of cognitive function and QoL were conducted at baseline (pre-test) and within one to two weeks after completing the programme (post-test). These assessments included –

- Addenbrooke's Cognitive Examination III (Tamil and English Literate version) (ACE III) (Mathuranath, Nestor, Berrios, Rakowicz, and Hodges, 2000): to assess level of cognitive function
- Quality of Life (QoL) (Patient and Caregiver Versions) (QoL-AD) (Logsdon, Gibbons, McCurry, and Teri, 1999): a self-report tool to assess the QoL of the client, both from their own perspective as well as the perspective of their family caregivers

Sessions were conducted according to the adapted manual. After each session feedback was collected verbally from participants and from written reports by the facilitators.

Results

As P1 progressed, some structural elements and sessions were found to need further modification, as they were unsuitable in practice. These modifications are described in Table 15.2.

Table 15.2 Modifications made after the initial pilot

Activity/Session	*Activity conducted*	*Reason for modification*	*Alternative Activity*
Group song	N/A	Participants found this childish as this is a practice very common in schools.	Playing music in the background after the session. This sometimes engaged the participants who would sing along.
Being Creative	Potting plants	Gardening proved to be very difficult to conduct at the centre and might not be feasible in other settings. Other activities like knitting, seasonal collages (Chennai does not have distinct seasons) were not culturally relevant.	There were other activities in the manual that we could draw on and some culturally relevant activities were added e.g., creating Rangolis, threading flowers to make small garlands, making cardboard houses, craft work etc.
Faces and Scenes	Discussion of characteristics of faces and scenes	Participants were not interested in discussing only the characteristics and features of the scenes and faces that were displayed.	Participants were asked to share information they knew about the different faces and scenes that were displayed and recollect memories of visiting the scenes and prominent incidents that occurred with the people that were displayed.
Using Money	Guessing the prices of products	Participants were not interested in guessing prices of objects.	Comparing prices of various objects and budgeting was a more familiar concept. An activity involving listing commonly purchased items as well as large investments (real estate, appliances etc.) and their average price during the period when the participants were young adults and comparing those prices to current prices and having a discussion, was added instead.

The modifications discussed in Table 15.2 were subsequently implemented in a P2. The programme did not require any further changes after P2, and all changes to the manual were finalised and written up.

Apart from the feasibility analyses, data on outcome measures were analysed to indicate the direction of change following participation in the CST programme. Demographic data and scores on outcome measures are shown in Table 15.3.

Participants were all male, and the mean age was 76.4 years. Data was collected on outcome measures of cognition and QoL (patient and caregiver perspectives). Table 15.3 illustrates that, on average, participants showed improvements on all measures. The largest mean difference from pre-test to post-test was

Table 15.3 Demographic details and results on outcome measures from P1 and P2

ID	*Sex*	*Occupation*	*Age*	*Years of Literacy*	*ACE III*			*QoL-AD (Client)*			*QoL-AD (Caregiver)*		
					Pre-Test	*Post-Test*	*D*	*Pre-Test*	*Post-Test*	*D*	*Pre-Test*	*Post-Test*	*D*
					P1								
CST01	M	Retired agricultural expert	84	20	76	82	6	39	43	4	24	43	19
CST02	M	Retired bank manager	60	17	71	79	8	45	48	3	38	48	10
CST03	M	Retired Businessman	81	10	81	87	6	26	DO	–	17	D.O	–
CST04	M	Businessman	78	5	D.O	D.O	–	29	DO	–	24	D.O	–
CST05	M	Publisher	83	16	57	D.O	–	41	DO	–	N.A	D.O	–
					P2								
CST06	M	Building supervisor	75	10	78	84	6	27	36	9	27	39	12
CST07	M	Molding Business	70	14	63	70	7	32	29	−3	19	37	18
CST08	M	Retired Teacher	75	12	82	71	−11	39	33	−6	NA	NA	–
CST09	M	Accounts supervisor	82	11	66	D.O.	–	52	D.O.	–	NA	D.O.	–
Mean			76.4	12.77	Mean D		3.6	Mean D		1.4	Mean D		14.75

ACE III – Addenbrooke's Cognitive Examination III

QoL-AD – Quality of Life-Alzheimer's Disease Scale

D – Difference

D.O. – Dropped Out

N.A – Not Available due to absence of Caregiver

observed in the caregivers' perception of the client's QoL with a mean increase of 14.75 points. This demonstrates that caregivers found the programme to be hugely beneficial in improving the QoL of the person with dementia at home. On average, participants self-reported QoL improved by 1.4 points.

On the measure of cognitive function, participants improved on average 3.6 points from pre-intervention to post-intervention. Decline in cognitive ability was found in only one of the seven participants across P1 and P2.

This preliminary analysis of outcome measures post-CST is encouraging in that participants generally demonstrated change in a positive direction. Further examination with larger sample sizes in randomised control trials (RCTs) is necessary to establish the full-scale efficacy of CST in this sociocultural setting.

Phase 5: synthesising stakeholder (participant and facilitator) feedback from the pilot and finalising the culturally adapted manual

Feedback was collected from participants, caregivers, and session facilitators at the end of both P1 and P2. The facilitators recorded participants' responses during each session. At the end of each pilot, unstructured interviews were conducted individually with the participants to seek general feedback about the overall experience. A survey was administered to caregivers after the programme for both pilots. Written feedback on each session was provided by the facilitators and assistants who delivered each round of the programme. Finally, all of the data collected was reviewed for challenges and positive experiences in conducting and participating in the CST sessions to find suggestions for improvement.

Participant feedback

Feedback from the participants on CST as an activity was largely positive. Most participants commented on the usefulness of the sessions in eliminating boredom, and providing them with a chance to socialise and engage with others, which they felt they were lacking at home. When asked what was enjoyable about the sessions, one participant commented –

> 'At home we are just idle, looking here and there, watching television. But here, it's a mix of . . . we get to know about something, we talk about it, discussions etc. I am enjoying it and it is very useful.'

The current affairs discussion session was among the more popular activities, as participants saw this as an opportunity to get to know people and their opinions on things of importance and relevance. Politics was an especially popular, albeit mildly controversial at times, topic among the participants.

Clients complained about the duration of the sessions, especially at the end of P1. The general consensus was their time spent at the sessions was too short, and that they felt like they were being 'chased away'.

> We are coming here at 11, having lunch at 2.00 and then going home immediately. This can be avoided. You can arrange the session for a full day; you can charge for it. More people can join the session.

Therefore, it may not be ideal for CST to be provided as an isolated intervention programme. In P2, which took place at the Centre for Active Ageing, clients were invited to participate in CST as part of their day-long attendance at the Centre. Predictably, there were no complaints of 'feeling rushed' at the end of P2, which demonstrates that it may be better to schedule CST as part of a day hospital or day centre setting so that clients can spend at least half the day (5–6 hours) together. For individuals who had little to no stimulation at home, participating in CST sessions was an opportunity to socialise and engage with people, which significantly helped them overcome feelings of loneliness and isolation. One participant commented –

> I enjoy it because I am meeting people with some common interest. Since I stay alone in my house, my wife passed away recently and I am virtually alone with three helpless women helping me in the house, so coming here is a kind of a diversion.

Participants also reported that they were concerned when the group members did not attend the sessions and when some withdrew from the programme. They wanted more people to be included in the group. This further supports the argument that CST would be better received in a larger facility that can accommodate more people for longer periods of time, rather than being conducted as a stand-alone activity. When asked if they would continue to participate in the programme, all participants answered firmly in the affirmative.

Caregiver feedback

Feedback from caregivers was collected through a written survey form, and was found to be largely positive. One caregiver who usually accompanied a participant to the sessions said –

> We both feel comfortable and good. We are having (a) chance to see and talk to new friends. Hoping that your well-designed programme will give us good result(s).

Caregivers were asked to rate changes seen in their loved ones. They all found that the language/communication, behaviour, and social interaction of the person with dementia had either improved or had remained stable post-CST. No decline was reported. Caregivers also rated quality of transport, venue, and staff friendliness positively. Caregivers were happy with how informed they felt about the programme and their loved one's participation. All caregivers wished their relative to continue participating in CST in the future.

At the end of P1, some caregivers raised the importance of the venue being accessible for older people, with lifts, railings, and elder-friendly toilets. P2 took place in a dementia-friendly environment and issues with the venue were not raised at the end of this programme.

Other suggestions from caregivers, specifically after P1, included conducting activities parallel to CST. One caregiver suggested –

> Try to arrange for bhajan classes, (and) yoga classes.

Bhajans are a popular community activity in India where people chant religious songs together. Yoga is also commonly practised in groups and can be good form of physical activity for the clients. The value of these suggestions may be explored in the future.

Facilitator feedback

Facilitators reported that delivering sessions was very enjoyable. The most successful session in both pilots was the 'Faces and Scenes' session. Facilitators from both groups felt that the session progressed seamlessly without requiring too much intervention from them. One facilitator recorded the following comment in her reports:

> You can see the faces of the participant light up when they recognise a picture. They also get so excited to exchange information about the picture with other participants who can relate to it more than we can. So, the sessions would have gone well even without us!

Other sessions that were a success were 'number games' where participants played bingo, 'word association', and 'team quiz' with facts on politics and history which really interested the participants.

In contrast, facilitators from both pilot programmes struggled to get the participants involved and interested in the 'being creative' session. Allowing the participants to choose activities did not work.

> They just tell us anything is fine (by them), and we have to end up choosing the activity ourselves.

'Being creative' was also the only session where recorded ratings of interest, enjoyment, mood, and communication were low. At the end of P2, one facilitator noted:

> We had to keep insisting they participate in the activity which we usually don't do. Even if we somehow get them to be interested, we can't sustain their attention long enough to complete the session. But they did co-operate and finish the task at hand, it was just more difficult than usual.

It is our contention that participants are not used to being involved in recreational activities that are creative in nature. These kinds of activities are usually associated with children and classrooms. It was thus difficult to convince the participants to enjoy these activities as they did not find them engaging. Creative sessions may require better planning and implementation in this culture.

Facilitators also noted how important the co-facilitator was in helping to prevent participants from feeling left out when one or more of the group members dominated sessions. It also helped in improving participation, communication, and interest in the activities being conducted.

Challenges and recommendations

Withdrawal from the programme

Withdrawal from the programme was seen as a critical challenge in implementing the CST. Due to the specific demographic of participants, illness and deterioration was the cause of dropouts in both sessions. Apart from this, difficulties in arranging transport, difficulty in travelling to the centre, or relocation to other cities were problematic.

The programme may be more successful in a clinical set-up that has a permanent client pool. Withdrawal from the programme did not go unnoticed by those who continued the programme, and absentee members were a cause of distress and confusion for some of them. Thus, care needs to be taken when including participants for the programme in the first place.

Language

Bilingualism and multilingualism proved to be a challenge, especially in P1. Although members were all familiar with Tamil, some participants often spoke a mix of both languages, which led others to feel less included if they were not as familiar with English. It was speculated that this might also have influenced two members to withdraw in P1, among other practical problems. In P2, this did not prove to be a problem as all members were more comfortable with Tamil. However, in bi/multilingual societies, it might be difficult to create groups that use only one language exclusively. Hence, language must be a prominent factor in selecting participants during the group formation stage.

Training and supervision

Facilitators faced some difficulty when it came to troubleshooting practical problems and managing conflicts that occurred in certain sessions. No formal training in delivering CST sessions was available to us. The facilitators trained themselves with advice from an experienced geriatric psychiatrist, and using the training videos and manual. Direct supervision by staff with experience in delivering CST would be useful to help with specific problems such as managing challenging behaviour, group dynamics, and planning suitable activities to meet group interests. However, this was not a major barrier, and problem solving for these issues was done on a trial and error basis. Access to continued supervision will significantly improve the quality and efficiency of delivering the programme.

Discharge

Planning discharge (post-maintenance cognitive stimulation therapy [MCST]) was found to be challenging. Services for people with dementia are few and are not well developed in Chennai, and in extension, India. At the end of CST and MCST programmes it would be very useful for participants to either continue activities at home or join other groups that might maximise the continued benefit of CST. Discontinuing a programme abruptly that has been a part of the client's schedule for over eight months can be quite unsettling. Clients are usually cognitively under stimulated and socially isolated at home, and may find the constant change in routine quite distressing. A day hospital/centre setting might be ideal for the delivery of CST as it could offer opportunities for socialising and stimulation. Training family members and other caregivers to deliver CST sessions at home may worth exploring in this setting.

Conclusion

Overall, delivering CST was found to be feasible in our setting. It was well accepted by service users from the pilots conducted. Improvements in cognition and QoL (as well as subjective reports of improvements in mood from participants who took part in the two pilots) are encouraging at this preliminary stage of evaluation. Research using robust clinical trial designs with large samples are required to establish the efficacy and cost-effectiveness of the programme in this setting. Furthermore, the culturally adapted manual is well worth being translated in other regional Indian languages for use as an alternative to pharmacological interventions in the management of mild-to-moderate dementia across the country. CST could also be tested as an intervention to prevent dementia in individuals at risk for dementia and cognitive decline.

References

Aguirre, E., Spector, A. and Orrell, M. (2014). Guidelines for adapting Cognitive Stimulation Therapy to other cultures. *Clinical Interventions in Aging*, pp. 1003–7.

Aguirre, E., Woods, R. T., Spector, A. and Orrell, M. (2013). Cognitive Stimulation for Dementia: A systematic review of the evidence of effectiveness from randomised controlled trails. *Aging Research Reviews*, 12(1), pp. 253–62.

Alzheimer's and Related Disorders Society of India. (2010). *The Demetia India Report 2010: Prevalence, Impact, Cost & Services for Dementia*, New Delhi: ARDSI.

Census of India. (2011). *District Census Handbook – Chennai*, Chennai: Census of India.

Central Statistics Office – Ministry of Statistics and Programme Implementation (Government of India). (2016). *Elderly in India – Profile and Programmes 2016*, New Delhi: Government of India.

Kandasamy, V. W. (1999). The game pallanguzhi – It's mathematical aspects. *Applied Science Periodical*, 1, pp. 74–5.

Knapp, M. et al. (2006). Cognitive Stimulation Therapy for people with dementia: Cost-effectiveness analysis. *The British Journal of Psychiatry : The Journal of Mental Science*, 188(6), pp. 574–80.

Logsdon, R. G., Gibbons, L. E., McCurry, S. M. and Teri, L. (1999). Quality of life in Alzheimer's Disease: Patient and caregiver reports. *Journal of Mental Health & Aging*, pp. 21–32.

Mathuranath, P. S. et al. (2000). A brief cognitive test battery to differentiate Alzheimer's disease and frontotemporal dementia. *Neurology*, pp. 1613–20.

Mathuranath, P. S. et al. (2005). Instrumental activities of daily living scale for dementia screening in elderly people. *International Psychogeriatrics*, pp. 461–74.

National Institute for Health and Clinical Excellence (2011). Donepezil, galantamine, rivastigmine and memantine for the treatment of Alzheimer's disease. Technology appraisal guidance [TA217]. London: NICE.

Spector, A. et al. (2003). Efficacy of an evidence based Cognitive Stimulation Therapy programme for people with dementia. *British Journal of Psychiatry*, pp. 248–54.

Spector, A., Gardner, C. and Orrell, M. (2011). The impact of Cognitive Stimulation Therapy groups on people with dementia: Views from participants, their carers and group facilitators. *Aging & Mental Health*, 15(8), pp. 945–9.

Takeda, M. et al. (2012). Non-pharmacological intervention for dementia patients. *Psychiatry and Clinical Neurosciences*, 66(1), pp. 1–7.

Yamaguchi, H., Maki, Y. and Yamagami, T. (2010). Overview of non-pharmacological intervention for dementia and principles of brain-activating rehabilitation. *Psychogeriatrics*, 10(4), pp. 206–13.

Chapter 16

Sub-Saharan Africa

Stella-Maria Paddick, Sarah H. Mkenda, Godfrey Mbowe, Aloyce Kisoli, William K. Gray, Catherine L. Dotchin, Adesola Ogunniyi, John Kissima, Olaide O. Olakehinde, Declare L. Mushi, Akeem Siwoku, Babatunde Adediran, and Richard W. Walker

The need for CST as a non-pharmacological intervention for dementia in sub-Saharan Africa

The majority of people with dementia live in low and middle income countries (LMICs) and population ageing in these regions is the largest contributor to the projected increases in dementia worldwide. Recent epidemiological projections suggest that by 2050 over 80% of people with dementia will live in LMICs as their populations continue to age (Wimo et al., 2013). In sub-Saharan Africa (SSA) an estimated 2.6 million older people currently have dementia and this number is projected to increase by 371% by 2030 (Prince et al., 2013). Our team previously reported a community door-to-door prevalence study of dementia in the Kilimanjaro region of Tanzania, finding an age-adjusted prevalence of 6.4% in people aged 70 years and over (Longdon et al., 2013). This is very similar to current prevalence in high income countries (HICs) such as the UK. Dementia in SSA was also associated with substantial carer burden (Dotchin et al., 2014), distressing behavioural and psychological symptoms (BPS) (Paddick et al., 2015), stigma, and lack of understanding (Mushi et al., 2014).

While the prevalence of dementia has increased, health services and interventions for people with dementia are almost completely absent in SSA, outside of large urban centres with neurological departments. In SSA, health services are scarce, and remain focused on communicable or infectious diseases, despite evidence of a shift in disease burden to non-communicable diseases associated with ageing, such as dementia, similar to that seen worldwide (Kowal et al., 2012, Beaglehole et al., 2011).

An additional problem in SSA is the large human resource gap. Across SSA there are estimated to be 200 times fewer trained mental health workers per 100,000 population when compared to HIC settings (Saxena et al., 2007). Specialist clinicians such as geriatricians, neurologists, and psychiatrists are also very few, especially outside large urban centres (Dotchin et al., 2012, Bower and Zenebe, 2005). For example, in Tanzania, there are a total of 15 registered psychiatrists for a total population of 50.8 million.

Cholinesterase inhibitors, which are medications used as cognitive enhancers for people with Alzheimer's disease dementia (ADD), are used widely in HICs due to evidence that they can improve symptoms for some people with dementia (Ballard et al., 2011). However, in SSA, use of these drugs for symptomatic treatment of dementia is unlikely to be helpful to most people with dementia. In Tanzania, these anti-dementia medications are not listed in the national formulary, meaning that they must be bought from private pharmacies, at a cost likely to be out of reach to most rural families. Additionally, the shortage of specialist clinicians means that these medications cannot be given safely at a population level, because there is no capacity for follow up and monitoring for side effects of these medications, which are experienced frequently by those receiving them.

The World Health Organisation (WHO) recommended strategy for addressing this resource gap is one of task-shifting (WHO, 2010). Task-shifting refers to the process of training non-specialist staff to carry out tasks usually performed by specialist workers. Despite the WHO strategy, few interventions for mental disorders have been trialled in LMIC countries using this approach (Van Ginneken et al., 2013). Awareness of dementia as a significant issue in LMICs is relatively recent and few interventional studies have taken place (Olayinka and Mbuyi, 2014). The only LMIC interventional trial using this task-shifting approach is a carer intervention. Existing studies are small, with methodological issues, and show limited evidence of scale-up and sustainability (Van Ginneken et al., 2013). Most interventions do not continue after their initial trial as a research study.

Since CST can be effectively delivered by non-specialist healthcare workers, or trained carers (Spector et al., 2006), there is clear potential for use in resource-limited settings. Despite this, CST has not previously been utilised or trialled in a LMIC setting, or in fact in SSA.

This work took place as part of the Identification and Interventions for Dementia in Elderly Africans (IDEA) study (ideastudy.org). This study was a three-year collaboration between Kilimanjaro Christian Medical University College (KCMUCo) in Tanzania, the University of Ibadan in Nigeria, and Newcastle University and Northumbria Healthcare NHS Trust in the UK. The study was funded through the Grand Challenges Canada (GCC) Grand Challenges in Mental Health programme. Our aim was to develop a sustainable and culturally appropriate intervention for dementia deliverable in a low-resource setting, by non-specialist healthcare workers.

Adaptation of CST for sub-Saharan Africa and development of CST-SSA

The formative method for adapting psychotherapy (FMAP) (Hwang, 2009) was used as the framework for CST adaptation. This collaborative and community-led adaptation method is recommended for the adaption of CST to other cultures (Aguirre et al., 2014); see Chapter 10 for more details. The FMAP consists of five phases: Phase I: generating knowledge and collaborating with stakeholders; Phase II: integrating generated information with theory and empirical and clinical knowledge; Phase III: reviewing and revising the initial culturally adapted intervention with stakeholders; Phase IV: testing the culturally adapted intervention; Phase V: finalising the culturally adapted intervention

Study sites

The IDEA study has two study sites; the Hai district of Tanzania, East Africa, and Lalupon, Oyo State, Nigeria, West Africa. Tanzania is a low income country (GNI per capita $630) and Nigeria is a lower middle income country (GNI $2710 per capita), (The World Bank, 2015). Hai district is located in the Kilimanjaro region in Northern Tanzania, where the local language is Swahili, although many older people only speak a tribal language. Subsistence level farming is the main occupation and source of income for most families, although some cash crops are grown in more fertile areas. The overall educational level of older adults is low, and over two-thirds of older women are illiterate (Longdon et al., 2013). Lalupon is located in the Lagelu local government area of Nigeria and has a population of 15,854. The population are Yoruba, whose main occupations are farming and trading. The study sites provided data on two distinct, but complimentary, rural populations with different health systems, languages, and lifestyles.

Preparatory phase

Issues related to the development of culturally appropriate interventions for people with dementia were discussed with key stakeholders at both sites. In Hai this took place during a community-based dementia prevalence study (Longdon et al., 2013), and in Nigeria this occurred during the Ibadan study of Ageing, and follow-up of the Indianapolis-Ibadan dementia project (Gureje et al., 2011; Ogunniyi et al., 2011). The need to educate people with dementia and their families about the causes of dementia and the possibility of intervention was highlighted during this process.

Community healthcare workers, mental healthcare workers, and academics from Nigeria and Tanzania were invited to a workshop held in Newcastle upon Tyne, UK from 13th-19th June 2013. At the start of the workshop, all participants underwent a one-day training session on CST and attended a month-long programme of dementia training from a multidisciplinary perspective, visiting clinics and nursing homes, and observing occupational therapy sessions.

Initial adaptation of the CST manual for sub-Saharan Africa (CST-SSA)

Team members from both Tanzania and Nigeria felt that the theoretical focus on respect and asking opinions rather than facts in CST was in agreement with SSA cultural views of older people, and that older people would find CST acceptable. A number of major issues requiring adaptation of the existing CST manual were nevertheless raised.

Content of individual sessions

In terms of individual session content, a number of common cultural and educational issues were noted. In Tanzania, privacy regarding family matters would be important to consider if leading discussions about family histories for example. In Nigeria, previous experience indicated that a healthcare examination such as blood pressure measurement would be expected by participants and that the drop-out rate would be high if this were not offered. At both sites, older people might have limited access to national news, and therefore current affairs sessions would need to be specific to the local area. In SSA, the illiteracy rate is currently 40% in adults (UNESCO, 2015), and greatest amongst older adults in rural areas. High proportions of participants at both sites were unlikely to have attended school meaning that tasks involving reading, writing, or drawing would be problematic. The need for visual and verbal stimuli to reflect experience of rural older people with limited experience beyond the local village was noted. Community healthcare workers were able to offer advice on whether illiterate, but cognitively intact older adults in their community would understand activities to the same extent as those with higher levels of education.

Practical issues in delivery of CST

Practical issues related to the CST programme design were raised. Since both sites were rural, and lacking public transport, travelling to sessions might involve significant cost and time. Similarly, in the rural Hai district of Tanzania, many villages are inaccessible during rainy season. In order to avoid disruption to sessions, timing would be crucial. The safety of participants returning home and the need to avoid being outside during evening rains was similarly important. Interventional studies in the UK have taken place in day centres and nursing homes; however, in rural SSA, few suitable large buildings exist other than religious buildings. It was felt culturally inappropriate to ask people to attend a building of a different faith than their own, and therefore village offices or health centres were the only possible options. Privacy and the need to avoid observation of the group by others was also a major challenge. Finally, in Tanzania, cultural norms are that all members of village communities attend significant events including meetings, burials, and marriages. It was agreed that the 14-session programme would need the flexibility to change session days in order to avoid these events.

This process resulted in production of a first draft of the adapted version of the CST manual for use in SSA (CST-SSA) developed by consensus of all members of the study team. CST-SSA was then piloted at both study sites. Pilots were held in Hai (n = 5) and Lalupon (n = 14) (Mkenda et al., 2016). Sessions generally ran well, and the pilot was used as an opportunity to train facilitators, test the assessment tools, and assess the logistics of running the sessions. Although few changes were made to the manual at this stage, issues with times and days of sessions, visual and hearing impairments, transport, and room hire were identified and strategies put in place in an effort to address them.

Implementation of CST-SSA; feasibility study

Following completion of the piloting phase and further changes to the manual as outlined above, a formal feasibility study and clinical effectiveness trial using a stepped-wedge design was conducted in rural Hai (Paddick et al., 2017). Recruitment to the Hai district CST trial took place during a two-stage community dementia screening programme. Detailed methods are published elsewhere (Gray et al., 2016; Collingwood et al., 2014). A total of 34 individuals (29 females) were recruited. Inclusion criteria were as follows; age 65 years or over, mild to moderate dementia of any subtype by Diagnostic and Statistical Manual of Mental Disorders Fourth Edition (DSM-IV) criteria (American Psychiatric Association, 2000), able to engage in group activity for up to an hour, able to understand simple instructions and communicate verbally; no agitation or psychosis or other behavioural issue likely to seriously disrupt the group. Individuals with sensory impairment were included as this was a common problem in Hai and representative of the local population. The median age of participants was 80 years, and 29.4% had some formal education (attended school for at least one year). No participant had a formal diagnosis of dementia prior to assessment by our research team during the trial recruitment and none were taking a cholinesterase inhibitor. This was because there were no specialist doctors locally who were able to provide a diagnosis or treatment.

The 34 participants were split into four CST groups (one group of 10 participants and three groups of eight participants). Two groups were then randomised to immediate start of the CST intervention and two to delayed start (eight weeks later), which acted as controls for the immediate start group in a stepped-wedge design.

This was primarily a feasibility study. Key outcomes in terms of the feasibility of conducting CST in this setting were session attendance, drop-out rate, and number of sessions started and completed on time. The primary clinical outcome was quality of life (QoL) measured by the Brief WHO Quality of Life (WHOQOL-Bref) scale. Secondary outcomes included cognition (assessed using an adaptation of the Alzheimer's Disease Assessment Scale-Cognitive (ADAS-Cog))(Paddick S-M et al., 2016), affective symptoms assessed with the Hospital Anxiety and Depression Scale (HADS)(Zigmond and Snaith, 1983). In addition, primary carers were asked to complete the WHOQOL-Bref, HADS, Zarit Caregiver Burden Scale (ZBI) and to rate neuropsychiatric symptoms with the Neuropsychiatric Inventory (NPI)(Cummings et al., 1994). The assessing team was blind to treatment group allocation.

Immediate start group assessments	Pre-CST/baseline assessment	Immediate post-CST assessment	Eight-weeks post-CST assessment
Delayed start group assessments	Baseline assessment	Pre-CST assessment	Immediate post-CST assessment
Time-point	T1	T2	T3
Week	1-2	10-11	18-19

Figure 16.1 Study assessment protocol

Assessments took place at baseline, following the first CST intervention, and at the end of the trial (see Figure 16.1). Data were analysed as a before and after study, with further analysis as a controlled trial in order to calculate the number needed to treat (NNT) for; (i) a four-point improvement in ADAS-Cog total score, and (ii) for absence of deterioration over the study period. This allowed direct comparison of our findings with other pharmacological and non-pharmacological treatment trials conducted in other settings (Spector et al., 2003; Livingston and Katona, 2000).

CST sessions

The CST-SSA programme took place between September and December 2014. CST sessions were led by two locally-based occupational therapists trained in the use of CST in the UK, and involved in the adaptation and pilot of CST-SSA (Mkenda et al., 2016).

Feasibility

Three consenting participants were randomised and completed all assessments, but did not attend any CST sessions. One subject appeared to have experienced further cognitive deterioration and refused to attend, and two were unable to attend for transportation and logistical reasons. Excluding these three participants, the overall attendance rate over the 56 sessions was 85%. Sessions were generally missed due to illness or family events such as weddings and burial ceremonies. The main obstacle to starting sessions on time was roads becoming difficult to drive on during the rainy session, although this was seen as acceptable and normal for the setting by participants. No one was lost to follow-up.

Clinical outcomes

Data comparing changes in clinical outcomes pre-CST, immediately post-CST, and at eight weeks post-CST (immediate start groups only (n = 16) are presented in Table 16.1. Our major finding was a significant improvement in cognition, measured using the ADAS-Cog. There was also significant improvement in the physical health domain of the WHOQOL-Bref. For primary carers, there were significant improvements in symptoms of anxiety and symptom burden measured using the NPI.

Data are presented in Table 16.2, for cognitive score at time point 1 (T1, see Figure 16.1) and time point 2 (T2). This analysis effectively treats the data as for a cluster randomised controlled trial (RCT), with the delayed start group acting as controls. T2 (outcome) scores were adjusted for group allocation, age, sex, education, and T1 (baseline) score using the analysis of covariance (ANCOVA) technique. There was a significant difference in T2 scores between the immediate start and delayed start groups across all three ADAS-Cog domains and in ADAS-Cog total score. The number needed to treat for a four-point improvement in the ADAS-Cog was 2.1 (~2), and to avoid a deterioration in cognition over the study period, NNT was 3.8 (~4).

Table 16.1 Change in clinical outcomes from pre- to post-intervention

	Pre-CST (n = 31)	*Immediately post-CST (n = 31)*	*Eight weeks post-CST (n = 16)*	*Significance of change pre-CST to immediately post-CST*
Patients				
WHOQOL: Physical (median, IQR)	11.4 (9.7 to 14.3)	13.1 (10.3 to 14.9)	13.7 (11.6 to 14.6)	**W = 199, Z = −2.048, p = .041**
WHOQOL: Psychological (median, IQR)	14.0 (12.7 to 15.3)	14.7 (12.7 to 16.0)	15.0 (13.5 to 16.0)	W = 52, Z = −0.626, p = .531
WHOQOL: Social (median, IQR)	16.0 (12.0 to 18.0)	16.0 (12.0 to 20.0)	16.0 (16.0 to 18.0)	W = 16, Z = −0.217, p = .829
WHOQOL: Environmental (median, IQR)	14.5 (12.5 to 16.0)	14.5 (13.0 to 16.5)	13.5 (12.5 to 15.0)	W = 108, Z = −1.300, p = .194
WHODAS 2.0 (median, IQR)	28.0 (23.0 to 35.3), 1 missing value	29.0 (20.0 to 37.0)	27 (20.25 to 34.75)	W = 28, Z = −0.337, p = .736
ADAS-Cog: Language (mean, SD)	7.6 (4.136)	5.4 (3.694)	6.2 (4.694)	**t = 3.814, p = .001**
ADAS-Cog: Memory/new learning (mean, SD)	15.5 (3.778)	12.5 (3.590)	11.4 (3.691)	**t = 4.979, p < .001**

(*Continued*)

Table 16.1 (Continued)

	Pre-CST (n = 31)	*Immediately post-CST (n = 31)*	*Eight weeks post-CST (n = 16)*	*Significance of change pre-CST to immediately post-CST*
ADAS-Cog: Praxis (mean, SD)	6.1 (1.640)	5.2 (1.726)	4.9 (1.628)	**t = 4.028, *p* < .001**
ADAS-Cog: Total (mean, SD)	29.3 (8.134)	23.1 (7.597)	22.5 (8.628)	**t = 5.864, *p* < .001**
HAD: Anxiety (median, IQR)	6.0 (4.0 to 12.0)	6.0 (2.0 to 9.0), 1 missing value	6.0 (3.3 to 9.8)	W = 116, Z = −1.399, *p* = .162
HAD: Depression (median, IQR)	9.0 (5.0 to 12.0)	9.5 (7.0 to 12.0), 1 missing value	10.5 (8.3 to 13.8)	W = 69, Z = −0.788, *p* = .431
Carers				
WHOQOL: Physical (median, IQR)	13.5 (13.0 to 15.5), 1 missing value	13.5 (12.5 to 14.5)	13.0 (12.5 to 13.9)	W = 47, Z = −0.636, *p* = .525
WHOQOL: Psychological (median, IQR)	14.7 (13.3 to 16.0), 1 missing value	14.0 (13.3 to 16.7)	14.7 (14.0 to 15.3)	W = 36, Z = −0.390, *p* = .696
WHOQOL: Social (median, IQR)	13.0 (10.7 to 16.0), 1 missing value	14.0 (12.0 to 16.0)	12.0 (12.0 to 14.0)	W = 87, Z = −1.175, *p* = .240
WHOQOL: Environmental (median, IQR)	11.5 (11.0 to 13.5), 1 missing value	13.0 (12.0 to 14.5)	13.3 (12.1 to 14.3)	W = 142, Z = −1.623, *p* = .105
HAD: Anxiety (median, IQR)	4.0 (2.0 to 5.3), 1 missing value	3.0 (1.0 to 5.0)	3.0 (2.0 to 5.0)	**W = 157, Z = −2.149, *p* = .032**
HAD: Depression (median, IQR)	11.0 (7.0 to 13.0), 1 missing value	12.0 (8.0 to 14.0)	12 (8.3 to 13.0)	W = 97, Z = −1.056, *p* = .291
Zarit Burden Inventory (median, IQR)	13.0 (9.8 to 20.3), 1 missing value	11.0 (8.0 to 17.0)	10.5 (7.3 to 12.0)	W = 162, Z = −1.950, *p* = .051
NPI: Total symptoms present/12 (median, SD)	3.0 (2.0 to 5.5), 2 missing value	1.0 (1.0 to 3.0)	3.0(1.0 to 5.8)	**W = 190, Z = −2.427, *p* = .015**
NPI: Distress (median, SD)	5.0 (1.5 to 10.0), 2 missing value	2.0 (1.0 to 4.0)	6.0 (2.3 to 9.0)	**W = 207, Z = −2.634, *p* = .008**
NPI: Severity (median, SD)	2.0 (0.0 to 6.0), 2 missing value	0.0 (0.0 to 1.0)	0.0 (0.0 to 3.5)	**W = 139, Z = −3.309, *p* = .001**

Key: WHOQOL= World Health Organisation Quality of Life assessment, WHODAS = World Health Organisation Disability Assessment Schedule, HAD = Hospital Anxiety and Depression Scale, NPI = Neuropsychiatric inventory, IQR = inter-quartile range, SD = standard deviation

Table 16.2 Comparison of immediate start and delayed start groups

	T1 score	*T2 score*	*Significance of difference*	*Significant other variables*
ADAS-Cog: Total				
Immediate start (mean, SD)	31.5 (8.358)	23.4 (8.560)	**F (1,27) = 7.076, *p* = .013**	ADAS-Cog at T1 (F (1,27) = 29.861, *p* < .001)
Delayed start (mean, SD)	27.4 (6.647)	26.6 (7.121)		
ADAS-Cog: Language				
Immediate start (mean, SD)	8.7 (4.757)	5.8 (4.612)	F (1,27) = 2.011, *p* = .168	ADAS-Cog Language at T1 (F (1,27) = 17.129, *p* < .001)
Delayed start (mean, SD)	5.9 (4.114)	6.4 (2.873)		
ADAS-Cog: Memory/new learning				
Immediate start (mean, SD)	16.4 (3.160)	12.6 (3.722)	**F (1,27) = 5.089, *p* = .032**	ADAS-Cog Memory at T1 (F (1,27) = 13.617, *p* = .001)
Delayed start (mean, SD)	15.4 (3.961)	14.4 (4.367)		
ADAS-Cog: Praxis				
Immediate start (mean, SD)	6.4 (1.544)	5.1 (1.668)	F (1,27) = 0.563, p = .460	ADAS-Cog praxis at T1 (F (1,27) = 13.239, *p* = .001)
Delayed start (mean, SD)	6.2 (1.724)	5.8 (1.618)		

Implementation of CST-SSA: benefits and challenges

The IDEA study has shown the promise of CST in terms of feasibility and clinical effectiveness. The reported improvement in cognition, measured with an adaptation of the ADAS-Cog, showed a NNT of two, higher than that reported in CST trials in the UK. Reasons for this are unclear and require further investigation, but the relatively high proportion of vascular cognitive impairment in this setting (Paddick et al., 2014) might indicate a greater rehabilitation potential. Additionally, in this cohort, the very low educational level and a lack of other healthcare services for people with dementia may mean that there is greater scope for cognitive improvement. The CST programme appeared feasible in terms of low drop-out rates, very high attendance, and successful completion of the programme. Patients and carers enjoyed the sessions and wanted them to continue, indicating a high degree of cultural acceptability.

There are a number of challenges to scaling-up CST on a population level in this setting. In terms of sustainability, the capacity for CST to be delivered by health workers locally in rural areas is crucial. Our initial feasibility study utilised senior occupational therapists (OTs) for delivery of sessions. Although the trial was successful, the longer-term cost and logistical difficulties of transporting specialist staff to remote areas may not be practical or sustainable. The challenge is therefore for specialist workers trained in CST to train primary health workers in rural areas in carrying out the intervention and providing support centrally for this to take place. A further challenge is in identification of people with dementia. Data from HIC settings suggests that over half of dementia cases remain undiagnosed, with only a very small minority of cases identified in most LMIC settings (Lang et al., 2017). Dementia is difficult to identify, even by experienced health professionals, in primary care unless a structured screening tool is used (Yokomizo et al., 2014). Such screening tools, validated in LMIC settings, are much needed. The IDEA study developed and validated a brief cognitive screening tool, the IDEA cognitive screen. It is likely that wider implementation and scale-up of CST will require simultaneous training in cognitive screening so that people likely to benefit from CST can be identified.

Future directions for CST-SSA

CST-SSA has now been integrated into university level OT training in Tanzania. It is hoped that this process is a first step towards making CST available in a wide range of healthcare settings. Annual CST workshops have taken place in the Kilimanjaro region with healthcare workers from many regions of Tanzania represented, with support from their Regional Medical Officer. Our IDEA study team continue to work together to move towards implementing CST in other areas of Tanzania delivered by non-specialist primary healthcare staff in a sustainable manner. In the long-term, we hope to roll-out CST-SSA to other parts of SSA.

A final consideration is provision of services for individuals with severe dementia, for whom CST may not yield benefits. Failure to consider interventions for this group is unacceptable. We have therefore piloted a carers educational manual to assist patients and families to manage the difficulties they face in management of severe dementia. All IDEA study materials are available online (ideastudy.org).

References

Aguirre, E., Spector, A. and Orrell, M. (2014). Guidelines for adapting Cognitive Stimulation Therapy to other cultures. *Clinical Interventions in Aging*, 9.

American Psychiatric Association. (2000). *DSM-IV-TR: Diagnostic and Statistical Manual of Mental Disorders, Text Revision*. Washington, DC: American Psychiatric Association, 75.

Ballard, C., Corbett, A. and Sharp, S. (2011). Aligning the evidence with practice: NICE guidelines for drug treatment of Alzheimer's disease. *Expert Review of Neurotherapeutics*, 11, 327–329.

Beaglehole, R., Bonita, R., Horton, R., Adams, C., Alleyne, G., Asaria, P., Baugh, V., Bekedam, H., Billo, N. and Casswell, S. (2011). Priority actions for the non-communicable disease crisis. *The Lancet*, 377, 1438–1447.

Bower, J. H. and Zenebe, G. (2005). Neurologic services in the nations of Africa. *Neurology*, 64, 412–415.

Collingwood, C., Paddick, S.-M., Kisoli, A., Dotchin, C. L., Gray, W. K., Mbowe, G., Mkenda, S., Urasa, S., Mushi, D. and Chaote, P. (2014). Development and community-based validation of the IDEA study Instrumental Activities of Daily Living (IDEA-IADL) questionnaire. *Global Health Action*, 7.

Cummings, J. L., Mega, M., Gray, K., Rosenberg-Thompson, S., Carusi, D. A. and Gornbein, J. (1994). The Neuropsychiatric Inventory: Comprehensive assessment of psychopathology in dementia. *Neurology*, 44, 2308–14.

Dotchin, C., Paddick, S.-M., Longdon, A., Kisoli, A., Gray, W., Dewhurst, F., Chaote, P., Dewhurst, M. and Walker, R. (2014). A comparison of caregiver burden in older persons and persons with Parkinson's disease or dementia in sub-Saharan Africa. *International Psychogeriatrics*, 26, 687–692.

Dotchin, C. L., Akinyemi, R. O., Gray, W. K. and Walker, R. W. (2012). Geriatric medicine: Services and training in Africa. *Age and Ageing*, doi:10.1093/ageing/afs119.

Gray, W. K., Paddick, S. M., Collingwood, C., Kisoli, A., Mbowe, G., Mkenda, S., Lissu, C., Rogathi, J., Kissima, J. and Walker, R. W. (2016). Community validation of the IDEA study cognitive screen in rural Tanzania. *International Journal of Geriatric Psychiatry*.

Gureje, O., Ogunniyi, A., Kola, L. and Abiona, T. (2011). Incidence of and risk factors for dementia in the Ibadan study of aging. *Journal of the American Geriatrics Society*, 59, 869–874.

Hwang, W.-C. (2009). The Formative Method for Adapting Psychotherapy (FMAP): A community-based developmental approach to culturally adapting therapy. *Professional Psychology: Research and Practice*, 40, 369.

Kowal, P., Chatterji, S., Naidoo, N., Biritwum, R., Fan, W., Ridaura, R. L., Maximova, T., Arokiasamy, P., Phaswana-Mafuya, N. and Williams, S. (2012). Data resource profile: The World Health Organization Study on global AGEing and adult health (SAGE). *International Journal of Epidemiology*, 41, 1639–1649.

Lang, L., Clifford, A., Wei, L., Zhang, D., Leung, D., Augustine, G., Danat, I. M., Zhou, W., Copeland, J. R. and Anstey, K. J. (2017). Prevalence and determinants of undetected dementia in the community: A systematic literature review and a meta-analysis. *BMJ Open*, 7, e011146.

Livingston, G. and Katona, C. (2000). How useful are cholinesterase inhibitors in the treatment of Alzheimer's disease? A number needed to treat analysis. *International Journal of Geriatric Psychiatry*, 15, 203–207.

Longdon, A. R., Paddick, S. M., Kisoli, A., Dotchin, C., Gray, W. K., Dewhurst, F., Chaote, P., Teodorczuk, A., Dewhurst, M. and Jusabani, A. M. (2013). The prevalence of dementia in rural Tanzania: A cross-sectional community-based study. *International Journal of Geriatric Psychiatry*, 28, 728–737.

Mkenda, S., Olakehinde, O., Mbowe, G., Siwoku, A., Kisoli, A., Paddick, S. M., Adediran, B., Gray, W. K., Dotchin, C. L., Adebiyi, A., Walker, R. W., Mushi, D. and Ogunniyi, A. (2016). Cognitive stimulation therapy as a low-resource intervention for dementia in sub-Saharan Africa (CST-SSA): Adaptation for rural Tanzania and Nigeria. *Dementia (London)*.

Mushi, D., Rongai, A., Paddick, S.-M., Dotchin, C., Mtuya, C. and Walker, R. 2014. Social representation and practices related to dementia in Hai District of Tanzania. *BMC Public Health*, 14, 260.

Ogunniyi, A., Lane, K., Baiyewu, O., Gao, S., Gureje, O., Unverzagt, F., Murrell, J., Smith-Gamble, V., Hall, K. and Hendrie, H. (2011). Hypertension and incident dementia in community-dwelling elderly Yoruba Nigerians. *Acta Neurologica Scandinavica*, 124, 396–402.

Olayinka, O. O. and Mbuyi, N. N. (2014). Epidemiology of dementia among the elderly in sub-Saharan Africa. *International Journal of Alzheimer's Disease*, 2014.

Paddick, S.-M., Kisoli, A., Mkenda, S., Mbowe, G., Gray, W. K., Dotchin, C., Ogunniyi, A., Kisima, J., Olakehinde, O., Mushi, D. and Walker, W. R. (2016). Adaptation and validation of the Alzheimer's Disease Assessment Scale – Cognitive (ADAS-Cog) in a low-literacy setting in sub-Saharan Africa. *Acta Neuropsychiatrica*, Accepted Article.

Paddick, S.-M., Longdon, A., Kisoli, A., Gray, W. K., Dotchin, C. L., Jusabani, A., Iqbal, A., Hughes, J., Teodorczuk, A. and Chaote, P. (2014). The prevalence of dementia subtypes in rural Tanzania. *The American Journal of Geriatric Psychiatry*, 22, 1613–1622.

Paddick, S.-M., Mkenda, S., Mbowe, G., Kisoli, A., Gray, W. K., Dotchin, C. L., Ternent, L., Ogunniyi, A., Kissima, J. and Olakehinde, O. (2017). Cognitive stimulation therapy as a sustainable intervention for dementia in sub-Saharan Africa: Feasibility and clinical efficacy using a stepped-wedge design. *International Psychogeriatrics*, 1–11.

Paddick, S. M., Kisoli, A., Longdon, A., Dotchin, C., Gray, W., Chaote, P., Teodorczuk, A. and Walker, R. (2015). The prevalence and burden of behavioural and psychological symptoms of dementia in rural Tanzania. *International Journal of Geriatric Psychiatry*, 30, 815–823.

Prince, M., Bryce, R., Albanese, E., Wimo, A., Ribeiro, W. and Ferri, C. P. (2013). The global prevalence of dementia: A systematic review and metaanalysis. *Alzheimer's & Dementia*, 9, 63–75. e2.

Saxena, S., Thornicroft, G., Knapp, M. and Whiteford, H. (2007). Resources for mental health: Scarcity, inequity, and inefficiency. *The Lancet*, 370, 878–889.

Spector, A., Thorgrimsen, L., Woods, B., Royan, L., Davies, S., Butterworth, M. and Orrell, M. (2003). Efficacy of an evidence-based Cognitive Stimulation Therapy programme for people with dementia: Randomised controlled trial. *British Journal of Psychiatry*, 183, 248–254.

Spector, A., Thorgrimsen, L., Woods, R. T. and Orrell, M. (2006). *Making a Difference: An Evidence-based Group Programme to Offer Cognitive Stimulation Therapy (CST) to People With Dementia.* Hawker Publications.

UNESCO. (2015). *Education Data 2015.* 2015 edition. Quebec, Canada: UNESCO.

Van Ginneken, N., Tharyan, P., Lewin, S., Rao, G. N., Meera, S. M., Pian, J., Chandrashekar, S. and Patel, V. (2013). Non-specialist health worker interventions for the care of mental, neurological and substance-abuse disorders in low-and middle-income countries. *The Cochrane Library*.

WHO. (2010). *mhGAP Intervention Guide for Mental, Neurological and Substance Use Disorders in Non-specialized Health Settings.*

Wimo, A., Jönsson, L., Bond, J., Prince, M. and Winblad, B. (2013). The worldwide economic impact of dementia 2010. *Alzheimer's & Dementia*, 9, 1–11.e3.

The World Bank. (2015). *Data: Countries and Economies.* Available: http://data.worldbank.org/country [Accessed 30th March 2015].

Yokomizo, J. E., Simon, S. S. and De Campos Bottino, C. M. (2014). Cognitive screening for dementia in primary care: A systematic review. *International Psychogeriatrics*, 26, 1783–1804.

Zigmond, A. S. and Snaith, R. P. (1983). The hospital anxiety and depression scale. *Acta Psychiatrica Scandinavica*, 67, 361–370.

Index

acetylcholinesterase inhibitors (ACHEIs): in China 227; MCST and 56, 59, 62–3, 64; in sub-Saharan Africa 254
'active ingredients' of NPT 23–4
adaption of CST to other cultures: bottom-up approach to 177–8, 180; Formative Method for Adapting Psychotherapy and 179–81; future of 190–1; generating knowledge and collaborating with stakeholders 181–2, 186–7, 238–9; in Germany 186–9; in India 238–49; integrating information with theory, empirical, and clinical knowledge 182–3, 187–8, 240–1; in New Zealand 211–12; overview 177–8; pilot testing 184–5, 189, 242–6; reviewing and revising 183–4, 188, 241–2; in sub-Saharan Africa 254–7; synthesising feedback and finalising intervention 185, 189, 246–9; theoretical methods for 178–9; top-down approach to 177, 180; in United States 216–18
ADAS-Cog (Alzheimer's Disease Assessment Scale-Cognition): MRI study of change in 163, 165–6, 167, 168; overview 115; pilot testing and 42, 44
adherence: to CST 93; to iCST 79, 82, 83–4, 144–6
Africa *see* sub-Saharan Africa
alertness, improvement in 140–1
Alzheimer's disease (AD): brain network connectivity in 154–5; cognitive benefits of CST for 169; cognitive interventions for 155–7; pathogenesis of 153; pharmacological therapies for 33; prevalence of 11
anti-N-methyl-D-aspartate receptor encephalitis 227
assessment for intervention for people with dementia and carers 114–16, 124; *see also* ADAS-Cog; QoL-AD

Behavioural Management Technique 196
benefits of CST 169
binding ties theory 131
biological studies, data from 15–16
bottom-up approach to cultural adaptation 177–8, 180
brain-derived neurotrophic factor (BDNF) 15
brain network connectivity: in Alzheimer's disease 154–5; CST and 160–1, 169
brain plasticity 13–14, 154
brain reserve 12–13, 154, 168
Breuil, V. 4, 43

caregiver burden 109
caregiving: defined 109; impact of 109
care homes: service evaluation of CST in 98–100; training of staff in 201–2
carers: adherence to iCST programme 79, 82, 83–4, 144–6; awareness of needs of persons with dementia 144; in China 227; CST training for 111–12, 116–17, 121–2; feedback from 247–8; iCST and 76, 79; as interventionists 84–5; interventions for people with dementia and 110–11, 116–17; outcomes for 81; outcomes of interventions for people with dementia and 117–25; rationale for including in CST 109–10; study of intervention for people with dementia and 112–14; *see also* quality of caregiving relationship
'ceiling effect' 82–3, 104
central executive network (CEN) 154, 155, 169

centres, variation in outcome between 44, 53–4, 55
change: in everyday life due to CST 139–44; mechanisms of 54–5
China: development of CST in 228–32; effectiveness and feasibility of CST in 232–4; need for CST in 227–8
cholinesterase inhibitors *see* acetylcholinesterase inhibitors
Cochrane reviews 20, 40, 49, 56, 57
CogEx (CST and physical exercise) 213
cognition-focused NPT *see* non-pharmacological therapies
cognitive rehabilitation (CR) 19, 20–2, 155–6
cognitive reserve 12–13, 154, 168, 170
cognitive stimulation (CS) 18
Cognitive Stimulation Therapy (CST): characteristics of 153; evidence for and future of 8–9; feasibility study and piloting of 42–3, 49–50; international translation and adaptation of 8; key principles of 6–7; overview 49; in UK 5, 8–9; worldwide impact of 189–90; *see also* adaption of CST to other cultures; experience of CST; implementation of CST; Maintenance CST (MCST) programme; neuropsychological aspects of CST; individual (one-on-one) CST (iCST) programme
cognitive training (CT) 18, 19–20, 155–6
communication, opportunities for 141–2
community-based integrated care centres in Japan 195
compensatory approach to CR 21
computer-based programmes 85
concentration, improvement in 140–1
control groups 26
cost-effectiveness of programmes 25
CR (cognitive rehabilitation) 19, 20–2, 155–6
cross-modality intervention, CST as 156
CS (cognitive stimulation) 18
CST *see* Cognitive Stimulation Therapy
CST-J *see* Japanese adaptation of CST
CST-SSA *see* sub-Saharan Africa
CT (cognitive training) 18, 19–20, 155–6
cultural adaptation *see* adaption of CST to other cultures
cultural adaptation process model 178
culture: defined 177; dementia and 179–80

default mode network (DMN) 154–5, 169
dementia: burden and aetiology of 11–13; causes of 12; in China 227–8; defined 179; diagnosis of 262; in India 237; in Japan 195; in low and middle income countries 253; in New Zealand 205; NICE guidelines for 5, 45; overview 146–7; positive approaches to 34–9; in sub-Saharan Africa 253–4; in United States 215; *see also* Alzheimer's disease
detection bias 63–4
development: of CST 3–4, 33–4, 40–1; of MCST 57
discharge planning 250
DMN (default mode network) 154–5, 169
domain-specific interventions, CT and CR as 155–6
donepezil 54

ecological validity model 178
email support 92
enjoyment of CST sessions 142–3
enrichment process theory 131, 147
executive dysfunction 197
exercise and CST: in New Zealand 213; in United States 220–1
experience of CST: carer adherence to intervention 144–6; changes in everyday life 139–44; concepts of mental stimulation 137–9; CST groups 133, 134, 135; data collection and analyses 135–6; iCST development phase and post-trial 133–6; in India 246–9; interventions 135; key topic questions 136; methods 133–5; overview 131–2, 146–9; thematic analysis results 136–46; in United States 222–3

family carers *see* carers
Family Planning Policy in China 227
focus groups 181–2, 238–9
Folsom, James 35
Formative Method for Adapting Psychotherapy (FMAP): CST guidelines and 179–81; in Germany 186–9; in India 238–49; in New Zealand 212; overview 196; phases of 181–5; in sub-Saharan Africa 254–5; *see also* adaption of CST to other cultures
format of CST 121, 125
France, cognitive stimulation programme in 3–4, 40, 45
frontotemporal lobar degeneration 11
functional connectivity analysis 160–1

galantamine 54
German adaptation of CST 186–9

human resource gap in sub-Saharan Africa 253–4

implementation of CST: in care homes, service evaluation of 98–100; in China 233–4; in India 249–50; in Japan 202–3; justification for outreach support options 89–90; in New Zealand 210–11; overview 103–5; in practice, study of 101–3; in sub-Saharan Africa 261–2; training and 89; in United States 215–16, 222–3; *see also* outreach support for implementation of CST
inclusion criteria 104
India: acceptability and feasibility of CST in 238; adaptation of CST for 237–8; dementia and ageing in 237; Formative Method for Adaptation Psychotherapy in 238–49; implementation of CST in 249–50
individual CST (iCST) programme: adherence to 79, 82, 83–4; assessment procedure 79–80; barriers to implementation of 148; in China 234; consent 80; development of 69–73; experience of 133–6, 146–9; features of 74; focus groups and interviews 71–2; future of 85; key principles of 76; methods 78–9; in New Zealand 212–13; outcome measures 80; overview 5; pilot study 72–3; pre-clinical phase of development 70; RCT of 77–80; reflections on trial of 82–5; results 81–2; session content 74–5; tailoring activities 75–6; thematic analysis results about experience of 136–46; in United States 218–19
induction period 241
International CST Centre, University College of London 69, 189–90
International Non-Pharmacological Therapies Project (INPTP) 19–20
interventionists, carers as 84–5
interventions: cultural adaptation of 177; Medical Research Council framework for evaluation of 39, 57, 69–70, 89; *see also specific interventions,* such as Reality Orientation
introductions, making 197–8

Japanese adaptation of CST (CST-J): activities featured in 185, 196–7; benefits and challenges of implementation 202–3; controlled clinical trial of 198–9; development of 196–8; impact to specific areas of cognitive function 199–201; need for 195–6; staff training in 201–3

language issues in India 249–50
Learning Therapy 195–6
Lewy body disease 11
local supervision for support 92–3
long-term care system in Japan 195
long-term impact of CST 56

Maintenance CST (MCST) programme: in China 234; development of 57; implementation of 104–5; methods 57–8; outcomes and assessments 58–9; overview 4–5; perceptions and considerations of 95–6; pilot study 56–7; quality of delivery 61–2; reflections on trial of 62–4; results 59–61; sample size 59; in United States 218
MCI (mild cognitive impairment) 14
Medical Research Council (MRC), framework for evaluation of interventions 39, 57, 69–70, 89; *see also* Formative Method for Adapting Psychotherapy
Medicare in United States 217
Memory Services National Accreditation Programme 189
Mental Capacity Act 80
mental stimulation: effects of 137–8; opportunities for 139–40; types of 138–9
mild cognitive impairment (MCI) 14
mindfulness 26
Mini-Mental State Examination (MMSE) 115
minority dementias 11–12
model of response to psychosocial interventions 16
MRI study of neuropsychological mechanisms of CST: data analysis 160–1; discussion of results of 168–70; methods 157–60; results 161–8
multi-sensory stimulation 4, 49

National Institute of Clinical Excellence (NICE) guidelines for dementia 5, 45
neuroimaging studies, data from 14–15, 26; *see also* MRI study of neuropsychological mechanisms of CST

neuroplasticity 13–14, 154
neuropsychological aspects of CST: brain and cognitive reserve and predictors of benefit 168; current evidence of 156–7; data analysis 160–1; MRI study of 157–60; overview 153; results of MRI study of 161–70
New Zealand: acceptability of CST in 207–8; adaption and feasibility of CST in 205–6; adaption of CST to Māori culture 211–12; CogEx intervention in 213; dementia and ageing in 205; facilitator training and evaluation in 208–10; feasibility study in 206–7; iCST in 212–13; implementation of CST in 210–11
NHS Institute for Innovations 189
NICE (National Institute of Clinical Excellence) guidelines for dementia 5, 45
Nigerian adaptation of CST 184, 185, 255
non-pharmacological therapies (NPT): 'active ingredients' of 23–4; cognition-focused 18–22; future of 25–7; overview 16–18; pattern and predictors of response to 22–3; in United States 215; *see also* psychological approaches
non-threatening environment of CST groups 143–4

online forum for support 92
Orrell, Martin 33–4, 216
outcomes: of CST-J on specific areas of cognitive function 199–201; of iCST 80–2; of MCST 58–62; of outreach support for CST 93–7
outcomes of CST: in China 233–4; combined interventions for people with dementia and carers 110–11, 117–25; iCST outcomes compared to 84; mechanisms of change 54–5; medication compared to 54; in New Zealand 206–7; overview 44–5, 53–4; in sub-Saharan Africa 258–61
outreach support for implementation of CST: in care homes 100; justification for 89–90; results of study of 94–8; study of 90–4

positive approaches to dementia 34–9
psychological approaches, methodology for evaluation of 39–40; *see also* non-pharmacological therapies; Reality Orientation; Reminiscence Therapy
psychosocial interventions 13, 16
psychotherapy adaptation and modification framework 179

QoL-AD (Quality of Life-Alzheimer's Disease Scale) 43, 115
quality of caregiving relationship 81, 83, 144, 147–8
quality of delivery of MCST 61–2
quality of life (QoL): iCST and 82, 83; MCST and 62, 63, 64
Quality of the Current Relationship in Caregiving (QCRC) scale 115–16

randomised controlled trials (RCTs): in China 232–4; history of 4–5; at Hospital Broca in Paris 3–4; of iCST 77–80; integrity of blinding process in 124; of intervention for people with dementia and carers 112–14; limitations and challenges of 55–6; of MCST 57–62; methods 50; multi-centre single-blind 43–4; outcomes 53–4; of outreach support for implementation of CST 90–8; results of 50–3
Reality Orientation (RO): components of 35–6; concerns about 37; CST as having roots in 45; development of 18, 35; effects of 49; in Germany 187–8; group-based programme for 41–3; historical perspective on 33; overview 3–4; power differential and 37–8; review of 40–1; UK controlled trials of 36–7
relationship-centred approach 84
Reminiscence Therapy (RT): CST and 49; historical perspective on 33; overview 3, 4, 38; review of 40; in United States 215
reserve: brain 12–13, 154, 168; cognitive 12–13, 154, 168, 170; concept of 153–4
restorative approach to CR 21
rivastigmine 54
RO *see* Reality Orientation
RT *see* Reminiscence Therapy

scaffolding process theory 131, 148
selective adaptation model 179
South Asian adaptation of CST 182, 184
Spector, Aimee 34, 92, 216, 217
Staff Training in Assisted Living Residences programme 215
stakeholders, identifying 181
Streater, Amy 92, 99, 216

sub-Saharan Africa (SSA): adaptation and development of CST for 254–7; feasibility study in 257–8; implementation of CST in 261–2; need for CST in 253; outcomes in 258–61; *see also* Nigerian adaptation of CST; Tanzanian adaptation of CST
supportive environment of CST groups 143–4
'switch on' phenomenon 207

tacrine 3, 33, 54
'Tacrine and psychological therapies in dementia: no contest?' (Orrell and Woods) 34
Tanzanian adaptation of CST 183, 184, 185, 255
task-shifting 254
top-down approach to cultural adaptation 177, 180
training: for care home staff 99; for carers 111–12, 116–17, 121–2; of facilitators in New Zealand 208–10; in iCST 79; in India 250; in Japan 201–3; outreach support package and 92–3; in United States 221–2
training manuals: in China 228–32; for CST 6, 8, 91; for CST-J 202; for CST-SSA 255–6; in India 241–2; translation of 188; in United States 218
transportation to CST programmes 218, 240

United States: adaption of CST to 216–18; implementation of CST in 215–16, 222–3; incorporation of exercise into CST in 220–1; MCST and iCST in 218–19; Saint Louis University CST education, training and research 221–2; studies of CST in rural hospital in 219–20
University College of London, International CST Centre at 69, 189–90

validation therapy 38
vascular disease 11, 26–7
voxel-based morphometry (VBM) analysis 160

Woods, Bob 33–4
World Alzheimer Report 8, 56, 190

yoga and CST 221